AIDS: Assessment, Prevention and Treatment

AIDS: Assessment, Prevention and Treatment

Editor: Evan Maverick

FOSTER ACADEMICS

www.fosteracademics.com

www.fosteracademics.com

FOSTER ACADEMICS

Cataloging-in-Publication Data

AIDS : assessment, prevention and treatment / edited by Evan Maverick.
p. cm.
Includes bibliographical references and index.
ISBN 978-1-63242-869-1
1. AIDS (Disease). 2. AIDS (Disease)--Diagnosis. 3. AIDS (Disease)--Prevention.
4. AIDS (Disease)--Treatment. I. Maverick, Evan
RC606.6 .A33 2020
616.979 2--dc23

Foster Academics,
118-35 Queens Blvd., Suite 400,
Forest Hills, NY 11375, USA

ISBN 978-1-63242-869-1 (Hardback)

Contents

Preface IX

Chapter 1 **Factors associated with viral non-suppression among adolescents living with HIV in Cambodia** 1
Kolab Chhim, Gitau Mburu, Sovannary Tuot, Ratana Sopha, Vohith Khol, Pheak Chhoun and Siyan Yi

Chapter 2 **Factors associated with pre-treatment HIV RNA: application for the use of abacavir and rilpivirine as the first-line regimen for HIV-infected patients in resource-limited settings** 11
Sasisopin Kiertiburanakul, David Boettiger, Oon Tek Ng, Nguyen Van Kinh, Tuti Parwati Merati, Anchalee Avihingsanon, Wing-Wai Wong, Man Po Lee, Romanee Chaiwarith, Adeeba Kamarulzaman, Pacharee Kantipong, Fujie Zhang, Jun Yong Choi, Nagalingeswaran Kumarasamy, Rossana Ditangco, Do Duy Cuong, Shinichi Oka, Benedict Lim Heng Sim, Winai Ratanasuwan, Penh Sun Ly, Evy Yunihastuti, Sanjay Pujari, Jeremy L. Ross, Matthew Law and Somnuek Sungkanuparph

Chapter 3 **HIV care in Yangon, Myanmar; successes, challenges and implications for policy** 18
Ne Myo Aung, Josh Hanson, Tint Tint Kyi, Zaw Win Htet, David A. Cooper, Mark A. Boyd, Mar Mar Kyi and Htin Aung Saw

Chapter 4 **CLINICAL outcomes and loss to follow-up among people living with HIV participating in the *NAMWEZA* intervention in Dar es Salaam, Tanzania** 24
Hellen N. Siril, Sylvia F. Kaaya, Mary Kay Smith Fawzi, Expeditho Mtisi, Magreat Somba, Japheth Kilewo, Ferdinand Mugusi, Anna Minja, Anna Kaale and Jim Todd

Chapter 5 **What influences quality of life in older people living with HIV?** 34
Jose Catalan, Veronica Tuffrey, Damien Ridge and Dana Rosenfeld

Chapter 6 **Late presentation increases risk and costs of non-infectious comorbidities in people with HIV** 43
Giovanni Guaraldi, Stefano Zona, Marianna Menozzi, Thomas D. Brothers, Federica Carli, Chiara Stentarelli, Giovanni Dolci, Antonella Santoro, Ana Rita Domingues Da Silva, Elisa Rossi, Julian Falutz and Cristina Mussini

Chapter 7 **The therapeutic landscape of HIV-1 via genome editing** 50
Alexander Kwarteng, Samuel Terkper Ahuno and Godwin Kwakye-Nuako

Chapter 8 **Validity assessment of the PROMIS fatigue domain among people living with HIV** 66
L. E. Gibbons, R. Fredericksen, D. S. Batey, L. Dant, T. C. Edwards, K. H. Mayer, W. C. Mathews, L. S. Morales, M. J. Mugavero, F. M. Yang, E. Paez, M. M. Kitahata, D. L. Patrick, H. M. Crane and P. K. Crane

Chapter 9 **Safety and immunogenicity of the quadrivalent human papillomavirus (qHPV) vaccine in HIV-positive Spanish men who have sex with men (MSM)** 77
Carmen Hidalgo-Tenorio, Jessica Ramírez-Taboada, Concepción Gil-Anguita, Javier Esquivias, Mohamed Omar-Mohamed-Balgahata, Antonio SamPedro, Miguel Lopez-Ruz and Juan Pasquau

Chapter 10 **Comparison of six methods to estimate adherence in an ART-naïve cohort in a resource-poor setting: which best predicts virological and resistance outcomes?** 88
Catherine Orrell, Karen Cohen, Rory Leisegang, David R. Bangsberg, Robin Wood and Gary Maartens

Chapter 11 **Distribution and fate of HIV-1 unintegrated DNA species** 99
Faysal Bin Hamid, Jinsun Kim and Cha-Gyun Shin

Chapter 12 **Bone mineral density in people living with HIV** 107
M. J. Kruger and T. A. Nell

Chapter 13 **Effect of *Moringa oleifera* Lam. leaf powder on the pharmacokinetics of nevirapine in HIV-infected adults** 124
Tsitsi G. Monera-Penduka, Charles C. Maponga, Alan R. Wolfe, Lubbe Wiesner, Gene D. Morse and Charles F. B. Nhachi

Chapter 14 **Immunological outcomes of Tenofovir versus Zidovudine-based regimens among people living with HIV/AIDS** 130
Teshale Ayele, Habtemu Jarso and Girma Mamo

Chapter 15 **Factors associated with loss to follow-up after occupational HIV exposure** 139
Nectarios Sophocles Papavarnavas, Kathryn Manning, Fahd Conrad, Milah Govender and Gary Maartens

Chapter 16 **HIV-1 drug-resistant mutations and related risk factors among HIV-1-positive individuals experiencing treatment failure in Hebei Province, China** 146
Xinli Lu, Hongru Zhao, Yuqi Zhang, Wei Wang, Cuiying Zhao, Yan Li, Lin Ma, Ze Cui and Suliang Chen*

Chapter 17 **A frailty index predicts post-liver transplant morbidity and mortality in HIV-positive patients** 159
Giovanni Guaraldi, Giovanni Dolci, Stefano Zona, Giuseppe Tarantino, Valentina Serra, Roberto Ballarin, Erica Franceschini, Mauro Codeluppi, Thomas D. Brothers, Cristina Mussini and Fabrizio Di Benedetto

Chapter 18 **Risk factors and outcomes for the Q151M and T69 insertion HIV-1 resistance mutations in historic UK data** 167
Oliver T. Stirrup, David T. Dunn, Anna Tostevin, Caroline A. Sabin, Anton Pozniak, David Asboe, Alison Cox, Chloe Orkin, Fabiola Martin and Patricia Cane

Chapter 19 **Geographic patterns of poor HIV/AIDS care continuum in District of Columbia** 181
Suparna Das, Jenevieve Opoku, Michael Kharfen and Adam Allston

Chapter 20 **Prevalence of lower limb deep venous thrombosis among adult HIV positive patients attending an outpatient clinic at Mulago Hospital** 190
Sosthene Tsongo Vululi, Samuel Bugeza, Muyinda Zeridah, Henry Ddungu, Akello Betty Openy, Mubiru Frank and Rosalind Parkes-Ratanshi

Chapter 21 **Social-support needs among adolescents living with HIV in transition from pediatric to adult care in Cambodia**.. 197
Graham Toth, Gitau Mburu, Sovannary Tuot, Vohith Khol, Chanrith Ngin, Pheak Chhoun and Siyan Yi

Chapter 22 **Validation of a questionnaire to monitor symptoms in HIV-infected patients during hepatitis C treatment** 208
Edward R. Cachay, Craig Ballard, Bradford Colwell, Francesca Torriani, Charles Hicks and Wm. Christopher Mathews

Permissions

List of Contributors

Index

Preface

This book has been an outcome of determined endeavour from a group of educationists in the field. The primary objective was to involve a broad spectrum of professionals from diverse cultural background involved in the field for developing new researches. The book not only targets students but also scholars pursuing higher research for further enhancement of the theoretical and practical applications of the subject.

Infection with the human immunodeficiency virus (HIV) causes a spectrum of conditions called as HIV/AIDS or human immunodeficiency virus infection and acquired immune deficiency syndrome. It is primarily caused by unprotected sex, hypodermic needles, contaminated blood transfusions, mother to child transmission during pregnancy, childbirth or breastfeeding. HIV/AIDS is diagnosed on the basis of laboratory testing and staged based on the presence of certain signs or symptoms. People infected with HIV usually develop specific antibodies within the first three to twelve weeks after the initial infection. The diagnosis is therefore done by PCR testing for HIV RNA or DNA, or by measuring p24 antigen or HIV-RNA. There is no definitive cure for the disease but it can be managed by highly active antiretroviral therapy that slows the progression of the disease and leads to a near-normal life expectancy. Disease in a newborn can be prevented by the application of mother and child antiretroviral medication. This book is compiled in such a manner, that it will provide in-depth knowledge about the assessment, prevention and treatment of AIDS. It includes some of the vital pieces of work being conducted across the world, on various topics related to HIV/AIDS. It includes contributions of experts and scientists, which will provide innovative insights into this disease.

It was an honour to edit such a profound book and also a challenging task to compile and examine all the relevant data for accuracy and originality. I wish to acknowledge the efforts of the contributors for submitting such brilliant and diverse chapters in the field and for endlessly working for the completion of the book. Last, but not the least; I thank my family for being a constant source of support in all my research endeavours.

Editor

1

Factors associated with viral non-suppression among adolescents living with HIV in Cambodia

Kolab Chhim[1], Gitau Mburu[2], Sovannary Tuot[1], Ratana Sopha[1], Vohith Khol[3], Pheak Chhoun[1] and Siyan Yi[1,4,5*]

Abstract

Background: Adolescents living with HIV on antiretroviral therapy (ART) have worse treatment adherence, viral suppression, and mortality rates compared to adults. This study investigated factors associated with viral non-suppression among adolescents living with HIV in Cambodia.

Methods: A cross-sectional study was conducted in August 2016 among 328 adolescents living with HIV aged 15–17 years who were randomly selected from 11 ART clinics in the capital city of Phnom Penh and 10 other provinces. Clinical and immunological data, including CD4 count and viral load, were obtained from medical records at ART clinics. Adolescents were categorized as having achieved viral suppression if their latest viral load count was < 1000 ribonucleic acid (RNA) copies/mL. Multivariate logistic regression analysis was performed to identify factors independently associated with viral non-suppression.

Results: The mean age of the participants was 15.9 years (SD = 0.8), and 48.5% were female. Median duration on ART was 8.6 (interquartile range = 6.0–10.6) years. Of total, 76.8% of the participants had achieved viral suppression. After adjustment for other covariates, the likelihood of having viral non-suppression remained significantly lower among adolescents who were: older/aged 17 (AOR = 0.46, 95% CI 0.21–0.98), had been on ART for more than 9 years (AOR = 0.35, 95% CI 0.19–0.64), had most recent CD4 count of > 672 (AOR = 0.47, 95% CI 0.26–0.86), had a relative as the main daily caregiver (AOR = 0.37, 95% CI 0.17–0.80), and did not believe that there is a cure for AIDS (AOR = 0.40, 95% CI 0.21–0.75) compared to their reference group. The likelihood of having viral non-suppression also remained significantly higher among adolescents who had first viral load > 628 RNA copies/mL (AOR = 1.81, 95% CI 1.05–4.08) and among those who were receiving HIV care and treatment from an adult clinic (AOR = 2.95, 95% CI 1.56–5.59).

Conclusions: The proportion of adolescents living with HIV with viral suppression in this study was relatively high at 76.8%, but falls short of the global target of 90%. Programs targeting younger adolescents and adolescents in transition from pediatric to adult care with a range of interventions including psychosocial support and treatment literacy could further improve viral suppression outcomes.

Keywords: Adolescents, Antiretroviral therapy (ART), HIV care and treatment, Viral suppression, Social determinants, Cambodia

*Correspondence: siyan@doctor.com

[1] KHANA Center for Population Health Research, No. 33, Street 71, Phnom Penh, Cambodia

Full list of author information is available at the end of the article

Background

Human immunodeficiency virus (HIV) is a leading cause of global burden of disease [1]. In recent years, significant progress has been made in increasing access to antiretroviral therapy (ART) for people living with HIV [2]. A key goal of ART is to suppress the replication of the virus. Suppressed viral replication facilitates restoration of the immune function and significantly reduces the risk of onward HIV transmission [3]. The World Health Organization (WHO) introduced viral load monitoring as a gold standard to follow up the treatment effectiveness in 2013 [4], and Cambodia adopted these guidelines in late 2015 [5]. The Cambodian national guidelines recommend that viral load testing be performed 6 months after ART initiation and repeated routinely once a year.

Despite the increasing access to ART, numerous studies have demonstrated suboptimal levels of viral suppression in different populations in many low-resource settings [1]. In particular, adolescents living with HIV tend to experience worse immunological and viral suppression outcomes compared to adults [6–9], which in turn contributes to their higher mortality [10, 11]. Indeed, HIV-related deaths among adolescents have tripled since 2000, making HIV the second leading cause of death among adolescents globally [12]. While health related data for this age group remain scarce, there is emerging evidence indicating that adolescents living with HIV have been facing challenges in accessing HIV services [13].

Studies from different settings have identified a wide range of factors that may determine HIV treatment outcomes among adolescents. These factors include sub-optimal disclosure of adolescents' HIV status [14, 15], poor linkage to care [10], attrition from care and treatment [16], poor transition from pediatric to adult services [17], challenges with adherence to ART [18], economic hardships [19, 20], and AIDS-related stigma [15, 21]. These factors commonly prevent attainment of optimal ART outcomes among this young population.

In Cambodia, 8512 children and adolescents are living with HIV and accessing care and treatment services from 37 ART clinics across the country [22]. Majority of them are infected through mother-to-child transmission [5]. According to the national guidelines, children and adolescents up to the age of 15 are recommended to receive HIV care and treatment services from pediatric ART clinics and to thereafter be transitioned to adult clinics. However, in practice, most adolescents living with HIV transition to adult care between 15 and 20 years of age [5]. Previous studies have indicated that, similar to the global situation, adolescents living with HIV in Cambodia face challenges related to transitioning into adult services [23], AIDS-related stigma and issues of confidentiality [24, 25], all of which affect HIV treatment outcomes. In addition, there is very limited information about viral suppression and its determinants among adolescents living with HIV in Cambodia.

Given the above concerns and data gaps, the objective of this study is to determine the prevalence rate of viral suppression and factors associated with viral non-suppression among adolescents living with HIV in Cambodia. This information will be critical in identifying program interventions that can be further strengthened to optimize ART outcomes among this population in Cambodia and other resource-limited settings.

Methods

Study design and population

This cross-sectional study was conducted in August 2016 as part of a larger study exploring challenges in transition into adult care among adolescents living with HIV in the capital city of Phnom Penh and 10 other provinces. Details of this study have been reported elsewhere [20, 26]. A structured questionnaire was used for face-to-face interviews complemented by routine clinical data retrieved from medical records in ART clinics. The study participants included adolescents living with HIV aged 15–17, who were receiving HIV care and treatment services from 11 ART clinics. In 2016, the number of adolescents living with HIV in 18 clinics represented approximately 90% of the total number of adolescents living with HIV in the country. The remaining 10% were distributed across 21 sites, each with less than 10 adolescents.

Participants were selected in three stages. First, a two-stage cluster sampling method was used to select clusters to sample participants from the selected clinics, using a methodology developed by the WHO [27]. A comprehensive list of all ART clinics in the country with adolescents living with HIV population estimates was created and used to select the clusters after excluding ART clinics with less than 10 adolescents. This left a universe of 598 adolescents receiving care and treatment from the 18 major ART clinics. To minimize costs of data collection, additional seven clinics with less than 20 adolescent clients aged 15–17 were excluded.

Second, the required sample size was determined taking into account population size, confidence interval, and estimated proportion of the population with the outcome of interest [28], which in this case is viral suppression. Assuming that 50% of adolescents had viral suppression, a finite population size of 598, a design effect of 1.4, and a 10% dropout or refusal rate, a minimum sample size of 310 was required for the study to measure variables among selected adolescents with a confidence interval of 4.3%.

Third, the number of participants recruited from each cluster was determined. Because the size of the ART clinics varies, the probability proportional to size sampling method [28] was used in order to ensure that adolescents in larger sites have the same probability of being included in the sample as those in smaller sites. Cumulative population size of each ART clinic was calculated, sampling interval was determined, and potential participants were randomly selected from the database using a random number table.

Finally, a list of selected adolescents was prepared and assigned with a unique identification number based on the clinic identification (ID) code. The selected adolescents were then contacted on the phone, screened for eligibility, and informed about the research objectives as well as place, date, and time of the interview by local study coordinators. Potential participants were included if they were aged between 15 and 17 years, receiving HIV care and treatment services from the selected ART clinics, able to communicate in Khmer, allowed by a parent or guardian to participate, able to present themselves on the day of the interview, and physically and mentally stable to assent and participate in the study. Recruitment continued until the required sample size for each cluster was achieved.

Variables and measurements

In reference to existing literature [29, 30], a structured questionnaire was developed. Socio-demographic characteristics included age, gender, schooling-related information, parental and caregiver information, and social support the adolescents or their family had received for health care. Clinical and immunological data were obtained from medical records at the clinic. These included CD4 count and viral load at the enrolment in the clinic and the most recent test, duration of receiving HIV care and treatment, type of ART clinic (pediatric or adult), current antiretroviral (ARV) regimen (first or second line), as well as ARV supply and arrangement. We also collected information on adolescents' preference, experience, and understanding in HIV care and treatment, HIV knowledge, coping strategies, and the maturity of the adolescents in dealing with HIV care and treatment.

Data collection training

Two teams of interviewers and coordinators were trained for two days on the study protocol, research ethics, confidentiality, and interview techniques. Tool pretesting was conducted among 20 adolescents living with HIV in an ART clinic in Phnom Penh, followed by revisions of contents and language based on feedback from the pre-test. Adolescents who participated in the pre-test were not included in the main study.

Data analyses

Epi Data version 3 (Odense, Denmark) was used for double data entry and coding. Descriptive analyses were conducted to determine proportions for categorical variables and means and standard deviation (SD) or median and interquartile range (IQR) for continuous variables. In accordance with the national guidelines [5], adolescents were categorized as having viral suppression if the viral load count was < 1000 ribonucleic acid (RNA) copies/mL at the latest viral load count, which differs from the definition used in high-income settings [31]. We used Chi square test (or Fisher's exact test when a cell count was smaller than five) for categorical variables and Student's t-test or Mann–Whitney Test as appropriate for continuous variables to compare variables among adolescents with and without viral suppression.

To identify factors associated with viral non-suppression, a multivariate logistic regression model was constructed. Age, gender, and all variables associated with viral non-suppression in bivariate analyses at a level of p-value < 0.05 were simultaneously included in the model, followed by a backward selection. p-values of < 0.05 were considered statistically significant. SPSS version 22 (IBM Corporation, New York, USA) was used for all statistical analyses.

Ethics statement

The National Ethics Committee for Health Research, Ministry of Health, in Cambodia approved the study protocol (Ref: 297NECHR). All participants were required to assent to the study, and a written informed consent from a parent or guardian was obtained before data collection. Interviews were conducted in private locations, and confidentiality was strictly protected by removing all personal identifiers from the sampling frame, questionnaires, and field notes. Each participant was assigned a unique code. Researchers and data collectors were carefully trained on ethical issues. All participants were provided with a token of US$5 for transportation and time compensation.

Results

Socio-demographic characteristics

Socio-demographic characteristics of participants are shown in Table 1. This study included 328 adolescents living with HIV with a mean age of 15.9 (SD = 0.8); of whom, 48.5% were female. Less than half (42.7%) reported currently living with their biological parents, and 50.9% reported that their mother was alive. More

Table 1 Socio-demographic characteristics of adolescents living with HIV with and without viral suppression

Socio-demographic characteristics	Total ($n=328$) n (%)	Latest viral load count	
		≥ 1000 RNA copies/mL ($n=76$) n (%)	<1000 RNA copies/mL ($n=252$) n (%)
Age group (in years)			
15	126 (38.4)	36 (47.4)	90 (35.7)
16	107 (32.6)	25 (32.9)	82 (32.5)
17	95 (29.0)	15 (19.7)	80 (31.7)
Male gender	169 (51.5)	38 (50.0)	131 (52.0)
Currently living with			
Parents	140 (42.7)	44 (57.9)	96 (38.1)
Grandparents	49 (14.9)	15 (19.7)	34 (13.5)
Relatives	106 (32.3)	11 (14.5)	95 (37.7)
In an orphanage	27 (8.2)	4 (5.3)	23 (9.1)
Other	6 (1.8)	2 (2.6)	4 (1.6)
Mother is still alive	167 (50.9)	33 (44.3)	134 (53.2)
Mother's level of formal education			
Lower than high school	97 (29.6)	31 (40.8)	66 (26.2)
High school or higher	61 (18.6)	12 (15.8)	49 (19.4)
No mother/don't know	170 (51.8)	33 (43.4)	137 (54.4)
Father is still alive	130 (39.6)	34 (44.7)	96 (38.1)
Father's level of formal education			
Lower than high school	58 (17.7)	21 (27.6)	37 (14.7)
High school or higher	68 (20.7)	13 (17.1)	55 (21.8)
No father/don't know	202 (61.6)	42 (55.3)	160 (63.5)
Main daily caregiver			
Parent	187 (57.0)	58 (76.3)	129 (51.2)
Grand parent	5 (1.5)	1 (1.3)	4 (4.6)
Sibling	24 (7.3)	3 (3.9)	21 (8.3)
Relatives	100 (30.5)	11 (14.5)	89 (35.3)
Orphanage/NGO staff	12 (3.7)	3 (3.9)	9 (3.6)
Main caregiver's education lower than high school	54 (27.7)	11 (32.4)	43 (26.7)
Your level of formal education			
Primary school or lower	92 (28.0)	25 (32.9)	67 (26.6)
Secondary school	168 (51.2)	37 (48.7)	131 (52.0)
High school or higher	68 (20.7)	14 (18.4)	54 (21.4)
Currently attending school			
Not currently in school	55 (16.8)	16 (21.1)	39 (15.5)
With disruption	75 (22.9)	18 (23.7)	57 (22.6)
Fulltime	198 (60.4)	42 (55.3)	156 (61.9)
Family received social support	114 (34.8)	23 (30.3)	91 (36.1)
Belonged to a support group	97 (29.6)	16 (21.1)	81 (32.1)
Type of ART site			
Pediatric	225 (68.6)	36 (47.4)	189 (75.0)
Adult	94 (28.7)	36 (47.4)	58 (23.0)
Other	9 (2.7)	4 (5.3)	5 (2.0)
Receiving first line ARV regimen	271 (82.6)	63 (82.9)	208 (82.5)

ART antiretroviral therapy, *CI* confidence interval, *HIV* human immunodeficiency virus, *NGO* non-governmental organization

than half (57.0%) reported that their parent was their main caregiver. In general, level of education of their parents was low, with less than half completing high school. Regarding their own education, 60.4% reported currently attending school full time, while 22.9% were in school but with interruption. About one-third (34.8%) reported that their family received social support for their health care, and 29.6% belonged to a patient support group. The majority (68.6%) were receiving HIV care and treatment from a pediatric ART clinic, and 82.6% were on first line ART regimen.

Compared to 15.8% among adolescents aged 17, 28.6% of adolescents aged 15 had a viral load ≥ 1000 RNA copies/mL ($p=0.03$). Almost one-third (31.4%) of adolescents living a biological parent had a viral load ≥ 1000 RNA copies/mL compared to 10.4% among adolescents living with a relative ($p<0.001$). Similarly, the proportion of adolescents having a viral load ≥ 1000 RNA copies/mL was significantly higher among adolescents having a parent as the main caregiver compared to that among adolescents having a relative as the main caregiver (31.0% vs. 11.0%, $p<0.001$). The proportion of adolescents having a viral load ≥ 1000 RNA copies/mL was also significantly higher among adolescents receiving HIV care in an adult clinic compared to that among adolescents receiving HIV care in a pediatric clinic (38.3% vs. 16.0%, $p<0.001$).

Medical history

Table 2 shows that, on average, the adolescents had been in HIV care for 10.1 (interquartile range [IQR] = 8.0–11.5) years and received ART for 8.6 (IQR = 6.0–10.6) years. Median CD4 count at the enrolment was 561 (IQR = 274–798) and at the most recent test was 672 (IQR = 483–827). Median viral load at the first test was 628 RNA copies/mL (IQR = 315–3427) and at the most recent test was 215 RNA copies/mL (IQR = 168–2153). Compared to adolescents with viral suppression, adolescents without viral suppression had received care services from an ART clinic (8.9 years vs. 10.4 years, $p=0.002$) and been on ART (6.9 years vs. 9.2 years, $p<0.001$) for a significantly shorter duration. Adolescents without viral suppression had significantly lower latest CD4 count (594 vs. 699, $p<0.001$) and higher first viral load count (7036 RNA copies/mL vs. 312 RNA copies/mL, $p<0.001$) than adolescents with viral suppression.

HIV knowledge

As shown in Table 3, HIV knowledge among adolescents living with HIV in this study was generally good, although room remains for improvement. For example, 42.1% of the participants agreed that there is a cure for AIDS. A considerable proportion of them believed that, if both partners are HIV-positive, they do not have to use a condom (38.1%); if people living with HIV take medicines, they do not have to use a condom (26.2%), and it is okay for people living with HIV to miss their medicines (13.1%). The proportion of adolescents having a viral load ≥ 1000 RNA copies/mL was significantly higher among adolescents who believed that there is a cure for AIDS compared to adolescents who did not believe this (33.3% vs. 13.9%, $p<0.001$).

Understanding of HIV care and treatment

Table 4 shows that the majority (68.0%) of participants preferred to receive HIV care and treatment services from a pediatric ART clinic; 47.9% preferred to discuss questions related to health, sexual life, or daily life with their family members; 72.0% could recognize when they are getting sick; 88.7% were somewhat prepared or very prepared to manage their treatment going forward; 80.5% knew when they need to call a doctor; and 54.0% were responsible for refilling their own medicines. Regarding adherence to ART, 23.8% found it difficult to remember to take medicines; 11.0% would stop taking medicines when they feel worse; and 14.0% had missed medicines in the past 4 days. The proportion of adolescents having a

Table 2 Medical history among adolescents living with HIV with and without viral suppression

Medical history	Total (*n* = 328)	Latest viral load count	
		≥ 1000 RNA copies/mL (*n* = 76)	< 1000 RNA copies/mL (*n* = 252)
Time since first ART clinic visit (in years)	10.1 (8.0–11.5)	8.9 (5.2–10.4)	10.4 (8.8–11.7)
Time since ART initiation (in years)	8.6 (6.0–10.6)	6.9 (0.1–12.5)	9.2 (1.2–14.3)
CD4 count at enrolment	561 (274–798)	567 (271–710)	561 (277–825)
Latest CD4 count	672 (483–827)	594 (376–723)	699 (529–858)
First viral load count (RNA copies/mL)	628 (315–34,427)	7036 (426–93,625)	312 (218–630)

Values are median (interquartile range)

ARV antiretroviral, *ART* antiretroviral therapy, *HIV* human immunodeficiency virus, *RNA* ribonucleic acid

Table 3 Assessment of HIV knowledge among adolescents living with HIV with and without viral suppression

HIV knowledge	Total ($n=328$) n (%)	Latest viral load count	
		≥ 1000 RNA copies/mL ($n=76$) n (%)	< 1000 RNA copies/mL ($n=252$) n (%)
HIV is a virus that attacks a person's immune system			
True	263 (80.2)	58 (76.3)	205 (81.3)
False	44 (13.4)	11 (14.5)	33 (13.1)
Don't know	21 (6.4)	7 (9.2)	14 (5.6)
The cells of immune system that fight infections are called CD4 cells			
True	203 (61.9)	44 (57.9)	159 (63.1)
False	22 (6.7)	4 (5.3)	18 (7.1)
Don't know	103 (31.4)	28 (36.8)	75 (29.8)
The amount of HIV in a person's blood is called viral load			
True	160 (48.8)	35 (46.1)	125 (49.6)
False	26 (7.9)	5 (6.6)	21 (8.3)
Don't know	142 (43.3)	36 (47.4)	106 (42.1)
There is a cure for AIDS			
True	138 (42.1)	46 (60.5)	92 (36.5)
False	165 (50.3)	23 (30.3)	142 (56.3)
Don't know	25 (27.6)	7 (9.2)	18 (7.1)
You can tell a person has HIV by looking at him or her			
True	46 (14.0)	11 (14.5)	35 (13.9)
False	269 (82.0)	63 (82.9)	206 (81.7)
Don't know	13 (4.0)	2 (2.6)	11 (4.0)
A person will stay healthy if their CD4 cells are high and their viral load is low			
True	284 (86.6)	68 (89.5)	216 (85.7)
False	23 (7.0)	4 (5.3)	19 (7.5)
Don't know	21 (6.4)	4 (5.3)	17 (6.7)
Even though a person with HIV may feel healthy, the virus can still be damaging his or her immune system			
True	248 (75.9)	64 (84.2)	184 (73.0)
False	65 (19.8)	10 (13.2)	55 (21.8)
Don't know	15 (4.6)	2 (2.6)	13 (5.2)
If both partners are HIV positive, they don't have to use a condom			
True	125 (38.1)	34 (44.7)	91 (36.1)
False	155 (47.3)	33 (44.3)	122 (48.4)
Don't know	48 (14.6)	9 (11.8)	39 (15.5)
If people living with HIV take medicines, they don't have to use a condom			
True	86 (26.2)	20 (26.3)	66 (26.2)
False	193 (58.8)	42 (55.3)	151 (59.9)
Don't know	49 (14.9)	14 (18.4)	35 (13.9)
It is okay for people living with HIV to miss their medicines			
True	43 (13.1)	13 (17.1)	30 (11.9)
False	274 (83.5)	61 (80.3)	213 (84.5)
Don't know	11 (3.4)	2 (2.6)	9 (3.6)

CI confidence interval, *HIV* human immunodeficiency virus, *OR* odds ratio

viral load ≥ 1000 RNA copies/mL was significantly higher among adolescents who responded that they preferred to discuss issues related to health, sexual life, or daily life with their family members compared to adolescents who preferred to discuss these issues with health care providers (29.9% vs. 17.9%, $p=0.02$).

Factors associated with viral non-suppression

Table 5 shows factors associated with viral non-suppression in a multivariate logistic regression model. After controlling for the effect of other covariates, the likelihood of having viral non-suppression remained significantly lower among adolescents who were aged 17 (AOR = 0.46, 95% CI 0.21–0.98), had been on ART for more than nine years (AOR = 0.35, 95% CI 0.19–0.64), had most recent CD4 count of >672 (AOR = 0.47, 95% CI 0.26–0.86), had a relative as the main caregiver (AOR = 0.37, 95% CI 0.17–0.80), and did not believe that there is a cure for AIDS (AOR = 0.40, 95% CI 0.21–0.75) compared to their reference group. The likelihood of having viral non-suppression remained significantly higher among adolescents who had first viral load >628 RNA copies/mL (AOR = 1.81, 95% CI 1.05–4.08) and were receiving HIV care and treatment from an adult ART clinic (AOR = 2.95, 95% CI 1.56–5.59).

Discussion

After an average of 8.6 years on ART, the rate of viral suppression among adolescents living with HIV in this study was considerably high at 76.8%. This observed level of viral suppression falls short of the UNAIDS's 90–90–90 global targets, but it is well within the range reported in other studies. In a recent review, eight studies reported that the proportion of adolescents with viral suppression at 12 months ranged from 27 to 89% [32]. Another review that included 11 cohort studies also reported viral suppression rates between 28 and 78% [3]. Apart from reporting the proportion of adolescents with suppressed viral loads, the present study also identified independent predictors of viral non-suppression, which have important implications for HIV clinical service delivery across the study sites.

Older age may predict viral suppression. This might be related to the increasing treatment experience among older long-term survivors as reported in other studies [33, 34]. In Cambodia, treatment regimen and formulations for people living with HIV aged over 14 years old are similar to that for adults as long as they weigh more than 35 kg [5]. Because adolescence is characterized by increasing cognition [35–37], the relationship between viral suppression and age among long-term survivors of HIV could be mediated

Table 4 Understanding of HIV care and treatment among adolescents living with HIV with and without viral suppression

Understanding in HIV care and treatment	Total ($n=328$) n (%)	Latest viral load count	
		≥ 1000 RNA copies/mL ($n=76$)	< 1000 RNA copies/mL ($n=252$)
		n (%)	n (%)
Preference in receiving HIV care and treatment services			
Pediatric ART clinic	217 (66.2)	44 (57.9)	173 (68.7)
Adult ART clinic	111 (38.8)	32 (42.1)	79 (31.3)
Preferred to discuss questions related to health, sexual life, or daily life with			
Health care providers	67 (20.4)	12 (15.8)	55 (21.8)
Counselors/peer educators	19 (5.8)	5 (6.6)	14 (5.6)
Friends	44 (13.4)	4 (5.3)	40 (15.9)
Family	157 (47.9)	47 (61.8)	110 (43.7)
Other	41 (12.5)	8 (10.5)	33 (13.1)
Could recognize when you are sick	236 (72.0)	177 (70.2)	59 (77.6)
Preparedness to manage your treatment going forward			
Very prepared	42 (12.8)	9 (11.8)	33 (13.1)
Somewhat prepared	249 (75.9)	57 (75.0)	192 (76.2)
Somewhat unprepared	21 (6.4)	9 (11.8)	12 (4.8)
Very unprepared	16 (4.9)	1 (1.3)	15 (6.0)
Know when you need to call a doctor	264 (80.5)	58 (76.3)	206 (81.7)
Responsible for making appointments	151 (46.0)	28 (36.8)	123 (48.8)
Responsible for refilling own medicines	177 (54.0)	35 (46.1)	142 (56.3)
Feel comfortable asking questions	44 (13.4)	10 (13.2)	34 (13.5)
Difficult to remember to take medicines	78 (23.8)	12 (15.8)	66 (26.2)
Stop taking medicines when you feel better	2 (0.6)	0 (0.0)	2 (0.8)
Stop taking medicines when you feel worse	36 (11.0)	12 (15.8)	24 (9.5)
Have missed medicines in the past 4 days	46 (14.0)	13 (17.1)	33 (13.1)

ART antiretroviral therapy, *HIV* human immunodeficiency virus

by the impact of self-efficacy and self-competency and risk-taking on ART adherence [3, 33]. Similar findings regarding age were also found in a study among people living with HIV in South Africa, whereby adolescents aged < 15 were more likely to have unsuppressed viral load (viral load > 400 RNA copies/mL) compared with older patients [38]. Indeed, studies have consistently reported that increasing age reduced odds of non-viral suppression in Uganda (≥ 1000 RNA copies/mL) [39] and in several countries across Europe (> 50 RNA copies/mL) [40].

Shorter duration on ART was associated with viral non-suppression, which is to be expected given the destruction of CD4 cells resulting from high viral replication. Although the relationship between viral non-suppression, immunological responses, and duration on ART is not always consistent [41], similar findings were reported in a South African study, which reported that adolescents who had been on ART between six and 12 months were more likely to have viral non-suppression (viral load > 400 RNA copies/mL) compared with those who had been on treatment longer [38]. In our study, a lower viral load at the time of initial clinic enrollment also predicted viral suppression, which is in line with mechanisms of ART action [3].

Preference for receiving HIV care and treatment from a pediatric ART clinic predicted viral suppression. This could be because of the existing familiarity and ability of pediatric providers to provide appropriate counseling to young people in Cambodia. According to the national monitoring data, the majority of the Cambodian adolescents living with HIV are perinatally infected [5], and this may lead to having close relationships and contacts with their pediatric providers. Previous studies in Cambodia have shown that adolescents highly value current relationships with pediatric health providers and do not trust adult providers to maintain confidentiality [24, 25].

We also found that the belief that there is no cure for AIDS predicted viral suppression. This could be an indication of the perception of the importance of ART, and

Table 5 Factors associated with viral non-suppression among adolescents living with HIV ($n=328$)

Variables in the model	Viral non-suppression[a]			
	OR (95% CI)	*p*-value	AOR (95% CI)	*p*-value[†]
Age group				
15	Reference		Reference	
16	0.76 (0.42–1.38)	0.37	0.80 (0.40–1.57)	0.51
17	0.47 (0.24–0.92)	0.03	0.46 (0.21–0.98)	0.04
Duration on ART[†] (years)				
≤9	Reference		Reference	
>9	0.26 (0.15–0.45)	<0.001	0.35 (0.19–0.64)	0.001
Most recent CD4 count[†]				
≤672	Reference		Reference	
>672	0.45 (0.26–0.77)	0.003	0.47 (0.26–0.86)	0.02
First viral load[†]				
≤628 RNA copies/mL	Reference		Reference	
>628 RNA copies/mL	2.04 (1.04–2.50)	0.02	1.92 (1.02–4.42)	0.04
Main daily care giver				
Parent	Reference		Reference	
Grand parent	0.56 (0.06–5.08)	0.60	0.72 (0.06–6.10)	0.80
Sibling	0.32 (0.09–0.11)	0.07	0.30 (0.07–1.18)	0.08
Relatives	0.28 (0.14–0.55)	<0.001	0.37 (0.17–0.80)	0.01
Orphanage/NGO staff	0.74 (0.19–2.84)	0.66	0.49 (0.10–2.32)	0.37
Receiving HIV care and treatment from:				
Pediatric ART clinic	Reference		Reference	
Adult ART clinic	3.26 (1.88–5.64)	<0.001	2.95 (1.56–5.59)	0.001
There is a cure for AIDS				
True	Reference		Reference	
False	0.32 (0.18–0.57)	<0.001	0.40 (0.21–0.75)	0.005
Receiving HIV care and treatment from:				
Pediatric ART clinic	Reference		Reference	
Adult ART clinic	3.26 (1.88–5.64)	<0.001	2.95 (1.56–5.59)	0.001

Age, gender, and all variables associated with viral non-suppression at a level of $p<0.05$ were simultaneously included in a multivariate logistic regression model

AOR adjusted odds ratio, *ART* antiretroviral therapy, *CI* confidence interval

[a] Viral load count of < 1000 RNA copies/mL

[†] Median value was used as a cutoff to categorize the variables

potentially the importance of adherence. It is also possible that this is a reflection of appropriate education and counseling, which may also reinforce adherence. Poor treatment literacy and comprehension of the benefits of ART as a curative intervention negatively affects adherence [42].

Several implications emanate from findings in this study. First, better evaluation of adherence among the 24.2% who were not virally suppressed is warranted. Second, practical interventions are needed to strengthen adherence among this subsample. These interventions need to be tailored to the individual needs of each adolescent, and a combination of multiple approaches may be necessary. For instance, focusing particularly on younger adolescents and adolescents in transition to adult clinic with a range of counseling and social support could improve their treatment outcomes. Data from this sample (published elsewhere) suggest that transition to adult clinic is an ongoing challenge [23].

Data from this study showed that more than 88.0% of the adolescents were somewhat prepared or very prepared to manage their own treatment, which reflects the strong self-preparedness and self-reliance for transition. One of the challenges encountered for transition is the preparedness at the adult provider side. This could have an implication on the observation that 68.0% of adolescents preferred to receive services at a pediatric ART clinic. Similarly, enhancing counseling and treatment literacy to improve adolescents' understanding of the importance of ART and the currently incurable nature of HIV could improve adherence to the treatment and viral suppression. For younger adolescents, the education and information could be reinforced with their main caregivers and themselves during routine patient support group sessions.

Study limitations

This study has a number of limitations, which should be taken into account while interpreting the above findings. First, due to the sampling strategy, the study only included adolescents who were currently on treatment. Adolescents who were lost to follow-up were not included, which could have resulted in overestimating the rate of viral suppression. Longitudinal follow up with multiple assessments of viral load trends may provide a better picture of virological response compared to the single latest viral load measurement used in this study. Second, the study relied on self-reported data, which may be affected by recall and social desirability bias [43]. Third, adolescents who accessed care from low volume sites providing care to less than 10 adolescents were excluded, which may bias the results given that volume of patients is a key determinant of provider competency [44] and patient outcomes [45]. Finally, due to a lack of genotype data for the sample, exploration of virological failure was not possible.

Conclusions

The proportion of adolescents living with HIV in this study who had viral load < 1000 RNA copies/mL was relatively high at 76.8%. However, this proportion falls short of the UNAIDS' 90% target for on-treatment viral suppression. Findings from this study indicate that programs targeting younger adolescents and adolescents in transition from pediatric to adult clinics with a range of interventions including psychosocial support and treatment counseling could further improve viral suppression outcomes among this young population.

Authors' contributions

SY, ST, and VK conceived the study. KC, PC, and ST were responsible for data collection training, data collection, and data entry. SY, KC, and RS analyzed data and interpreted the findings. SY, KC, GM, and RS wrote the manuscript. All authors provided critical inputs for the writing. All authors read and approved the final manuscript.

Author details

[1] KHANA Center for Population Health Research, No. 33, Street 71, Phnom Penh, Cambodia. [2] Division of Health Research, Lancaster University, Lancaster, UK. [3] National Center for HIV/AIDS, Dermatology and STD, Phnom Penh, Cambodia. [4] Saw Swee Hock School of Public Health, National University of Singapore and National University Health System, Singapore, Singapore. [5] Center for Global Health Research, Touro University California, Vallejo, CA, USA.

Acknowledgements

The authors thank staff members of participating ART clinics, implementing partners, community support volunteers as well as all study participants and their family for their excellent contribution to the data collection. The authors' views expressed in this manuscript do not necessarily reflect the views of UNICEF Cambodia or the authors' affiliated institutions.

Competing interests

The authors declare that they have no competing interests.

Funding

Data used for this analysis were collected as part of a larger study funded by UNICEF Cambodia.

References

1. The Global Burden of Disease Study (GBD 2015) HIV Collaborators. Estimates of global, regional, and national incidence, prevalence, and mortality of HIV, 1980–2015: the global burden of disease study 2015. Lancet HIV. 2016;3(8):e361–87. https://doi.org/10.1016/s2352-3018(16)30087-x.
2. UNAIDS—the Joint United Nations Programme on HIV/AIDS. Global AIDS update. Geneva: UNAIDS; 2016.
3. Agwu AL, Fairlie L. Antiretroviral treatment, management challenges and outcomes in perinatally HIV-infected adolescents. J Int AIDS Soc. 2013;16:18579. https://doi.org/10.7448/IAS.16.1.18579.
4. World Health Organization (WHO). Consolidated guidelines on the use of antiretroviral drugs for treating and preventing HIV infection: recommendations for a public health approach. Geneva: WHO; 2013.
5. National Center for HIV/AIDS Dermatology and STD (NCHADS). National HIV clinical management guidelines for adults and adolescent, 4th revision. Phnom Penh: NCHADS; 2015.
6. Jobanputra K, Parker LA, Azih C, Okello V, Maphalala G, Kershberger B, et al. Factors associated with virological failure and suppression after enhanced adherence counselling, in children, adolescents and adults on antiretroviral therapy for HIV in Swaziland. PLoS ONE. 2015;10(2):e0116144. https://doi.org/10.1371/journal.pone.0116144.
7. Cruz ML, Cardoso CA, Darmont MQ, Souza E, Andrade SD, D'Al Fabbro MM, et al. Viral suppression and adherence among HIV-infected children and adolescents on antiretroviral therapy: results of a multicenter study. J Pediatr (Rio J). 2014;90(6):563–71. https://doi.org/10.1016/j.jped.2014.04.007.
8. Zanoni BC, Mayer KH. The adolescent and young adult HIV cascade of care in the United States: exaggerated health disparities. AIDS Patient Care STDS. 2014;28(3):128–35. https://doi.org/10.1089/apc.2013.0345.
9. Nachega JB, Hislop M, Nguyen H, Dowdy DW, Chaisson RE, Regensberg L, et al. Antiretroviral therapy adherence, virologic and immunologic outcomes in adolescents compared with adults in southern Africa. J Acquir Immune Defic Syndr. 2009;51(1):65–71. https://doi.org/10.1097/QAI.0b013e318199072e.
10. Idele P, Gillespie A, Porth T, Suzuki C, Mahy M, Kasedde S, et al. Epidemiology of HIV and AIDS among adolescents: current status, inequities, and data gaps. J Acquir Immune Defic Syndr. 2014;66(Suppl 2):S144–53. https://doi.org/10.1097/QAI.0000000000000176.
11. UNAIDS—the Joint United Nations Programme on HIV/AIDS. Global report. UNAIDS report on the global AIDS epidemic 2013. Geneva: UNAIDS; 2013.
12. World Health Organization (WHO). Health for the world's adolescents: a second chance in the second decade. Geneva: WHO; 2014.
13. World Health Organization (WHO). Consolidated guidelines on the use of antiretroviral drugs for treating and preventing HIV infection: recommendations for a public health approach. 2nd ed. Geneva: WHO; 2016.
14. Mburu G, Hodgson I, Kalibala S, Haamujompa C, Cataldo F, Lowenthal ED, et al. Adolescent HIV disclosure in Zambia: barriers, facilitators and outcomes. J Int AIDS Soc. 2014;17:18866. https://doi.org/10.7448/IAS.17.1.18866.
15. Siu GE, Bakeera-Kitaka S, Kennedy CE, Dhabangi A, Kambugu A. HIV serostatus disclosure and lived experiences of adolescents at the transition clinic of the infectious diseases clinic in Kampala, Uganda: a qualitative study. AIDS Care. 2012;24(5):606–11. https://doi.org/10.1080/09540121.2011.630346.

16. Ryscavage P, Macharia T, Patel D, Palmeiro R, Tepper V. Linkage to and retention in care following healthcare transition from pediatric to adult HIV care. AIDS Care. 2016;28(5):561–5. https://doi.org/10.1080/09540121.2015.1131967.
17. Dahourou DL, Gautier-Lafaye C, Teasdale CA, Renner L, Yotebieng M, Desmonde S, et al. Transition from paediatric to adult care of adolescents living with HIV in sub-Saharan Africa: challenges, youth-friendly models, and outcomes. J Int AIDS Soc. 2017;20(Suppl 3):21528. https://doi.org/10.7448/IAS.20.4.21528.
18. Kim SH, Gerver SM, Fidler S, Ward H. Adherence to antiretroviral therapy in adolescents living with HIV: systematic review and meta-analysis. AIDS. 2014;28(13):1945–56. https://doi.org/10.1097/qad.0000000000000316.
19. Abubakar A, Van de Vijver FJ, Fischer R, Hassan AS, Gona JK, Dzombo JT, et al. 'Everyone has a secret they keep close to their hearts': challenges faced by adolescents living with HIV infection at the Kenyan coast. BMC Public Health. 2016;16:197. https://doi.org/10.1186/s12889-016-2854-y.
20. Cluver LD, Toska E, Orkin FM, Meinck F, Hodes R, Yakubovich AR, et al. Achieving equity in HIV-treatment outcomes: can social protection improve adolescent ART-adherence in South Africa? AIDS Care. 2016;28(Suppl 2):73–82. https://doi.org/10.1080/09540121.2016.1179008.
21. Bailey H, Cruz MLS, Songtaweesin WN, Puthanakit T. Adolescents with HIV and transition to adult care in the Caribbean, Central America and South America, Eastern Europe and Asia and Pacific regions. J Int AIDS Soc. 2017;20(Suppl 3):21475. https://doi.org/10.7448/IAS.20.4.21475.
22. National Center for HIV/AIDS, Dermatology and STD (NCHADS). Diagnosis and treatment for HIV infected infant, children and adolescents in Cambodia. Phnom Penh: NCHADS; 2013.
23. Yi S, Ngin C, Pal K, Khol V, Tuot S, Sau S, et al. Transition into adult care: factors associated with level of preparedness among adolescents living with HIV in Cambodia. AIDS Res Ther. 2017;14(1):33. https://doi.org/10.1186/s12981-017-0159-6.
24. National Center for HIV/AIDS, Dermatology and STD (NCHADS). Factors affecting the transition from paediatric to adult HIV care services among children living with HIV aged 12–17 in Cambodia. Phnom Penh: NCHADS; 2012.
25. Seng SDT, Welle E, Mok S, Soch K, Tep S, et al. Stigma and discrimination as factors affecting the transition from paediatric to adult HIV care services by children living with HIV aged 12–17 in Cambodia: a qualitative exploratory study. In: International AIDS Conference, Melbourne, Australia; 2014.
26. Toth G, Mburu G, Tuot S, Khol V, Ngin C, Chhoun P, et al. Social-support needs among adolescents living with HIV in transition from pediatric to adult care in Cambodia: findings from a cross-sectional study. AIDS Res Ther. 2018;15(1):8. https://doi.org/10.1186/s12981-018-0195-x.
27. Henderson RH, Sundaresan T. Cluster sampling to assess immunization coverage: a review of experience with a simplified sampling method. Bull World Health Organ. 1982;60(2):253–60.
28. Skinner J. Probability proportional to size (PPS) sampling. London: Wiley; 2006.
29. Sharma N, Willen E, Garcia A, Sharma TS. Attitudes toward transitioning in youth with perinatally acquired HIV and their family caregivers. J Assoc Nurses AIDS Care. 2014;25(2):168–75. https://doi.org/10.1016/j.jana.2013.01.007.
30. Bakeera-Kitaka S, Nabukeera-Barungi N, Nostlinger C, Addy K, Colebunders R. Sexual risk reduction needs of adolescents living with HIV in a clinical care setting. AIDS Care. 2008;20(4):426–33. https://doi.org/10.1080/09540120701867099.
31. Poveda E, Crespo M. Hot News: impact of low-level viremia on treatment outcomes during ART—is it time to revise the definition of virological failure? AIDS Rev. 2018;20(1):71–2.
32. Ferrand RA, Briggs D, Ferguson J, Penazzato M, Armstrong A, MacPherson P, et al. Viral suppression in adolescents on antiretroviral treatment: review of the literature and critical appraisal of methodological challenges. Trop Med Int Health. 2016;21(3):325–33. https://doi.org/10.1111/tmi.12656.
33. Mburu G, Hodgson I, Teltschik A, Ram M, Haamujompa C, Bajpai D, et al. Rights-based services for adolescents living with HIV: adolescent self-efficacy and implications for health systems in Zambia. Reprod Health Matters. 2013;21(41):176–85. https://doi.org/10.1016/S0968-8080(13)41701-9.
34. Battles HB, Wiener LS. From adolescence through young adulthood: psychosocial adjustment associated with long-term survival of HIV. J Adolesc Health. 2002;30(3):161–8.
35. Gibb DM, Goodall RL, Giacomet V, McGee L, Compagnucci A, Lyall H, et al. Adherence to prescribed antiretroviral therapy in human immunodeficiency virus-infected children in the PENTA 5 trial. Pediatr Infect Dis J. 2003;22(1):56–62.
36. Choudhury S, Blakemore SJ, Charman T. Social cognitive development during adolescence. Soc Cogn Affect Neurosci. 2006;1(3):165–74. https://doi.org/10.1093/scan/nsl024.
37. Lowenthal ED, Bakeera-Kitaka S, Marukutira T, Chapman J, Goldrath K, Ferrand RA. Perinatally acquired HIV infection in adolescents from sub-Saharan Africa: a review of emerging challenges. Lancet Infect Dis. 2014;14(7):627–39. https://doi.org/10.1016/S1473-3099(13)70363-3.
38. Joseph D, Abrahams Z, Feinberg M, Prins M, Serrao C, Medeossi B, et al. Factors associated with recent unsuppressed viral load in HIV-1-infected patients in care on first-line antiretroviral therapy in South Africa. Int J STD AIDS. 2018;29(6):603–10. https://doi.org/10.1177/0956462417748859.
39. Bulage L, Ssewanyana I, Nankabirwa V, Nsubuga F, Kihembo C, Pande G, et al. Factors associated with virological non-suppression among HIV-positive patients on antiretroviral therapy in Uganda, August 2014–July 2015. BMC Infect Dis. 2017;17(1):326. https://doi.org/10.1186/s12879-017-2428-3.
40. Collaboration of Observational HIV Epidemiological Research Europe (COHERE) Study Group, Sabin CA, Smith CJ, d'Arminio Monforte A, Battegay M, Gabiano C, et al. Response to combination antiretroviral therapy: variation by age. AIDS. 2008;22(12):1463–73. https://doi.org/10.1097/qad.0b013e3282f88d02.
41. Fokam J, Billong SC, Jogue F, Ndiang SMT, Motaze ACN, Paul KN, et al. Immuno-virological response and associated factors amongst HIV-1 vertically infected adolescents in Yaounde-Cameroon. PLoS ONE. 2017;12(11):e0187566. https://doi.org/10.1371/journal.pone.0187566.
42. Veinot TC, Flicker SE, Skinner HA, McClelland A, Saulnier P, Read SE, et al. "Supposed to make you better but it doesn't really": HIV-positive youths' perceptions of HIV treatment. J Adolesc Health. 2006;38(3):261–7. https://doi.org/10.1016/j.jadohealth.2005.03.008.
43. Nieuwkerk PT, Oort FJ. Self-reported adherence to antiretroviral therapy for HIV-1 infection and virologic treatment response: a meta-analysis. J Acquir Immune Defic Syndr 2005;38(4):445–8.
44. Rackal JM, Tynan AM, Handford CD, Rzeznikiewiz D, Agha A, Glazier R. Provider training and experience for people living with HIV/AIDS. Cochrane Database Syst Rev. 2011;6:CD003938. https://doi.org/10.1002/14651858.cd003938.pub2.
45. Sangsari S, Milloy MJ, Ibrahim A, Kerr T, Zhang R, Montaner J, et al. Physician experience and rates of plasma HIV-1 RNA suppression among illicit drug users: an observational study. BMC Infect Dis. 2012;12:22. https://doi.org/10.1186/1471-2334-12-22.

2

Factors associated with pre-treatment HIV RNA: application for the use of abacavir and rilpivirine as the first-line regimen for HIV-infected patients in resource-limited settings

Sasisopin Kiertiburanakul[1*], David Boettiger[2], Oon Tek Ng[3], Nguyen Van Kinh[4], Tuti Parwati Merati[5], Anchalee Avihingsanon[6], Wing-Wai Wong[7], Man Po Lee[8], Romanee Chaiwarith[9], Adeeba Kamarulzaman[10], Pacharee Kantipong[11], Fujie Zhang[12], Jun Yong Choi[13], Nagalingeswaran Kumarasamy[14], Rossana Ditangco[15], Do Duy Cuong[16], Shinichi Oka[17], Benedict Lim Heng Sim[18], Winai Ratanasuwan[19], Penh Sun Ly[20], Evy Yunihastuti[21], Sanjay Pujari[22], Jeremy L. Ross[23], Matthew Law[2], Somnuek Sungkanuparph[1] and on behalf of the TREAT Asia HIV Observational Databases (TAHOD)

Abstract

Background: Abacavir and rilpivirine are alternative antiretroviral drugs for treatment-naïve HIV-infected patients. However, both drugs are only recommended for the patients who have pre-treatment HIV RNA <100,000 copies/mL. In resource-limited settings, pre-treatment HIV RNA is not routinely performed and not widely available. The aims of this study are to determine factors associated with pre-treatment HIV RNA <100,000 copies/mL and to construct a model to predict this outcome.

Methods: HIV-infected adults enrolled in the TREAT Asia HIV Observational Database were eligible if they had an HIV RNA measurement documented at the time of ART initiation. The dataset was randomly split into a derivation data set (75% of patients) and a validation data set (25%). Factors associated with pre-treatment HIV RNA <100,000 copies/mL were evaluated by logistic regression adjusted for study site. A prediction model and prediction scores were created.

Results: A total of 2592 patients were enrolled for the analysis. Median [interquartile range (IQR)] age was 35.8 (29.9–42.5) years; CD4 count was 147 (50–248) cells/mm^3; and pre-treatment HIV RNA was 100,000 (34,045–301,075) copies/mL. Factors associated with pre-treatment HIV RNA <100,000 copies/mL were age <30 years [OR 1.40 vs. 41–50 years; 95% confidence interval (CI) 1.10–1.80, $p = 0.01$], body mass index ≥30 kg/m^2 (OR 2.4 vs. <18.5 kg/m^2; 95% CI 1.1–5.1, $p = 0.02$), anemia (OR 1.70; 95% CI 1.40–2.10, $p < 0.01$), CD4 count ≥350 cells/mm^3 (OR 3.9 vs. <100 cells/mm^3; 95% CI 2.0–4.1, $p < 0.01$), total lymphocyte count ≥2000 cells/mm^3 (OR 1.7 vs. <1000 cells/mm^3; 95% CI 1.3–2.3, $p < 0.01$), and no prior AIDS-defining illness (OR 1.8; 95% CI 1.5–2.3, $p < 0.01$). Receiver-operator characteristic (ROC) analysis yielded area under the curve of 0.70 (95% CI 0.67–0.72) among derivation patients and 0.69 (95% CI 0.65–0.74) among validation patients. A cut off score >25 yielded the sensitivity of 46.7%, specificity of 79.1%, positive predictive value

*Correspondence: sasisopin.kie@mahidol.ac.th
[1] Department of Medicine, Faculty of Medicine Ramathibodi Hospital, Mahidol University, 270 Rama VI Road, Bangkok 10400, Thailand
Full list of author information is available at the end of the article

of 67.7%, and negative predictive value of 61.2% for prediction of pre-treatment HIV RNA <100,000 copies/mL among derivation patients.

Conclusion: A model prediction for pre-treatment HIV RNA <100,000 copies/mL produced an area under the ROC curve of 0.70. A larger sample size for prediction model development as well as for model validation is warranted.

Keywords: Abacavir, HIV RNA, Model, Prediction, Rilpivirine

Background

Antiretroviral therapy (ART) for the treatment of human immunodeficiency virus (HIV) infection has dramatically reduced HIV-associated morbidity and mortality and has transformed HIV infection into a manageable chronic condition [1, 2]. Furthermore, early ART is highly effective in preventing HIV transmission to sexual partners [3]. More than 25 antiretroviral drugs (ARV) in 6 classes are approved for treatment of HIV infection [4]. Selection of an ARV regimen should be individualized on the basis of efficacy, adverse effects, pill burden, dosing frequency, drug–drug interactions, comorbid conditions, and cost [4, 5].

The initial ARV regimen for a treatment-naïve HIV-infected patient generally consists of 2 nucleoside/nucleotide reverse transcriptase inhibitors, usually abacavir (ABC) plus lamivudine (3TC) or tenofovir disoproxil fumarate plus emtricitabine (TDF/FTC), plus a drug from 1 of 3 drug classes: an integrase strand transfer inhibitor, a non-nucleoside reverse transcriptase inhibitor (NNRTIs), or a boosted protease inhibitor [4, 5]. ABC is usually preferred over TDF for individuals with chronic kidney disease and/or those at risk of osteoporosis and fractures [4, 5]. However, ABC is recommended for patients who are HLA-B*5701 allele negative and have a pre-treatment HIV RNA <100,000 copies/mL [6], except when used with dolutegravir (DTG) and 3TC in the same regimen [4, 5].

Rilpivirine (RPV) is a recently approved NNRTI available at relatively low cost in Thailand (7 USD per month) and other countries. The advantages of RPV are once-daily dosing and very small pill size. In addition, RPV is associated with fewer treatment discontinuations for central nervous system adverse effects, fewer lipid effects, and fewer rashes when compared with efavirenz (EFV) [7, 8]. Nevertheless, RPV has a higher rate of virological failure when compared to EFV, especially in the first 48 weeks of treatment [7]. RPV is thus recommended as an alternative option for treatment naïve HIV-infected patients with a pre-treatment HIV RNA <100,000 copies/mL and CD4 count >200 cells/mm^3 [4, 5].

Testing of HIV RNA levels is recommended during initial patient visits by treatment guidelines in developed countries [4, 5]. In resource-limited settings, pre-treatment HIV RNA is not routinely performed and not widely available [9, 10]. This limits the use of ABC and RPV as a component of the first-line ARV regimen. If a clinical prediction tool based on routinely collected data could accurately predict whether pre-treatment HIV RNA was <100,000 copies/mL, this could be applied into clinical practice. The aims of this study are to determine factors associated with pre-treatment HIV RNA <100,000 copies/mL and to construct prediction tools that predict a pre-treatment HIV RNA <100,000 copies/mL. This prediction tool might support the use of ABC and RPV as part of first-line regimens for selected treatment-naïve HIV-infected individuals in resource-limited settings with limited access to HIV RNA testing.

Patients and methods

Our study population consisted of HIV-infected patients enrolled in the TREAT (Therapeutics Research, Education, and AIDS Training) Asia HIV Observational Database (TAHOD). The characteristics of this cohort have been described previously. Briefly, TAHOD is a prospective multi-center, observational study of patients with HIV and aims to assess HIV disease natural history in treated and untreated patients in the Asia and Pacific region [11]. We included patients enrolled in the cohort from 23 clinical sites throughout 13 countries in the Asia Pacific region since September 2003. The date of data censoring for the analysis of this study was 31 March 2015.

HIV-infected adults enrolled in TAHOD were eligible if they had an HIV RNA measurement documented at or around the time of ART initiation (pre-treatment HIV RNA). The window period of pre-treatment HIV RNA measurement was between 3 months prior to 1 day after the date of starting ART. ART was defined as a regimen containing $\geq$3 ARVs. Those exposed to mono or dual therapy prior to starting combination ART were excluded. Baseline was defined as the date of ART initiation. At baseline, co-variables included age, sex, HIV exposure, hepatitis B and C serology (ever positive), time since diagnosis of HIV infection, HIV subtype, and AIDS diagnosis prior to baseline. The window period of the following co-variables was between 3 months prior to 3 months after the date of ART initiation; body mass index (BMI), anemia (hemoglobin <13 g/dL for men, <12 g/dL for women), total lymphocyte count, CD4 count, CD8 count, CD4:CD8 ratio, and syphilis serology [Rapid plasma reagin (RPR), Venereal Disease Research Laboratory (VDRL) or *Treponema pallidum* particle agglutination assay (TPHA)].

Statistical analysis

The dataset was randomly split into a derivation data set (containing data from 75% of all eligible patients) and validation data set (containing data from 25% of all eligible patients) using the PROC SURVEYSELECT command in SAS version 9.4 (SAS Institute Inc., Cary, North Carolina, USA). The study endpoint was pre-treatment HIV RNA <100,000 copies/mL. Factors associated with this endpoint were evaluated by logistic regression adjusted for study site. Co-variables were considered for inclusion in the multivariate model if one or more categories exhibited a p-value <0.1. They were retained in the multivariate model if one or more categories exhibited a p-value <0.05. Missing categories, where present, were included in all models but odds ratios (OR) were not shown.

Prediction scores were created by multiplying the OR for each multivariate co-variable category by 10 and subtracting 1 [12]. Scores were rounded to the nearest 0.5 points. Some categories among the variables including in the multivariate model gave similar OR and were therefore collapsed together for the prediction tool.

The discrimination was evaluated using the area under the receiver-operator characteristic (AUROC) curve [13]. We used data of patients that had data available on all variables including in the prediction model. The optimum cut-off point for the score was evaluated by sensitivity, specificity, positive predictive value, and negative predictive value. Stata version 14.1 (StataCorp, College Station, Texas, USA) was used for all statistical analysis.

Results

A total of 2592 patients were included in our derivation analysis. Median [interquartile range (IQR)] age was 35.8 (29.9–42.5) years, 56.2% had heterosexual HIV exposure, median (IQR) BMI was 21.1 (19.0–23.4) kg/m^2, median duration of HIV diagnosis was 4.3 (1.4–29.2) months, and 34.5% had prior AIDS-defining illness. Median CD4 count was 147 (50–248) cells/mm^3 and median pre-treatment HIV RNA was 100,000 (34,045–301,075) copies/mL. For other laboratory investigations, 49.3% had anemia, 10.8% had positive HBsAg, 8.3% had positive anti-HCV, 19.6% had positive syphilis serology, and 75.1% had HIV infection with CRF01_AE subtype. Baseline characteristics of the patients are shown in Table 1.

Factors that statistically significantly associated with pre-treatment HIV RNA <100,000 copies/mL in the derivation patients by multivariate logistic regression,

Table 1 Baseline characteristics of 2592 HIV-infected patients

Baseline characteristics	Value[a]
Median (IQR) age, years	35.8 (29.9–42.5)
Male	1883 (72.6)
HIV exposure	
Heterosexual	1456 (56.2)
Homosexual	778 (30.0)
Intravenous drug use	93 (3.6)
Other	265 (10.2)
Median (IQR) body mass index, kg/m^2	21.1 (19.0–23.4)
Missing	683 (26.4)
Anemia	
No, n (% tested)	1208 (50.7)
Yes, n (% tested)	1176 (49.3)
Unknown	208 (8.0)
Hepatitis B surface antigen	
Negative, n (% tested)	1925 (89.2)
Positive, n (% tested)	232 (10.8)
Unknown	435 (16.8)
Hepatitis C antibody	
Negative, n (% tested)	1844 (91.7)
Positive, n (% tested)	168 (8.3)
Unknown	580 (22.4)
Syphilis serology	
Negative, n (% tested)	825 (80.4)
Positive, n (% tested)	201 (19.6)
Unknown	1566 (60.4)
Median (IQR) duration of HIV diagnosis, months	4.3 (1.4–29.2)
Missing	29 (1.1)
HIV subtype	
CRF01_AE, n (% tested)	796 (75.1)
B, n (% tested)	173 (16.3)
Other, n (% tested)	91 (8.6)
Unknown	1532 (59.1)
Median (IQR) HIV RNA, copies/mL	100,000 (34,045–301,075)
Median (IQR) CD4 count, cells/mm^3	147 (50–248)
Missing	106 (4.1)
Median (IQR) CD8 count, cells/mm^3	753 (485–1103)
Missing	1268 (48.9)
Median (IQR) CD4:CD8 ratio	0.19 (0.09–0.32)
Missing	1268 (48.9)
Median (IQR) total lymphocyte count, cells/mm^3	1472 (1000–2005)
Missing	286 (11.0)
Prior AIDS illness	
No	1698 (65.5)
Yes	894 (34.5)

IQR interquartile range

[a] Values are n (% total) unless otherwise specified

were age <30 years [OR 1.40 vs. 41–50 years; 95% confidence interval (CI) 1.10–1.80, $p = 0.01$], body mass index ≥30 kg/m^2 (OR 2.4 vs. <18.5 kg/m^2; 95% CI 1.1–5.1, $p = 0.02$), anemia (OR 1.70; 95% CI 1.40–2.10, $p < 0.01$], CD4 count ≥350 cells/mm^3 (OR 3.9 vs. <100 cells/mm^3; 95% CI 2.0–4.1, $p < 0.01$), total lymphocyte count ≥2000 cells/mm^3 (OR 1.7 vs. <1000 cells/mm^3; 95% CI 1.3–2.3, $p < 0.01$), and no prior AIDS-defining illness (OR 1.8; 95% CI 1.5–2.3, $p < 0.01$) (Table 2).

Clinical prediction tool scores for pre-treatment HIV RNA <100,000 copies/mL are shown in Table 3. Scores were +3.5 for age ≤30 years, +2.5 for BMI of 18.5–29.9 kg/m^2 or +14.5 for BMI of ≥30 kg/m^2, +7.0 for non-anemia, +17.0 for CD4 count ≥200 cells/mm^3 or +5.5 for 100–199 cells/mm^3, and +8.5 for no prior AIDS-defining illness. The possible maximum score was 50.5.

AUROC analysis was 0.70 (95% CI 0.67–0.72) among the derivation patients (Fig. 1) and 0.69 (95% CI 0.65–0.74) among validation patients.

A cut off total score >25 yielded sensitivity of 46.7 and 47.4%, specificity of 79.1 and 77.1%, positive predictive value of 67.7 and 64.2%, and negative predictive value of 61.2 and 63.0% for pre-treatment HIV RNA <100,000 copies/mL among the derivation patients and validation patients, respectively (Tables 4, 5). In contrast a cut off score >5 yielded the highest sensitivity of 91.1 and 91.9% and lowest specificity of 24.8 and 24.1% among derivation patients and validation patients, respectively (Tables 4, 5). We also conducted a sensitivity analysis using other prediction models, e.g. using total lymphocyte count instead of CD4 count and restriction analysis only among patients with CD4 count >200 cells/mm^3, however these models did not perform better.

Discussion

Plasma HIV RNA is one laboratory test used to stage HIV disease and to assist in the selection of ARV drug regimens [4, 5]. If treatment-naïve HIV-infected patients have a pre-treatment HIV RNA >100,000 copies/mL, the following regimens are not recommended; ABC/3TC with EFV or atazanavir/ritonavir (ATV/r) or raltegravir (RAL), RPV-based regimens, and darunavir/r (DRV/r) plus RAL [4, 5]. The main reason is being the higher rates of virologic failure observed in patients who received these particular drugs [7]. In addition, patients with pre-treatment HIV RNA >100,000 copies/mL or CD4 count <200 cells/μL are a subset of patients who may experience suboptimal virologic suppression if the regimen consists of ABC or PRV [5].

To our knowledge, this is the first study on prediction tool of pre-treatment HIV RNA <100,000 copies/mL in treatment-naïve HIV-infected patients that aims to facilitate the use of ABC and RPV as one of ARV in the first-line ART in resource-limited settings. We found some clinical and laboratory factors statistically significantly associated with pre-treatment HIV RNA <100,000 copies/mL. Our prediction tool of pre-treatment HIV RNA <100,000 copies/mL performed AUROC curve of 0.70. A cut off score >25 yielded the highest specificity of 79.0% for predicting pre-treatment HIV RNA <100,000 copies/mL.

Few studies focus on the association between HIV RNA levels and HIV-related outcomes. The results from some previous studies showed that HIV RNA level is rarely directly associated with the type of opportunistic infection [14] or HIV disease progression [15]. One study demonstrated a significant correlation between HIV RNA level and wasting syndrome in naïve HIV-infected patients, with HIV RNA levels in patients with wasting syndrome, significantly higher than those without the condition [16].

We also found six independent factors associated with pre-treatment HIV RNA <100,000 copies/mL: age, BMI, anemia, CD4 count, total lymphocyte count, and prior AIDS-defining illness. For example, patients with age ≤30 years had higher odds of 1.4 of having pre-treatment HIV RNA <100,000 copies/mL compared to patients 41–50 years old. Furthermore, patients with baseline CD4 count 100–199 cells/mm^3 had higher odds of 1.6 of having pre-treatment HIV RNA <100,000 copies/mL compared to patients with baseline CD4 count <100 cells/mm^3. These factors might be easily applied in the assessment of patients in resource-limited settings because they are patients' clinical characteristics and routine baseline laboratory investigations.

The AUROC curve is a single index for measuring the performance a test and can be used to estimate the discriminating power of a test. The AUROC of a 'perfect' test would be 1.00, that of a useless test, 0.50 [13, 17]. The AUROC for the pre-treatment HIV RNA model applied to the derivation population was 0.70. The AUROC curve when the model was applied to the validation population was 0.69, indicating some loss of discriminating power when applied to the new population. The score >5 showed the highest sensitivity but lowest specificity. With prediction of pre-treatment HIV RNA <100,000 copies/mL, higher specificity is required to minimize false positive results. Using a score >25 for prediction of pre-treatment HIV RNA yielded specificity approximately 80% and positive predictive value almost 70% and might be more appropriate. Additional data variables and/or an increased number of the patients might be needed to improve this prediction model and enhance its performance.

This study had some limitations. First, some patients must be excluded from the regression analysis and from

Table 2 Factors associated pre-treatment HIV RNA <100,000 copies/mL in derivation population

Factors	Number of patients	Patients (% total) with HIV RNA <100,000 copies/mL	Univariate OR (95% CI)	p-value	Multivariate OR (95% CI)	p- value
Years of age[b]						
≤30	656	360 (54.9)	1.6 (1.2–2.0)	<0.01	1.4 (1.1–1.8)	0.01
31–40	1057	514 (48.6)	1.2 (0.9–1.4)	0.15	1.1 (0.9–1.4)	0.40
41–50	600	273 (45.5)	1.0		1.0	
>50	279	131 (47.0)	1.0 (0.8–1.4)	0.85	1.0 (0.7–1.4)	0.96
Sex[b]						
Male	1883	908 (48.2)	1.0			
Female	709	370 (52.2)	1.2 (1.0–1.5)	0.02		
HIV exposure						
Heterosexual	1456	688 (47.3)	1.0			
Homosexual	778	422 (54.2)	1.3 (1.0–1.6)	0.03		
Intravenous drug use	93	41 (44.1)	0.9 (0.6–1.4)	0.54		
Other	265	127 (47.9)	0.9 (0.7–1.3)	0.70		
Body mass index (kg/m^2)[b]						
<18.5	366	134 (36.6)	1.0		1.0	
18.5–24.9	1289	648 (50.3)	1.7 (1.3–2.2)	<0.01	1.3 (1.0–1.7)	0.07
25.0–29.9	213	112 (52.6)	1.8 (1.3–2.6)	<0.01	1.2 (0.8–1.7)	0.47
≥30.0	41	29 (70.7)	4.1 (2.0–8.4)	<0.01	2.5 (1.2–5.2)	0.02
Unknown	683	355 (52.0)	–		–	
Anemia[b]						
No	1208	741 (61.3)	2.7 (2.3–3.3)	<0.01	1.7 (1.4–2.1)	<0.01
Yes	1176	442 (37.6)	1.0		1.0	
Unknown	208	95 (45.7)	–		–	
Hepatitis C antibody						
Negative	1844	916 (49.7)	1.0			
Positive	168	73 (43.5)	0.8 (0.6–1.1)	0.15		
Unknown	580	289 (49.8)	–			
Month since HIV diagnosis						
<6	1384	614 (44.4)	1.0			
6–18	338	189 (55.9)	1.6 (1.3–2.1)	<0.01		
>18	841	461 (54.8)	1.5 (1.3–1.8)	<0.01		
Unknown	29	14 (48.3)	–			
CD4 count (cells/mm^3)[b]						
≥350	219	147 (67.1)	4.8 (3.4–6.7)	<0.01	2.9 (2.0–4.1)	<0.01
200–349	694	456 (65.7)	4.2 (3.4–5.3)	<0.01	2.7 (2.1–3.4)	<0.01
100–199	617	308 (49.9)	2.1 (1.7–2.6)	<0.01	1.6 (1.2–2.0)	<0.01
<100	956	318 (33.3)	1.0		1.0	
Unknown	106	49 (46.2)	–		–	
Total lymphocyte count (cells/mm^3)[a]						
≥2000	593	325 (54.8)	2.9 (2.2–3.7)	<0.01	1.7 (1.3–2.3)	
1500–1999	529	303 (57.3)	2.9 (2.3–3.7)	<0.01	1.8 (1.4–2.4)	
1000–1499	627	331 (52.8)	2.3 (1.8–2.9)	<0.01	1.6 (1.3–2.1)	<0.01
<1000	557	180 (32.3)	1.0		1.0	
Unknown	286	139 (48.6)	–		–	
Prior AIDS-defining illness[a]						
None known	1698	987 (58.1)	3.0 (2.5–3.6)	<0.01	1.8 (1.5–2.3)	<0.01
Yes	894	291 (32.6)	1.0		1.0	

OR odds ratio, *CI* confidence interval

[a] Multivariate result shows effect size when replacing CD4 count

[b] Included in the final model

Table 3 Clinical prediction tool scores for each variable for pre-treatment HIV RNA <100,000 copies/mL

Variables	Score
Age ≤30 years	+3.5
Age >30 years	0
Body mass index <18.5 kg/m^2	0
Body mass index 18.5–29.9 kg/m^2	+2.5
Body mass index ≥30 kg/m^2	+14.5
Anemic	0
Non-anemic	+7.0
CD4 count ≥200 cells/mm^3	+17.0
CD4 count 100–199 cells/mm^3	+5.5
CD4 count <100 cells/mm^3	0
No prior AIDS-defining illness	+8.5
Prior AIDS-defining illness	0
Maximum score	50.5

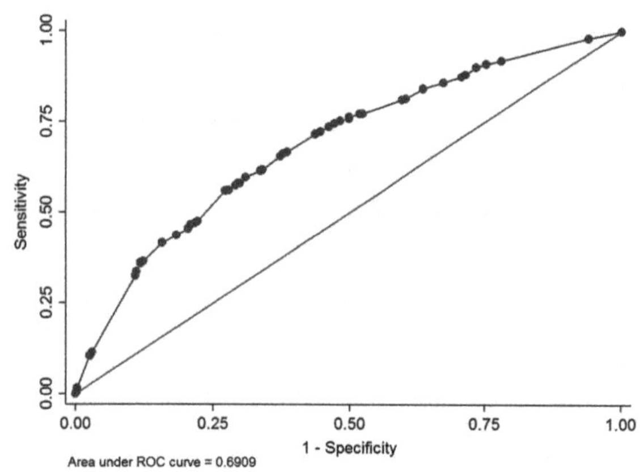

Fig. 1 Receiver-operator characteristic curve for predicting pre-treatment HIV RNA <100,000 copies/mL among derivation patients with data on all included variables (n = 1757)

the prediction tool due to missing data. Second, the performance of the model described by the AUROC of 0.70 might be associated with the small sample size of the study population among derivation and validation group.

Table 5 Sensitivities, specificities, positive predictive values, and negative predictive values of clinical prediction tool for pre-treatment HIV RNA <100,000 copies/mL among validation patients with data on all included variables (n = 587)

CPT score	N (%)	N (%) tests avoided	Sensitivity (%)	Specificity (%)	PPV (%)	NPV (%)
>25.0	201 (39.5)	386 (75.8)	47.4	77.1	64.2	63.0
>20.0	264 (51.9)	323 (63.5)	61.0	68.9	62.9	67.2
>15.0	355 (69.7)	232 (45.6)	75.4	52.4	57.7	71.1
>10.0	421 (82.7)	166 (32.6)	84.6	39.4	54.6	74.7
>5.0	489 (96.1)	98 (19.3)	91.9	24.1	51.1	77.6

CPT clinical prediction tool, *PPV* positive predictive value, *NPV* negative predictive value

In conclusion, in situations where HIV RNA cannot be obtained prior to ART initiation due to high costs or limited availability, certain risk factors and models for predicting pre-treatment HIV RNA <100,000 copies/mL might be useful to predict pre-treatment HIV RNA and afford opportunities for ABC and RPV initiation among naïve HIV-infected patients. A larger sample size with greater data variety would be warranted for prediction model construction as well as for model validation. Pre-treatment HIV RNA should be performed before ABC and RPV initiation if it is available and affordable.

Abbreviations

ART: antiretroviral therapy; HIV: human immunodeficiency virus; ARV: antiretroviral drugs; ABC: abacavir; 3TC: lamivudine; TDF: tenofovir disoproxil fumarate; FTC: emtricitabine; NNRTI: non-nucleoside reverse transcriptase inhibitors; DTG: dolutegravir; RPV: rilpivirine; EFV: efavirenz; TREAT: Therapeutics Research, Education, and AIDS Training; TAHOD: TREAT Asia HIV Observational Database; BMI: body mass index; RPR: rapid plasma regain; VDRL: Venereal Disease Research Laboratory; TPHA: *Treponema pallidum* particle agglutination assay; OR: odds ratio; AUROC: area under the receiver-operator characteristic; IQR: interquartile range; CI: confidence interval; ATV/r: atazanavir/ritonavir; RAL: raltegravir; DRV/r: darunavir/r; CPT: clinical prediction tool; PPV: positive predictive value; NPV: negative predictive value.

Authors' contributions

SK and SS initiated concept ideas. SK, OTN, NVK, TPM, AA, WWW, MPL, RC, AK, PK, FZ, JYC, NK, RD, DDC, SO, BS, WR, PSL, EY and SP contributed data for the analysis. DB performed the statistical analysis. All authors commented on the draft manuscript. All authors read and approved the final manuscript.

Table 4 Sensitivities, specificities, positive predictive values, and negative predictive values of clinical prediction tool for pre-treatment HIV RNA <100,000 copies/mL among derivation patients with data on all included variables (n = 1757)

CPT score	N (%)	N (%) tests avoided	Sensitivity (%)	Specificity (%)	PPV (%)	NPV (%)
>25.0	586 (37.7)	1171 (75.3)	46.7	79.1	67.7	61.2
>20.0	764 (49.1)	993 (63.8)	58.0	70.2	64.7	64.0
>15.0	1018 (65.4)	739 (47.5)	72.3	55.5	60.4	68.1
>10.0	1239 (79.6)	518 (33.3)	81.3	39.6	55.9	69.3
>5.0	1456 (93.6)	301 (19.3)	91.1	24.8	53.2	74.8

CPT clinical prediction tool, *PPV* positive predictive value, *NPV* negative predictive value

Author details

[1] Department of Medicine, Faculty of Medicine Ramathibodi Hospital, Mahidol University, 270 Rama VI Road, Bangkok 10400, Thailand. [2] The Kirby Institute, University of New South Wales, Sydney, Australia. [3] Tan Tock Seng Hospital, Singapore, Singapore. [4] National Hospital of Tropical Diseases, Hanoi, Vietnam. [5] Department of Medicine, Faculty of Medicine, Udayana University & Sanglah Hospital, Bali, Indonesia. [6] HIV-NAT/Thai Red Cross AIDS Research Centre, Bangkok, Thailand. [7] Taipei Veterans General Hospital, Taipei, Taiwan. [8] Queen Elizabeth Hospital, Hong Kong, China. [9] Research Institute for Health Sciences, Chiang Mai, Thailand. [10] University Malaya Medical Centre, Kuala Lumpur, Malaysia. [11] Chiangrai Prachanukroh Hospital, Chiang Rai, Thailand. [12] Beijing Ditan Hospital, Capital Medical University, Beijing, China. [13] Division of Infectious Diseases, Department of Internal Medicine, Yonsei University College of Medicine, Seoul, South Korea. [14] Chennai Antiviral Research and Treatment Clinical Research Site (CART CRS), YRGCARE Medical Centre, VHS, Chennai, India. [15] Research Institute for Tropical Medicine, Manila, Philippines. [16] Bach Mai Hospital, Hanoi, Vietnam. [17] National Center for Global Health and Medicine, Tokyo, Japan. [18] Hospital Sungai Buloh, Sungai Buloh, Malaysia. [19] Faculty of Medicine, Siriraj Hospital, Mahidol University, Bangkok, Thailand. [20] National Center for HIV/AIDS, Dermatology & STDs, University of Health Sciences, Phnom Penh, Cambodia. [21] Faculty of Medicine Universitas Indonesia, Dr. Cipto Mangunkusumo General Hospital, Jakarta, Indonesia. [22] Institute of Infectious Diseases, Pune, India. [23] TREAT Asia, amfAR, The Foundation for AIDS Research, Bangkok, Thailand.

Acknowledgements

PS Ly* and V Khol, National Center for HIV/AIDS, Dermatology & STDs, Phnom Penh, Cambodia; FJ Zhang*, HX Zhao and N Han, Beijing Ditan Hospital, Capital Medical University, Beijing, China; MP Lee* †, PCK Li, W Lam and YT Chan, Queen Elizabeth Hospital, Hong Kong, China; N Kumarasamy*, S Saghayam and C Ezhilarasi, Chennai Antiviral Research and Treatment Clinical Research Site (CART CRS), YRGCARE Medical Centre, VHS, Chennai, India; S Pujari*, K Joshi, S Gaikwad and A Chitalikar, Institute of Infectious Diseases, Pune, India; TP Merati*, DN Wirawan and F Yuliana, Faculty of Medicine Udayana University & Sanglah Hospital, Bali, Indonesia; E Yunihastuti*, D Imran and A Widhani, Faculty of Medicine Universitas Indonesia - Dr. Cipto Mangunkusumo General Hospital, Jakarta, Indonesia; S Oka*, J Tanuma and T Nishijima, National Center for Global Health and Medicine, Tokyo, Japan; JY Choi*, Na S and JM Kim, Division of Infectious Diseases, Department of Internal Medicine, Yonsei University College of Medicine, Seoul, South Korea; BLH Sim*, YM Gani, and R David, Hospital Sungai Buloh, Sungai Buloh, Malaysia; A Kamarulzaman*, SF Syed Omar, S Ponnampalavanar and I Azwa, University Malaya Medical Centre, Kuala Lumpur, Malaysia; R Ditangco*, E Uy and R Bantique, Research Institute for Tropical Medicine, Manila, Philippines; WW Wong*‡, WW Ku and PC Wu, Taipei Veterans General Hospital, Taipei, Taiwan; OT Ng*, PL Lim, LS Lee and PS Ohnmar, Tan Tock Seng Hospital, Singapore; A Avihingsanon*, S Gatechompol, P Phanuphak and C Phadungphon, HIV-NAT/Thai Red Cross AIDS Research Centre, Bangkok, Thailand; S Kiertiburanakul*, S Sungkanuparph, L Chumla and N Sanmeema, Faculty of Medicine Ramathibodi Hospital, Mahidol University, Bangkok, Thailand; R Chaiwarith*, T Sirisanthana, W Kotarathititum and J Praparattanapan, Research Institute for Health Sciences, Chiang Mai, Thailand; P Kantipong* and P Kambua, Chiangrai Prachanukroh Hospital, Chiang Rai, Thailand; W Ratanasuwan* and R Sriondee, Faculty of Medicine, Siriraj Hospital, Mahidol University, Bangkok, Thailand; KV Nguyen*, HV Bui, DTH Nguyen and DT Nguyen, National Hospital for Tropical Diseases, Hanoi, Vietnam; DD Cuong*, NV An and NT Luan, Bach Mai Hospital, Hanoi, Vietnam; AH Sohn*, JL Ross* and B Petersen, TREAT Asia, amfAR—The Foundation for AIDS Research, Bangkok, Thailand; DA Cooper, MG Law*, A Jiamsakul* and DC Boettiger, The Kirby Institute, UNSW Australia, Sydney, Australia. *TAHOD Steering Committee member; †Steering Committee Chair; ‡co-Chair.

Competing interests

The authors declare that they have no competing interests.

Funding

The TREAT Asia HIV Observational Database is an initiative of TREAT Asia, a program of amfAR, The Foundation for AIDS Research, with support from the US National Institutes of Health's National Institute of Allergy and Infectious Diseases, the Eunice Kennedy Shriver National Institute of Child Health and Human Development, the National Cancer Institute, the National Institute of Mental Health, and the National Institute on Drug Abuse, as part of the International Epidemiologic Databases to Evaluate AIDS (IeDEA; U01AI069907). The Kirby Institute is funded by the Australian Government Department of Health and Ageing, and is affiliated with the Faculty of Medicine, UNSW Australia. The content of this publication is solely the responsibility of the authors and does not necessarily represent the official views of any of the governments or institutions mentioned above.

Presentation

Parts of this manuscript were presented at the 27th European Congress of Clinical Microbiology and Infectious Diseases (Vienna), May 22–25, 2017 [abstract 784].

References

1. Taddei TH, Lo Re V 3rd, Justice AC. HIV, aging, and viral coinfections: taking the long view. Curr HIV/AIDS Rep. 2016;13:269–78.
2. Kiertiburanakul S, Luengroongroj P, Sungkanuparph S. Clinical characteristics of HIV-infected patients who survive after the diagnosis of HIV infection for more than 10 years in a resource-limited setting. J Int Assoc Physicians AIDS Care (Chic). 2012;11:361–5.
3. Cohen MS, Chen YQ, McCauley M, Gamble T, Hosseinipour MC, Kumarasamy N, et al. Antiretroviral therapy for the prevention of HIV-1 transmission. N Engl J Med. 2016;375:830–9.
4. Panel on antiretroviral guidelines for adults and adolescents. Guidelines for the use of antiretroviral agents in HIV-1-infected adults and adolescents. Department of Health and Human Services. http://www.aidsinfo.nih.gov/ContentFiles/AdultandAdolescentGL.pdf. Accessed 14 Sep 2016.
5. Günthard HF, Saag MS, Benson CA, del Rio C, Eron JJ, Gallant JE, et al. Antiretroviral drugs for treatment and prevention of HIV infection in adults: 2016 recommendations of the International Antiviral Society—USA panel. JAMA. 2016;316:191–210.
6. Sax PE, Tierney C, Collier AC, Fischl MA, Mollan K, Peeples L, et al. Abacavir–lamivudine versus tenofovir–emtricitabine for initial HIV-1 therapy. N Engl J Med. 2009;361:2230–40.
7. Cohen CJ, Molina JM, Cassetti I, Chetchotisakd P, Lazzarin A, Orkin C, et al. Week 96 efficacy and safety of rilpivirine in treatment-naive, HIV-1 patients in two phase III randomized trials. AIDS. 2013;27:939–50.
8. Tebas P, Sension M, Arribas J, Duiculescu D, Florence E, Hung CC, et al. Lipid levels and changes in body fat distribution in treatment-naive, HIV-1-Infected adults treated with rilpivirine or efavirenz for 96 weeks in the ECHO and THRIVE trials. Clin Infect Dis. 2014;59:425–34.
9. Manosuthi W, Ongwandee S, Bhakeecheep S, Leechawengwongs M, Ruxrungtham K, Phanuphak P, et al. Guidelines for antiretroviral therapy in HIV-1 infected adults and adolescents 2014 Thailand. AIDS Res Ther. 2015;12:12.
10. World Health Organization. Consolidated guidelines on HIV prevention, diagnosis, treatment and care for key populations. 2016. http://apps.who.int/iris/bitstream/10665/128048/1/9789241507431_eng.pdf?ua=1&ua=1. Accessed 8 Jan 2017.
11. Zhou J, Kumarasamy N, Ditangco R, Kamarulzaman A, Lee CK, Li PC, et al. The TREAT Asia HIV Observational Database: baseline and retrospective data. J Acquir Immune Defic Syndr. 2005;38:174–9.
12. Moons KG, Harrell FE, Steyerberg EW. Should scoring rules be based on odds ratios or regression coefficients? J Clin Epidemiol. 2002;55:1054–5.
13. Hanley JA, McNeil BJ. The meaning and use of the area under a receiver operating characteristic (ROC) curve. Radiology. 1982;143:29–36.
14. Kimmel AD, Goldie SJ, Walensky RP, Losina E, Weinstein MC, Paltiel AD, et al. Optimal frequency of CD4 cell count and HIV RNA monitoring prior to initiation of antiretroviral therapy in HIV-infected patients. Antivir Ther. 2005;10:41–52.
15. Rodríguez B, Sethi AK, Cheruvu VK, Mackay W, Bosch RJ, Kitahata M, et al. Predictive value of plasma HIV RNA level on rate of CD4 T-cell decline in untreated HIV infection. JAMA. 2006;296:1498–506.
16. Utama MS, Merati TP. Association of opportunistic infections with HIV-RNA and CD4 cell count in pre ARV and ARV failure at the care support treatment clinic of Sanglah Hospital, Bali. J Epidemiol Res. 2016;2:13–7.
17. Kummar R, Indrayan A. Receiver operating characteristic (ROC) curve for medical researchers. Indian Pediatr. 2011;48:277–89.

3

HIV care in Yangon, Myanmar; successes, challenges and implications for policy

Ne Myo Aung[1*†], Josh Hanson[1,2,3†], Tint Tint Kyi[4], Zaw Win Htet[5], David A. Cooper[3], Mark A. Boyd[3,6], Mar Mar Kyi[1] and Htin Aung Saw[1]

Abstract

Background: Approximately 0.8% of adults aged 18–49 in Myanmar are seropositive for Human Immunodeficiency Virus (HIV). Identifying the demographic, epidemiological and clinical characteristics of people living with HIV (PLHIV) is essential to inform optimal management strategies in this resource-limited country.

Methods: To create a "snapshot" of the PLHIV seeking anti-retroviral therapy (ART) in Myanmar, data were collected from the registration cards of all patients who had been prescribed ART at two large referral hospitals in Yangon, prior to March 18, 2016.

Results and discussion: Anti-retroviral therapy had been prescribed to 2643 patients at the two hospitals. The patients' median [interquartile range (IQR)] age was 37 (31–44) years; 1494 (57%) were male. At registration, injecting drug use was reported in 22 (0.8%), male-to-male sexual contact in eleven (0.4%) and female sex work in eleven (0.4%), suggesting that patients under-report these risk behaviours, that health care workers are uncomfortable enquiring about them or that the two hospitals are under-servicing these populations. All three explanations appear likely. Most patients were symptomatic at registration with 2027 (77%) presenting with WHO stage 3 or 4 disease. In the 2442 patients with a CD4+ T cell count recorded at registration, the median (IQR) count was 169 (59–328) cells/mm^3. After a median (IQR) duration of 359 (185–540) days of ART, 151 (5.7%) patients had died, 111 (4.2%) patients had been lost to follow-up, while 2381 were alive on ART. Tuberculosis (TB) co-infection was common: 1083 (41%) were already on anti-TB treatment at registration, while a further 41 (1.7%) required anti-TB treatment during follow-up. Only 21 (0.8%) patients were prescribed isoniazid prophylaxis therapy (IPT); one of these was lost to follow-up, but none of the remaining 20 patients died or required anti-TB treatment during a median (IQR) follow-up of 275 (235–293) days.

Conclusions: People living with HIV in Yangon, Myanmar are generally presenting late in their disease course, increasing their risk of death, disease and transmitting the virus. A centralised model of ART prescription struggles to deliver care to the key affected populations. TB co-infection is very common in Myanmar, but despite the proven efficacy of IPT, it is frequently not prescribed.

Keywords: HIV, Myanmar, Anti-retroviral therapy, Tuberculosis, Isoniazid prophylaxis therapy, Key affected populations, Resource limited settings

Background

Myanmar is a country at a critical point in its history. After five decades of military rule, the newly elected government faces enormous challenges in improving the health, welfare and prosperity of its people [1, 2]. The human immunodeficiency virus (HIV) epidemic is one of the country's greatest health concerns: in 2015, 0.8% of the country's adults aged 18–49 were seropositive [3]. Myanmar's health system remains poorly resourced and under-equipped to achieve the UNAIDS "90–90–90" target or the ambitious Sustainable Development Goal of ending the AIDS epidemic by 2030 [4, 5]. HIV prevalence is highest in people

*Correspondence: drnaymyoaung@gmail.com
†Ne Myo Aung and Josh Hanson contributed equally to this work
[1] Department of Medicine, University of Medicine 2, Yangon, Myanmar
Full list of author information is available at the end of the article

who inject drugs (PWID), men who have sex with men (MSM) and female sex workers (FSW) [6]. However, it is frequently challenging for Myanmar health services to reach these key affected populations (KAPs) and ensure that they are receiving optimal care [6].

One of the key aspects of the country's response to the HIV epidemic has been a rapid scale up of anti-retroviral therapy (ART). In 2015, 111,563 individuals—representing an estimated 50% of the people living with HIV (PLHIV)—were receiving ART and the rollout has accelerated since [6]. All PLHIV in Myanmar receiving ART have basic demographic, epidemiological and clinical data collected prospectively and entered into the National AIDS Programme's "Patient HIV Care and Antiretroviral Treatment (ART) Record", commonly referred to as "The White Card". The White Card records a patient's gender, age, address and marital and employment status. It documents their referral origin, their risk factors for infection, the CD4+ count, the WHO disease stage and the presence or history of tuberculosis. It also records the prescribed ART regimen and if a patient dies or is lost to follow up.

These simple data provide a useful insight into the characteristics of the PLHIV receiving ART, and therefore might inform approaches for the optimal delivery of care. Just as importantly, the absence of key populations in these data might highlight PLHIV who are not receiving ART, permitting policy makers to develop strategies to reach under-serviced populations, improving the health of these often vulnerable populations, and also preventing ongoing transmission [6–8].

This study examined White Card data collected at two large ART prescribing centres to create a "snapshot" of the HIV epidemic in Myanmar. It was hoped that this might both identify the successes of the current programme and the challenges that remain.

Methods

The White Cards of all PLHIV commencing ART between the 6th June 2001 and the 18th March 2016 at two Yangon hospitals—Waibargi Hospital (a specialist infectious disease hospital) and Insein General Hospital (a tertiary referral general hospital)—were reviewed. These data were de-identified and transferred from the hospital databases into an electronic database (Microsoft Excel); statistical analysis was performed using statistical software (Stata, version 10). Death was either witnessed in hospital or reported by the next of kin. If there was no contact for 3 months after the last outpatient visit, the patient was defined as lost to follow up. Groups were analysed using the Kruskal–Wallis and Chi squared tests. Multivariate analysis was performed using backwards stepwise logistic regression, with only variables that were significant in univariate analysis at a significance level of <0.05 selected for multivariate analysis. Ethical approval for the study was granted by the Human Research Ethics Committees of the University of Medicine 2, Yangon and the Menzies School of Health Research, Darwin, Australia. The Committees waived the requirement for informed consent as the publication of retrospective, aggregated, de-identified data was felt to pose negligible risk to the participants.

Results

There were 2643 patients with a completed white card at the two hospitals, 1674 at Waibargi Hospital and 969 at Insein General Hospital; their characteristics are presented in Tables 1 and 2. The median [interquartile range (IQR)] age of the patients was 37 (31–44) years; 1494 (57%) patients were male. Most patients were referred after having presented with symptoms to the outpatient department (1959 patients, 74%) or after an inpatient admission (449 patients, 17%); 68 patients (2.6%) presented for voluntary testing while only two patients (0.1%) were referred from a drug treatment service.

All patients had data collected on risk factors for infection: 2271 (86%) were recorded as having acquired the infection heterosexually, 82 (3.1%) were recorded as having acquired the infection from a blood transfusion. Only 22 (0.8%) were documented to have acquired the infection through injecting drug use, while male-to-male sexual contact was reported in eleven (0.4%) and eleven (0.4%) reported that they were female sex workers. Of the 2643 patients, 1545 (58%) were married; 664 (43%) had an HIV positive spouse, while in 207 (13%) cases the spouse was negative and in 674 (44%) the HIV status of the spouse was unknown. Waibargi Hospital looked after a greater number of patients from outside the Yangon region: 30% versus 4.5% at Insein General Hospital ($p < 0.001$).

Patients generally presented late in the course of the disease: 2027 (77%) presented with WHO stage 3 or 4 disease. In the 2442 patients with a CD4+ T-cell count recorded at registration, the median (IQR) CD4+ count was 169 (59–328) cells/mm^3. Tuberculosis was common in the cohort: 1083 (41%) were already on treatment for tuberculosis at the time of registration, while a further 41 (1.7%) required treatment for tuberculosis after registration. Despite the high rate of tuberculosis, only 21 patients in the cohort were prescribed isoniazid prophylaxis therapy (IPT) during the study period. There were 2627 patients with data available regarding co-trimoxazole prophylaxis (CPT), 2125 (81%) of whom received this therapy during the study period, including 1158 (85%) of the 1358 patients with a CD4+ count of <200 cells/mm^3.

Table 1 Characteristics of the patients at the two study sites

Variable	All n = 2643	Waibargi Hospital n = 1674	Insein Hospital n = 969	p^
Age	37 (31–44)	38 (32–45)	35 (29–41)	<0.001
Gender (% male)	1494 (57%)	1011 (60%)	483 (50%)	<0.001
Unemployed	917 (35%)	453 (27%)	464 (48%)	<0.001
Living in the same region[a]	2042 (80%)	1117 (70%)	925 (95%)	<0.001
CD4+ at registration	169 (59–328)	159 (50–332)	185 (74–323)	0.03
WHO stage at registration	3 (3–3)	3 (3–4)	3 (1–3)	<0.001
Prescribed TDF + FTC + EFV	2280 (86%)	1420 (85%)	860 (89%)	0.005
CD4+ change after ART (cells/mm^3)	148 (46–263)	141 (44–258)	166 (52–276)	0.19
Required anti-tuberculosis treatment	1124 (43%)	691 (41%)	433 (45%)	0.09
Isoniazid prophylaxis therapy	21 (0.8%)	0	21 (2%)	<0.001
Co-trimoxazole prophylaxis therapy	2125 (81%)	1254 (76%)	871 (90%)	<0.001
Died	151 (5.7%)	116 (7.3%)	35 (3.7%)	<0.001
Lost to follow up	111 (4.2%)	89 (5.3%)	22 (2.3%)	<0.001

All numbers represent median and interquartile range or absolute number (percentage)

WHO World Health Organization, *TDF* tenofovir disoproxil fumarate, *FTC* emtricitabine, *EFV* efavirenz, *ART* anti-retroviral therapy

^ Comparison between the study sites using Kruskal–Wallis or Chi squared test

[a] 75 patients did not have an address recorded; all were at Waibargi Hospital

Table 2 Comparison between patients who had died or who were alive on ART at the end of the study period

Variable	All n = 2643	Died n = 151[a]	Alive on ART n = 2381[a]	p^
Age	37 (31–44)	40 (33–45)	37 (31–44)	0.001
Gender (% male)	1494 (57%)	96 (64%)	1327 (56%)	0.06
Unemployed	917 (35%)	64 (42%)	814 (34%)	0.04
Living in a different region[b]	526 (20%)	43 (30%)	462 (20%)	0.005
CD4 + count at registration (cells/mm^3)	169 (59–328)	45 (23–127)	183 (65–337)	<0.001
WHO stage at registration	3 (3–3)	4 (3–4)	3 (2–3)	0.0001
On treatment for tuberculosis	1124 (43%)	99 (66%)	971 (41%)	<0.001
Isoniazid prophylaxis therapy[c]	21 (0.8%)	0	20 (0.8%)	0.26
Co-trimoxazole prophylaxis therapy[d]	2125 (81%)	136 (93%)	1904 (80%)	<0.001

All numbers represent median and interquartile range or absolute number (percentage)

^ Comparison between survivors and those that died using Kruskal–Wallis or Chi squared test

[a] Does not include the 111 patients in the cohort lost to follow up

[b] 75 patients did not have an address recorded; 6 patients who died and 69 still alive

[c] One patient lost to follow up

[d] 2627 (99%) had data regarding co-trimoxazole prescription

In the 2450 patients for whom the exact date of ART commencement was available, it was initiated at a median (IQR) of 21 (9–42) days after the HIV diagnosis was recorded. One hundred and seven (4.4%) PLHIV started ART on the same day that the diagnosis was recorded. The most commonly prescribed antiretroviral (ART) regimen was tenofovir, emtricitabine and efavirenz, with 2280 (86%) receiving this combination. In the 1247 patients with a recorded follow up CD4+ T-cell count at least 90 days after registration, there was a median increase in the CD4 count of 150 (47–263) cells/mm^3; 192 (15.1%) had a fall in their CD4+ count.

At the time of data analysis, a median (IQR) of 359 (185–540) days after patient registration, 151 (5.7%) patients had died, 111 (4.2%) had been lost to follow up and 2381 (90.1%) were alive and taking ART (Table 1). In multivariate analysis, the independent predictors of death were a CD4 + count at registration of <200 cells/ mm^3 (odds ratio (OR) 6.4, 95% confidence interval (CI) 3.5–11.6, $p < 0.0001$); treatment at Waibargi Hospital (OR (95% CI) 1.9 (1.2–2.8), $p = 0.004$); unemployment (OR (95% CI) 1.8 (1.3–2.7) $p = 0.002$); age >40 years (OR (95% CI) 1.6 (1.1–2.4) $p = 0.008$) and a requirement for TB therapy (OR (95% CI) 1.6 (1.1–2.4) $p = 0.02$). The only variable associated with loss to follow up in either univariate or multivariate analysis was treatment at Waibargi Hospital (OR (95% CI) 2.4 (1.5–3.9), $p < 0.001$). All 21 patients receiving IPT were being treated at IGH. Of these 21, one was subsequently lost to follow up but none of the remaining 20 died or required TB treatment during the follow up period.

Discussion

People living with human immunodeficiency virus at these two large treatment centres in Myanmar are presenting late in their disease course. The resulting delay in initiating ART increases their risk of disease and death and the likelihood of transmitting the virus [8, 9]. Tuberculosis co-infection is very common, but despite the proven efficacy of IPT [10]—and a strong recommendation for its prescription in WHO guidelines [11]—it was prescribed rarely in this cohort. The greatest burden of HIV in Myanmar is among PWID, MSM and FSW [6], however, very few patients in this cohort reported these risk behaviours at registration. This suggests that either these large ART prescribing centres are not servicing these KAPs, patients avoid acknowledging these risk behaviours or that health care workers are uncomfortable enquiring about them. All three explanations appear likely.

The late presentation of Myanmar PLHIV in this series resembles the findings in studies in other resource-limited settings [12–16]. Late presentation is not restricted to patients with HIV infection in a country whose public health care system is critically under-resourced [2]. In a 2012 WHO report, Myanmar was the country with the lowest government spending per person per year on health [17] and it is sobering to reflect that these data were collected in Yangon, one of the better resourced regions in the country [18]. Meanwhile, 70% of the population reside in rural areas, where resources and access to skilled health personnel are far more limited [2] and it is these areas—particularly the North and East of the country—where the HIV burden is greatest and programmes for PLHIV less developed [19–22].

The high prevalence of TB in this cohort emphasises the importance of integrating TB and HIV services [23] and brings into sharp relief the very low rates of IPT prescription, although the fact that co-trimoxazole was prescribed commonly demonstrates that there is no reluctance to prescribe prophylaxis per se [24]. Anecdotally, many Myanmar clinicians express concerns about the possibility of IPT leading to the development of resistance or adverse drug reactions, but there is no reason to think that this would occur at a higher rate than in other countries with a high TB prevalence where IPT has shown unequivocal benefit [25, 26]. While the number of patients prescribed IPT in our sample is too small to draw any broad conclusions, it may reassure sceptical Myanmar clinicians that no patients receiving IPT died or required TB treatment during follow-up. In a country where PLHIV are still presenting with advanced immunodeficiency, it is hoped that there is less resistance to the rollout of expanded prophylaxis regimens which have recently been shown to reduce mortality and hospitalisation without increased serious adverse events [27].

The majority of new HIV infections in Myanmar are in PWID (HIV prevalence in this population in 2014: 23.1%), MSM (HIV prevalence in 2014: 6.6%), and FSW (HIV prevalence in 2014: 6.3%) [6], but stigma and discrimination against these populations in Myanmar impose substantial barriers to their access to HIV prevention and care [28]. Both Waibargi and IGH are large hospitals running extremely busy, open-plan outpatient departments. While it appears likely that patients are under-reporting these risk behaviours and/or clinicians are under-documenting them, neither hospital provides an ideal setting for their disclosure. Unfortunately, this is a situation that is replicated around the country; it is estimated that a significant proportion of the KAPs are not being reached by the National AIDS Programme (NAP) and its partners, and an even smaller proportion are being tested for HIV [28].

People who inject drugs are a particularly challenging group to reach, reflected by the fact that this group accounted for 39% of all new infections in 2014 [6]. The fact that the rates of injecting drug use are highest in remote—and sometimes politically unstable—areas in the North of the country adds another layer of complexity to service delivery. However, there are positives: there has been a significant scaling-up of harm reduction activities, including the provision of methadone maintenance therapy and the possession of hypodermic needles is no longer illegal. Meanwhile, supportive drop-in-centres (DICs) continue to be the mainstay of prevention efforts targeting MSM and FSW, providing education, free condoms and outreach programmes. While support groups have been shown to reduce mortality and improve clinical outcomes [29], they undoubtedly improve the quality of life of many MSM and FSW who would otherwise feel ostracised in what remains a conservative country. Some of these DICs also offer onsite health care services and ART access.

The finding that outcomes were worse at Waibargi Hospital—a specialist infectious disease hospital—than IGH—a general hospital—is likely explained by the fact that Waibargi Hospital manages cases that are more complex than IGH. Indeed IGH refers its complicated patients with multiple comorbidities to Waibargi Hospital. Waibargi Hospital also receives more referrals from outside the Yangon region, which hinders optimal follow up care and almost certainly contributes to that hospital's higher rate of loss to follow up. The association between unemployment—a marker of socioeconomic disadvantage—and death is unsurprising, although the high rate of unemployment in the cohort emphasises the bidirectional relationship between HIV and poverty [30].

There are positives in these data: almost 85% of patients who were prescribed ART had an increase in their CD4+ count and even with high rates of advanced symptomatic disease, overall survival and retention in care was relatively good when compared to other series from low and middle income countries [13, 15, 31, 32]. However, the reality is that Myanmar's HIV program is grossly underfunded [33]. Total spending for HIV in Myanmar was approximately USD 84.1 million in 2015—an increase from USD 68.9 million in 2014—but this programme is heavily reliant on the Global Fund, and current funding levels are insufficient to reach Myanmar's stated objectives [34].

One of the greatest issues in the management of HIV in Myanmar is the profoundly under-developed state of laboratory services [35]. The clinical management of other common diseases in Myanmar—such as malaria—requires less laboratory support [36, 37]; however, this is assuredly not the case with HIV. The absence of viral load testing in the public health system precludes early recognition of poor adherence, drug malabsorption and viral resistance, but despite data to support its cost-effectiveness [38], there are enormous challenges in implementing viral load testing in resource-limited settings when even basic laboratory services are lacking [39, 40].

Our study has limitations. Although the data are collected from two of the largest ART prescribing centres in Myanmar's biggest city, they are not necessarily generalisable to the entire country. There are NGOs that target—and undoubtedly reach—KAPs more effectively and IPT is a key component of the care provided by these services. The data presented here are retrospective and relatively basic; to guide policy in the future, it will be important to collect detailed data prospectively and to link these data with the delivery of services and clinical outcomes. It will be essential to have robust quality assurance mechanisms to ensure that the collected data are complete, timely and accurate if they are to inform optimal policy.

The Myanmar National AIDS Programme (NAP) plans to increase access to public sector ART. It aims to achieve this through further decentralisation of HIV testing and ART prescription, transitioning to a "Test-and-Treat" strategy and expanded co-operation with non-government organisations [6]. There is a particular focus on improving the prevention of mother-to-child transmission, and the integration of TB and HIV services. There is the recognition that the strengthening of laboratory capacity is essential if these ambitious plans are to be to implemented [34]. The NAP acknowledges a failure to reach KAPs and it is hoped that the strengthening of community-based support groups and the integration of harm reduction strategies into community-based settings may improve the delivery of care to these vulnerable populations.

Conclusions

People living with human immunodeficiency virus at two of the largest ART prescription centres in Myanmar are presenting late in their disease course, increasing their risk of death and disease and the likelihood of viral transmission. Although retention rates and survival were relatively good at these centres, a centralised model of ART prescription is struggling to deliver care to the KAPs that bear the greatest burden of disease in the country. While TB co-infection is very common in Myanmar, IPT is frequently not prescribed despite its proven efficacy. Sustained political and financial commitment, health system strengthening, reliable data collection and flexible, evidence-based health policies are required to build on recent progress in the care of PLHIV in the country.

Abbreviations

ART: anti-retroviral therapy; DIC: drop in centre; EFV: efavirenz; FSW: female sex workers; FTC: emtricitabine; HIV: human immunodeficiency virus; IGH: Insein General Hospital; IPT: isoniazid prophylaxis therapy; IQR: interquartile range; KAP: key affected populations; MSM: men who have sex with men; NAP: National AIDS Programme; NGO: non-government organisation; PLHIV: people living with human immunodeficiency virus; PWID: people who inject drugs; TB: tuberculosis; TDF: tenofovir disoproxil fumarate; USD: United States dollars; WHO: World Health Organization.

Authors' contributions

NMA oversaw the data collection, data entry and was primarily responsible for coordinating the study in Myanmar. JH performed the statistical analysis and wrote the first draft. TTK supervised patient care and data entry. ZWH assisted with data entry and statistical analysis. MMK and HAS supervised patient care and data entry. DAC MAB and HAS revised the manuscript. All authors read and approved the final manuscript.

Author details

[1] Department of Medicine, University of Medicine 2, Yangon, Myanmar. [2] Menzies School of Health Research, Darwin, Australia. [3] The Kirby Institute, Sydney, Australia. [4] Department of Medical Care, Ministry of Health, Nay Pyi Taw, Myanmar. [5] Insein General Hospital, Yangon, Myanmar. [6] University of Adelaide, Adelaide, Australia.

Acknowledgements
The authors thank Dr. Pyae Phyo Maung, Dr. Htet Lwin Oo, Dr. Kaung Chit San, Dr. Kyaw Zin Aung, Dr. Kaung Myat and Dr. Si Hlaing Moe who assisted with data collection.

Competing interests
The authors declare that they have no competing interests.

Funding
JH (fellowship 1054195) is supported by the National Health and Medical Research Council of Australia, but this body did not provide any direct funding for the study. It played no role in the collection, analysis and interpretation of data, the writing of the manuscript, or in the decision to submit the manuscript for publication.

References

1. http://hdr.undp.org/en/countries/profiles/MMR. Accessed 15 Dec 2016.
2. Saw YM, Win KL, Shiao LW, Thandar MM, Amiya RM, Shibanuma A, Tun S, Jimba M. Taking stock of Myanmar's progress toward the health-related Millennium Development Goals: current roadblocks, paths ahead. Int J Equity Health. 2013;12:78.
3. HIV and AIDS estimates, Myanmar http://www.unaids.org/en/regions-countries/countries/myanmar. Accessed 15 Dec 2016.
4. Murray CJ. Shifting to sustainable development goals—implications for Global Health. N Engl J Med. 2015;373(15):1390–3.
5. Joint United Nations Programme on HIV/AIDS, Joint United Nations Programme on HIV/Aids. 90-90-90: an ambitious treatment target to help end the AIDS epidemic. Geneva: UNAIDS; 2014.
6. Global AIDS Response Progress Report Myanmar. National AIDS Programme, Ministry of Health, Republic of the Union of Myanmar; 2015.
7. McKinney MM, Marconi KM, Cleary PD, Kates J, Young SR, O'Neill JF. Delivering HIV services to vulnerable populations: an evaluation and research agenda. Public Health Rep. 2002;117(2):114–22.
8. Cohen MS, Chen YQ, McCauley M, Gamble T, Hosseinipour MC, Kumarasamy N, Hakim JG, Kumwenda J, Grinsztejn B, Pilotto JH, et al. Antiretroviral therapy for the prevention of HIV-1 transmission. N Engl J Med. 2016;375:830–9.
9. Grinsztejn B, Hosseinipour MC, Ribaudo HJ, Swindells S, Eron J, Chen YQ, Wang L, Ou SS, Anderson M, McCauley M, et al. Effects of early versus delayed initiation of antiretroviral treatment on clinical outcomes of HIV-1 infection: results from the phase 3 HPTN 052 randomised controlled trial. Lancet Infect Dis. 2014;14(4):281–90.
10. Briggs MA, Emerson C, Modi S, Taylor NK, Date A. Use of isoniazid preventive therapy for tuberculosis prophylaxis among people living with HIV/AIDS: a review of the literature. J Acquir Immune Defic Syndr. 2015;68(Suppl 3):S297–305.
11. Guidelines for intensified tuberculosis case-finding and isoniazid preventive therapy for people living with HIV in resource-constrained settings. World Health Organization; 2011.
12. Gelaw YA, Senbete GH, Adane AA, Alene KA. Determinants of late presentation to HIV/AIDS care in Southern Tigray Zone, Northern Ethiopia: an institution based case-control study. AIDS Res Ther. 2015;12:40.
13. Lawn SD, Harries AD, Anglaret X, Myer L, Wood R. Early mortality among adults accessing antiretroviral treatment programmes in sub-Saharan Africa. Aids. 2008;22(15):1897–908.
14. Lahuerta M, Ue F, Hoffman S, Elul B, Kulkarni SG, Wu Y, Nuwagaba-Biribonwoha H, Remien RH, El Sadr W, Nash D. The problem of late ART initiation in Sub-Saharan Africa: a transient aspect of scale-up or a long-term phenomenon? J Health Care Poor Underserved. 2013;24(1):359–83.
15. Brinkhof MW, Boulle A, Weigel R, Messou E, Mathers C, Orrell C, Dabis F, Pascoe M, Egger M. Mortality of HIV-infected patients starting antiretroviral therapy in sub-Saharan Africa: comparison with HIV-unrelated mortality. PLoS Med. 2009;6(4):e1000066.
16. Kiertiburanakul S, Boettiger D, Lee MP, Omar SF, Tanuma J, Ng OT, Durier N, Phanuphak P, Ditangco R, Chaiwarith R, et al. Trends of CD4 cell count levels at the initiation of antiretroviral therapy over time and factors associated with late initiation of antiretroviral therapy among Asian HIV-positive patients. J Int AIDS Soc. 2014;17:18804.
17. WHO Global Health Expediture Atlas. In.: World Health Organization; 2012.
18. Yangon Region Profile [http://www.unicef.org/myanmar/Yangon_Region_Profile_30-07-15.pdf]. Accessed 15 Dec 2016.
19. Shan State Profile [http://www.unicef.org/myanmar/Shan_State_Profile_30-07-15.pdf]. Accessed 15 Dec 2016.
20. Kachin State Profile [http://www.unicef.org/myanmar/Kachin_State_Profile_30-07-15.pdf]. Accessed 15 Dec 2016.
21. Beyrer C, Razak MH, Labrique A, Brookmeyer R. Assessing the magnitude of the HIV/AIDS epidemic in Burma. J Acquir Immune Defic Syndr. 2003;32(3):311–7.
22. Williams B, Baker D, Buhler M, Petrie C. Increase coverage of HIV and AIDS services in Myanmar. Confl Health. 2008;2:3.
23. Lawn SD, Meintjes G, McIlleron H, Harries AD, Wood R. Management of HIV-associated tuberculosis in resource-limited settings: a state-of-the-art review. BMC Med. 2013;11:253.
24. Suthar AB, Vitoria MA, Nagata JM, Anglaret X, Mbori-Ngacha D, Sued O, Kaplan JE, Doherty MC. Co-trimoxazole prophylaxis in adults, including pregnant women, with HIV: a systematic review and meta-analysis. Lancet HIV. 2015;2(4):e137–50.
25. Rangaka MX, Wilkinson RJ, Boulle A, Glynn JR, Fielding K, van Cutsem G, Wilkinson KA, Goliath R, Mathee S, Goemaere E, et al. Isoniazid plus antiretroviral therapy to prevent tuberculosis: a randomised double-blind, placebo-controlled trial. Lancet. 2014;384(9944):682–90.
26. Danel C, Moh R, Gabillard D, Badje A, Le Carrou J, Ouassa T, Ouattara E, Anzian A, Ntakpe JB, Minga A, et al. A trial of early antiretrovirals and isoniazid preventive therapy in Africa. N Engl J Med. 2015;373(9):808–22.
27. Hakim VM, Szubert AJ, Siika A, Mallewa J, Agutu C, Pett SL, Bwakura-Dangarembizi M, Lugemwa A, Kaunda S, Karoney M, Maitland K, Griffiths A, Kityo C, Mugyenyi P, Prendergast AJ, Walker AS, Gibb DM, REALITY Trial Team Zimbabwe. Ministry of Health and Child Welfare.: Enhanced infection prophylaxis reduces mortality in severely immunosuppressed HIV-infected adults and older children initiating antiretroviral therapy in Kenya, Malawi, Uganda and Zimbabwe: the REALITY trial. In: 21st International AIDS Conference (AIDS 2016): Durban; 2016.
28. National Guidelines. A Core Package for HIV Prevention Amongst Key Populations in Myanmar. Department of Health, Republic of the Union of Myanmar, National AIDS Control Programme; 2014.
29. Bateganya MH, Amanyeiwe U, Roxo U, Dong M. Impact of support groups for people living with HIV on clinical outcomes: a systematic review of the literature. J Acquir Immune Defic Syndr. 2015;68(Suppl 3):S368–74.
30. Rodrigo C, Rajapakse S. Current Status of HIV/AIDS in South Asia. J Glob Infect Dis. 2009;1(2):93–101.
31. Bachani D, Garg R, Rewari BB, Hegg L, Rajasekaran S, Deshpande A, Emmanuel KV, Chan P, Rao KS. Two-year treatment outcomes of patients enrolled in India's national first-line antiretroviral therapy programme. Natl Med J India. 2010;23(1):7–12.
32. Fregonese F, Collins IJ, Jourdain G, Lecoeur S, Cressey TR, Ngo-Giang-Houng N, Banchongkit S, Chutanunta A, Techapornroong M, Lallemant M. Predictors of 5-year mortality in HIV-infected adults starting highly active antiretroviral therapy in Thailand. J Acquir Immune Defic Syndr. 2012;60(1):91–8.
33. Piot P, Abdool Karim SS, Hecht R, Legido-Quigley H, Buse K, Stover J, Resch S, Ryckman T, Mogedal S, Dybul M, et al. Defeating AIDS–advancing global health. Lancet. 2015;386(9989):171–218.
34. Burma. Country Operational Plan. Strategic Direction Summary. http://www.pepfar.gov/documents/organization/257661.pdf. Accessed 15 Dec 2016.
35. Kyaw LL, Nozaki I, Wada K, Oo KY, Tin HH, Yoshihara N. Ensuring accurate testing for human immunodeficiency virus in Myanmar. Bull World Health Organ. 2015;93(1):42–6.
36. Kaung M, Kyi TT, Aung NM, Kyaw MP, Min M, Htet ZW, Anstey NM, Kyi MM, Hanson J. The prognostic utility of bedside assessment of adults hospitalised with malaria in Myanmar: a retrospective analysis. Malar J. 2015;14:63.
37. Aung NM, Kaung M, Kyi TT, Kyaw MP, Min M, Htet ZW, Anstey NM, Kyi MM, Hanson J. The safety of a conservative fluid replacement strategy in adults hospitalised with malaria. PLoS ONE. 2015;10(11):e0143062.
38. Phillips A, Shroufi A, Vojnov L, Cohn J, Roberts T, Ellman T, Bonner K, Rousseau C, Garnett G, Cambiano V, et al. Sustainable HIV treatment in Africa through viral-load-informed differentiated care. Nature. 2015;528(7580):S68–76.

4

CLINICAL outcomes and loss to follow-up among people living with HIV participating in the *NAMWEZA* intervention in Dar es Salaam, Tanzania

Hellen N. Siril[1,2*], Sylvia F. Kaaya[1], Mary Kay Smith Fawzi[3], Expeditho Mtisi[4], Magreat Somba[4], Japheth Kilewo[5], Ferdinand Mugusi[6], Anna Minja[4], Anna Kaale[4] and Jim Todd[7,8,9]

Abstract

Background: Psychosocial factors have been linked with loss to follow-up (LTFU) and clinical outcomes among people living with HIV (PLH), however little is known about the effect of psychosocial support on LTFU among PLH in treatment and care. The purpose of this study was to explore the effect of *NAMWEZA* ("Yes, together we can") friends' psychosocial support intervention on clinical outcomes and LTFU among PLH. *NAMWEZA* is based on a novel program using "appreciative inquiry", positive psychology approaches to empower, promote positive attitudes and foster hope.

Methods: PLH participating in the *NAMWEZA* intervention in HIV care clinics in Dar es Salaam Tanzania were compared with non-exposed PLH obtained from facilities that routinely collect clinical information and both followed longitudinally for 24 months. Baseline sociodemographic, clinical measures (CD4 cell count, hemoglobin (HGB), weight), and LTFU measures were collected. Chi square, Fisher's exact tests, and t-tests were used to compare the frequencies for categorical variables and the means of continuous variables from the intervention and the comparison groups to identify variables that were significantly different across the two groups. Random effects models were performed to examine the bivariate associations between the intervention status and clinical outcomes.

Results: At the end of 24 months of follow-up mean CD4 count and HGB levels increased significantly in both intervention and comparison groups ($p = 0.009$ and $p < 0.0001$, respectively). Weight increased significantly only in the intervention group ($p = 0.003$). Cumulative LTFU was three times higher in the comparison compared to the intervention ($p < 0.001$) group. Having a low CD4 count, extremes of weight, low HGB, younger age, and male gender were significantly associated with LTFU among the unexposed group, while being on ART for duration of 12 months or more was protective against LTFU in those intervened.

Conclusion: Among PLH on ART, exposed or not exposed to *NAMWEZA* intervention, clinical care outcomes improved over time. LTFU was much higher in the comparison group with factors commonly known to predict LTFU only apparent in the comparison group. *NAMWEZA* could be a promising peer-facilitated model to reduce LTFU among PLH in care that can be integrated in ART services; however, more research is needed to evaluate its longer term effects.

*Correspondence: neemasiril@gmail.com
[2] Management and Development for Health (MDH), Plot number 802, Mwai Kibaki Road, 255 Dar es Salaam, Tanzania
Full list of author information is available at the end of the article

Keywords: Psychosocial, NAMWEZA, HIV/AIDS, ART, LTFU, PLH, Dar es Salaam, Tanzania

Background

Although there has been increased public and patients' awareness of the benefits of antiretroviral therapy (ART) globally [1], in many countries attrition from ART care programs has been high, with loss to follow-up (LTFU) of patients listed as a leading cause [2–6]. However, ART can only be effective, resulting in virological suppression, if PLHs are highly adherent (commonly described as taking equal to or over 95% of ART medication) [7]. This level of drug adherence is very difficult to attain for PLH who are unable to sustain scheduled clinic follow-up visits, as studies indicate that the majority of patients with LTFU stop their ART. Stopping ART has been reported to quickly increase the risk of developing high serum viral load and other adverse health consequences [2, 5, 8, 9] including ART drug resistance, progression of HIV to AIDS, premature mortality, and re-infection, or infection of others with resistant strains [2–4, 10, 11].

In sub-Saharan Africa, LTFU is a factor reported to account for attrition from most ART programs than other causes [12–14] and varies for different groups of PLH. For instance LTFU ranges from 19 to 89% among women accessing Prevention of Mother-To-Child HIV transmission (PMTCT) services and 22% among HIV infected children [15]. In Tanzania, where this study was conducted, LTFU among PLH enrolled in ART care programs is estimated to be 49% and it varies with duration in ART care. About 18 and 36% of PLH in Tanzania are reported to be LTFU at the end of their first and third year respectively after starting ART. A report published by the Ministry of Health and Social Welfare in 2012 indicated that attrition of patients due to death accounted for only a small percent of PLH that was lost from ART treatment (5–8%). Most attrition was due to other unknown causes resulting in the majority of the LTFU [14, 16].

Some of the factors reported to contribute to LTFU from ART care in Tanzania include individual factors such as advanced clinical and immunological disease stage, younger age, malnutrition, low education, depression, and poor psychological support [17–21]. The World Health Organization (WHO) reported other individual risk factors for LTFU from ART care commonly reported from resource-limited countries, including feeling better, pill burden, treatment fatigue, work as well as home responsibilities, and migration—mobile populations ('silent transfers')—to other ART service providers [22]. Likewise system/infrastructural factors contributing to LTFU from ART care have been reported from East Africa. These include longer turnaround time of laboratory tests, drug stock outs, and clinics operating for less than 4 days a week [23] LTFU therefore results from complex individual and programmatic/system challenges facing PLH and ART programs that require greater effort to adapt effective interventions to maximize the benefit of ART programs for PLH and the role of ART as an HIV transmission prevention approach [3, 20, 24, 25].

Although a number of studies have reported LTFU and other ART treatment outcomes among PLH in Tanzania, most did not include assessments of additional interventions provided to PLH apart from routine ART care. Thus there is still limited information on effective interventions for PLH in care and receiving ART for reducing LTFU and improving other HIV treatment outcomes [8, 14]. In particular, those that influence psychological factors that have been reported to predict HIV risk behaviors, poor adherence, low retention and poor treatment outcomes among PLH [26]. Providing psychological counselling, offering psychoeducation, facilitating psychosocial support and providing support to PLH to reduce psychosocial challenges including depression, anxiety, relationship/family turmoil and poor communication have been reported to increase adherence to ART [21, 27–30]; however, not much has been reported on how psychosocial interventions may impact LTFU and other HIV treatment outcomes in Tanzania.

The primary objective of our study was to examine associations between exposure to the *NAMWEZA* intervention and HIV clinical outcomes as well as LTFU. In addition, factors associated with LTFU were assessed among PLH in Dar es Salaam, Tanzania.

Methods

Study design

We conducted a prospective cohort study involving 416 HIV infected adult participants exposed to the *NAMWEZA* intervention and 408 HIV-positive unexposed 'comparison group'. The data for this analysis was collected from January 2012 to December 2013 and were obtained from NAMWEZA intervention electronic records and National HIV care electronic database known as *CTC2* available at each of participating sites.

Eligibility criteria

Both *NAMWEZA* exposed and unexposed participants were eligible if HIV infected, 18 years of age and above, living in the catchment area of the HIV care and treatment center (CTC), registered for HIV care and treatment at the study CTCs, initiated on ART and had used ART for at least 3 months (enrolment criteria for both NAMWEZA exposed and controls), and resident in the Kinondoni District. The ART regimen and other standard HIV related health care services were provided similarly between the two groups. Exclusion from the study occurred if poor health prohibited participant's recruitment, if they had not started ART and for the NAMWEZA exposed, if unable to provide informed consent for participation, and not planning to remain resident for at least 2 years in the Kinondoni District.

Methods of follow up

Both the intervention and control participants were seen monthly at the clinic for routine ART care during the time period of follow-up (January 2012 to December 2013). HIV care included adherence counseling, seeing a physician for any health concerns, providing laboratory tests as scheduled and any other tests that a physician might feel the patient needs at that visit. Each clinic has trained and experienced community based health workers (CHWs) who tracked missing PLH. At the time of the study, data were collected prospectively from the clinical databases. The CHW worked with the clinic data clerks under the supervision of the clinic nurse in-charge to obtain daily lists of PLH who miss their scheduled clinic visits. After obtaining the list, they followed up the missing patients through phone calls (1 week after missing a scheduled clinic visit) and a home visit 2 weeks after a missed clinic appointment if phone calls were unsuccessful and or the patient didn't come to the clinic. The CHW provided reports that were entered into the CTC2 database daily to update patients' vital status (i.e. not ascertained, ascertained alive or died). The CHW continued to track those not found for three or more months after which if vital status could not be ascertained they are declared LTFU.

Exposure variable

NAMWEZA, pronounced as two linked words *NAM-WEZA* (Yes I can!), is an intervention that includes 10 once weekly structured sessions aimed at empowering PLH to become HIV prevention change agents in their communities. Psychosocial issues related to relationships and living with HIV as well as change agent's communication skills building occurred using an Appreciative Inquiry (AI) approach. The AI model engages stakeholders in self-determined change and was first used to change organizational/system behavior. It involves searching for the best in people, and the world around and systematic discovery of what gives a system 'life' when it is most effective and capable in economic, ecological, and human terms. Participants receive training sessions that targets developing the art and practice of asking questions that strengthen an individual or a system's capacity to heighten positive potential [31, 32]. The AI model components used in the process of delivery of *NAMWEZA* group sessions, included strategies that built participants skills to ask reflective and appreciative questions about what is working well in themselves, people's lives specifically their social network members and through the answers, identify and affirm abilities in self and others; and using dreams about the future and backlighting to focus action plans for change in the here and now. Participants used appreciative inquiry to explore their abilities potentials, dream for and draw feasible action plans for the future including abilities to access and manage microfinancing keep healthy relationships, Burgan for safer sexual practices, and handling HIV infection and disclosure. Also *NAMWEZA* fostered resilience and social support through building participant's communication skills in the use of "I" rather than "You" statements to improve clarity and reduce conflict when communicating with others. All sessions include repeated exercises and role plays practiced during the sessions, with each session building on the previous one. Participants were encouraged to practice the skills of each session at home and give feedback before the beginning of the next session. This approach aims to increase self-confidence and self-esteem as a way of exploring, highlighting, and developing skills as resources within each session theme [33]. The thematic content of *NAMWEZA* included themes that ranged from exploring love, relationships, sex, and feelings in session 1 to action planning in a closing session 10 (see Table 1).

Sessions were highly participatory and active learning occurred with the opportunity to practice learned skills and provide feedback in subsequent sessions. Training occurred in age and gender specific groups (women <35 years of age; men $\leq$35 years; women $\geq$35 years; and men $\geq$35) to foster group cohesion through shared experiences. Groups were facilitated by trained peer PLH. *NAMWEZA* exposed participants attended 1–10 sessions, with an average of 7.7 sessions; while the comparison group did not attend any sessions. All the sessions were available to all participants, who were informed of the dates and times and expected to attend all the 10 sessions. In addition, both the *NAMWEZA* exposed PLH and the comparison group received routine ART care including monthly prescriptions for medications, as well as other aspects of clinical care and ART adherence counseling sessions.

Outcome variables

Loss to follow-up (LTFU), immunological (CD4), and other clinical outcomes including weight, hemoglobin

Table 1 Summary of the contents of each NAMWEZA Training Session

Session 1	An introductory session: which include welcoming the participants, setting ground rules participants sharing life stories and group lived values, the story of the 5th province, whom do you hear calling your name and an introduction of appreciative inquiry in communication, how to spot abilities of others, dreaming positively for future, and how to be wise
Session 2	Titled Love relationship and emotions: include more training to use appreciative inquiry in communication, exploring values of love and how to view emotions from self and others (anger, sadness), as an invitation and a communication instead of an attack, and how to communicate back
Session 3	Titled Valuing others and self: include sharing experiences that influence life, how we value ourselves, how we value our own words and imagined negotiation
Session 4	Titled Happiness, safer sexual relationships, healthy living; include drawing a map of safer and happy living, appreciative inquiry, following direction education and discussions on HIV transmission and prevention myths and facts about HIV, following directions, positive networking and condom use
Session 5	Titled Developing assertiveness skills; revisions and role plays on appreciative inquiry, ability spotting, exploring hopes and fear, taking control during communications by using proper posture, eye contact and voice tones, I see, I feel, I want, putting things into practice drawing bodies as roadmap for sexually learning
Session 6	Titled Deepening and expanding assertiveness skills: More revision and role plays on appreciative inquiry, ability spotting, wider assertive skills building including manipulative how to manage an ambiguous situation, pushing the line during communication and entrepreneurial future
Session 7	Titled Disclosure 1; of an HIV positive status; confidentiality, appreciative inquiry, good care giver, human rights, telling and listening, how to become a good listener
Session 8	Titled Disclosure 2; challenges and positive possibilities, taking care of self, how to tell family and close relatives, sexual partners, supporting each other and spiders web
Session 9	Titled Visualizing; targets on focusing the participants to explore, reflect skills and resources in them and others, and create a microeconomic plan. This involve visualizing and drawing hoped for community/work, Appreciative inquiry exploring income generating skills including how to access and manage microfinances
Session 10	Titled The future; This is the final session that focuses on what has been learned during the all the other sessions by revisiting the tree of life and future possibilities for advocacy. Participants revisit and add on the previously tree of live adding their abilities and building on dreams and creating action plans for the future, mental gifts, tree of abilities and how to move in the community

level, and number of scheduled clinic visits attended were examined. For this study a patient was LTFU if he/she did not attend three scheduled clinic visits in three consecutive months with no reported/documented death or transfer out [34].

Data collection

Outcome data were obtained from the CTC electronic database which contains routinely collected clinical data for PLH accessing care at each of the participating sites. Data for sociodemographic measures, duration on ART, and all outcome variables including CD4, weight, and hemoglobin levels; as well LTFU measures were extracted from the database at 8, 16, and 24 months of follow-up.

Data analysis

Descriptive statistics for sociodemographic factors and clinical variables were estimated at baseline, including frequencies for categorical data as well as means and standard deviations for continuous variables. Chi square, Fisher's exact tests, and t-tests were used to compare the frequencies for categorical variables and the means of continuous variables from the intervention and the comparison groups to identify variables that were significantly different from the two groups. Random effects models were performed to examine the bivariate associations between the intervention status and clinical outcomes, including CD4 cell count, weight change, HGB levels, and LTFU. In the multivariate models variables that had a p value of 0.2 or less at baseline for the intervention and comparison groups were controlled for. In addition, a missing variable indicator was included to address missing data and logistic regression models were used to predict factors associated with LTFU for intervention and comparison groups. A Kaplan–Meier survival curve was used to estimate retention among the intervention and comparison groups. We also examined factors associated with LTFU using Cox proportional hazards regression models. SAS statistical software (version 9.3) was used for the analysis [35].

Results

All 450 HIV-positive participants of *NAMWEZA* intervention were eligible to participate. Thirty-four (7.5%) of the exposed participants had absent or incomplete clinical information and were dropped from the analysis. The final number of participants in the intervention group included in this study was 416 (92%). A total of 408 PLH were identified from the CTC2 database based on the same eligibility criteria.

At baseline, only gender and age variables were statistically significant different from the intervention and comparison groups (p = 0.03 and <0.0001, respectively). The other demographic characteristics were not significantly different (Table 2). Seventy-two percent and 77% of the participants from intervention and comparison groups respectively were females. The mean age was 46 and 37 year for intervention and comparison groups, respectively. About half (49%) of intervention and slightly above 50% (52%) of the comparison group, reported to be living with a sexual partner in a marital or cohabiting relationship. Majority of the participants in both the intervention and comparison groups reported that they were self-employed; 38 and 41% respectively, followed by those who were employed (35 and 36%) respectively, a few were house wives/husbands (9 and 11%) respectively and unemployed were 15% in the intervention and 16% in the comparison group (Tables 2, 3).

For the clinical outcome variables baseline CD4 cell count in the intervention and control groups was 308 and 270 cells/mm^3, respectively; and mean hemoglobin (HGB) levels were 9 g/dl for the intervention and 10 g/dl for the comparison group. The mean body weight of the participants was 61 and 60 kg in the intervention and control groups respectively. Similar to most demographic variables, the clinical parameters were not significantly different in the two groups (Table 3).

Table 2 Baseline sociodemographic characteristics for PLH receiving HIV treatment in Dar es Salaam, Tanzania

Characteristic	Comparison group, N = 408 n (%)/mean (SD)	Intervention, N = 416 n (%)/mean (SD)	p value
District of residence			
Kinondoni	387 (95.3)	412 (99.8)	
Ilala	10 (2.5)	1 (0.24)	0.0897[1]
Temeke	9 (2.2)	0 (0.0)	
Sex			
Male	92 (23.0)	116 (28.0)	0.0301[2]
Female	316 (77.0)	300 (72.0)	
Mean age	37 (9.1)	46 (9.7)	<0.0001[2]
Age groups in years			<0.0001[2]
<30	30 (11.3)	30 (7.2)	
≥30	236 (88.7)	386 (92.8)	
Marital status[a]			
Lives with partner (married or cohabiting)	208 (52.0)	205 (49.2)	0.3000[2]
Single (never married or widowed)	192 (48.0)	203 (48.7)	
Employment status			
Employed	142 (34.8)	148 (35.6)	
Self-employed	166 (40.7)	156 (37.5)	0.6510[2]
House wife/house husband	35 (8.6)	45 (10.8)	
Unemployed	65 (15.9)	67 (16.1)	

[1] p value obtained from Fisher's exact test

[2] p value was obtained from Chi Square test

[a] A total of eight participants from the comparison group and eight from the intervention with missing data were omitted

Table 3 Baseline clinical characteristics for PLH receiving ART care in Dar es Salaam, Tanzania

Characteristics	Comparison	Intervention	p value[1]
Mean CD4 (SD)	270 (173.4)	308 (184.1)	0.76
Immune suppression			
Severe immunosuppression (CD4 < 200)	116 (28.5)	96 (23.1)	0.09
Moderate immune suppression (CD4 = 200 to <350)	119 (29.2)	138 (33.2)	
Not immune suppressed (CD4 ≥ 350)	173 (42.4)	182 (43.8)	
Mean hemoglobin (SD)	10 (2.1)	9 (1.9)	0.09
Low hemoglobin(anemia) mean (SD)	11 (2.6)	5 (1.2)	
Severe anemia (<8.5)	60 (14.7)	52 (12.5)	0.03
Moderate anemia (8.6 to <10)	179 (43.9)	278 (88.8)	
Mild anemia (10 to <12)	122 (29.9)	81 (19.5)	
No anemia (>12)	44 (9.0)	91 (22.0)	
Mean weight (kg) (SD)	60 (11.9)	61 (12.7)	0.33
Weight groups (kg)			0.21
<45	72 (18.6)	21 (5.1)	
45–60	88 (21.6)	50 (12.0)	
>60	227 (55.6	341 (82.0)	
Mean duration on ART at baseline, mean (SD)	18 (17.0)	20 (16.0)	0.23

N-intervention group = 412 and 367 control group: A total of 21 participants in the comparison group and 4 in the intervention had missing data and were omitted

[1] p-value was obtained from Chi Square test

The mean duration on ART medication was 20 months in the intervention and 18 months in the comparison group (p = 0.23). The median follow up time was 20.2 months in the intervention and 23.3 months in the intervention group (Table 6). The average number of routine clinic visit made was significantly higher at 22.8 visits in the intervention group, compared to 16.9 visits in the comparison group (p = 0.003) (Table 6).

Multivariate analyses showed that CD4 counts increased significantly in both the intervention and comparison groups over time (p = 0.0024 and 0.047, respectively). However, women in both groups had significantly faster rates of CD4 count increase of about 41 cells/mm^3 per month compared to men (p = 0.005) (Table 4). Over time, participants in the intervention group had significantly higher weight gain of (0.270 kg per month compared to 0.140 kg in the comparison group (p = 0.003). At the end of follow-up, the proportion of PLH who

Table 4 Univariate and multivariate analyses of intervention vs. comparison group

Covariate of interest	Univariate		Multivariate	
	Effect estimate	p value	Effect estimate	p value[1]
CD4 count (cells/mm^3)				
Intervention vs. comparison	24.6 (−37.02, 86.23)	0.4337	26.9 (−36.31, 90.19)	0.4036
CD4 change over time				
Intervention	2.9 (1.19, 4.64)	0.0009	2.7 (0.96, 4.45)	0.0024
Comparison group	2.8 (0.84, 4.75)	0.0051	2.8 (0.87, 4.79)	0.047
Age			−0.58 (−1.72, 0.56)	0.3196
Gender			40.56 (12.41, 68.72)	0.0048
Weight (kg)				
Intervention vs. comparison	0.9 (−6.97, 8.71)	0.8270	−2.64 (−9.91, 4.620)	0.4757
Weight change over time				
Intervention	0.14 (−0.073, 0.35)	0.2000	0.27 (0.09, 0.44)	0.0025
Comparison group	0.15 (−0.03, 0.31)	0.0968	0.14 (−0.34, 0.31)	0.1234
Age			0.08 (−0.01, 0.17)	0.0681
Gender			−0.79 (−3.04, 1.46)	0.4892
Hemoglobin (HGB) (in g/dl)				
Intervention vs. comparison HGB change over time	0.12 (−1.60, 2.05)	0.8109	0.23 (−1.61, 2.06)	0.7268
Intervention	0.03 (−0.02, 0.09)	0.2726	0.031 (−0.02, 0.09)	0.0429
Comparison group	0.02 (−0.01, 0.05)	0.1154	0.020 (−0.01, 0.05)	0.0437
Age (in years)			0.01 (−0.01, 0.03)	0.2026
Gender			−0.61 (−1.05, −0.18)	0.006
Lost to follow-up				
Intervention vs. comparison	0.62 (0.51, 0.76)	<0.0001	0.64 (0.52, 0.78)	<0.001
LTFU change over time				
Intervention	0.92 (0.91, 0.93)	<0.0001	1.01 (1.01, 1.03)	0.0033
Comparison group	0.93 (0.51, 0.76)	<0.0001	0.92 (0.92, 0.93)	<0.001
Age			0.99 (1.00, 1.001)	0.1737
Gender			0.95 (0.89, 1.02)	0.3169

[1] p value obtained from random effects model

were LTFU was significantly lower in intervention (4.8%) compared to (14.7%) in the control group ($p = 0.002$) (Table 6). More PLH were retained in the intervention compared to the control group as depicted by the Kaplan–Meier curve in Fig. 1. In the intervention group, the proportion of LTFU was significantly higher (57%) among the participants who attended 1–6 *NAMWEZA* training sessions than those who attended 7–10 sessions (43%), $p = 0.033$ (Table 6).

For LTFU, five out of the six factors that were associated with LTFU, were only significant in the control participants, but not the intervention group participants. These included: low CD4; PLH with severe immune suppression (CD4 < 200 cells/mm^3 had higher risk of LTFU ($p < 0.0001$); extremes in weight, where those with extreme low or high weights (<45 and >60 kg) were at higher risk of LTFU ($p = 0.02$); low hemoglobin; participants with lower hemoglobin levels (<10 mg/dl) showed higher risk of LTFU ($p = 0.01$). Male gender was associated with higher risk of LTFU ($p = 0.04$) and younger age (<40 years) was associated with higher LTFU risks ($p = 0.03$). In the intervention group, PLH with longer duration of ART use, experienced less LTFU ($p < 0.0001$), while in the comparison group, persons with longer duration on ART were at higher risk of LTFU ($p < 0.0001$) (see Tables 5, 6).

Discussion

This study examined associations between exposure to a peer facilitated psychosocial intervention and clinical outcomes among PLH receiving ART. Participants exposed to the *NAMWEZA* intervention saw significant improvement in clinical outcomes that were not seen among those who did not receive the *NAMWEZA* intervention. Weight gain, CD4 counts, and hemoglobin all significantly increased among *NAMWEZA* participants, whereas smaller non-significant gains were seen in the comparison group. The *NAMWEZA* intervention had

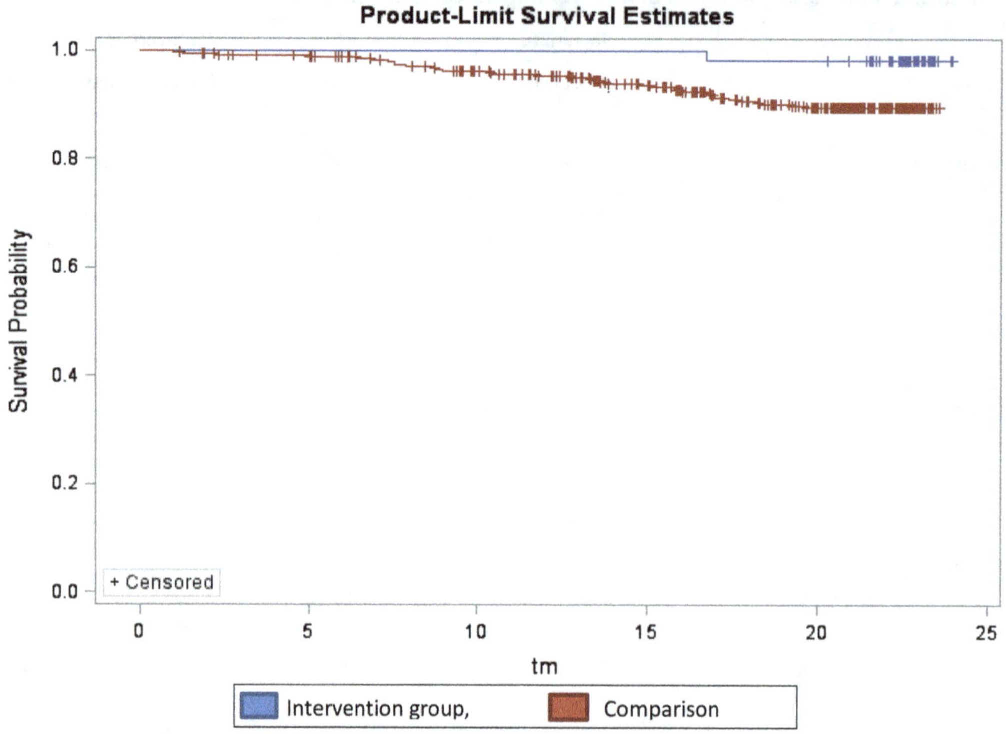

Fig. 1 Kaplan Meier curve; showing LTFU in the intervention group (*blue*) and Comparison group (*red*)

lower LTFU rates and participants were more likely to remain in treatment. The *NAMWEZA* protective effects against LTFU had a dose–response effect with lower rates observed among those who attended more of the *NAMWEZA* sessions.

In studies that have reported ART clinical outcomes among PLH, low CD4, younger age, male gender, low HGB, and weight were commonly reported to be associated with LTFU [8, 14, 24, 36]. In this study these risk factors for LTFU were all independently significantly associated with LTFU among PLH in the comparison group but were not found for intervention group participants. These findings are similar to other studies reporting ART treatment outcomes and rates of LTFU [8, 14, 36]. In addition, the cumulative rates of LTFU were three times higher in the comparison group as compared to the intervention group. This is also reflected in the average number of clinic visits which was significantly lower among the comparison group.

This variation could be related to the effect of exposure to the psychosocial intervention (*NAMWEZA*) in addition to routine ART care, and suggests that *NAMWEZA* may have had an effect on reducing LTFU in HIV care. Such interventions could be considered for integration within the ART care and treatment clinics to reduce LTFU.

The observed increase in CD4 counts and hemoglobin levels in both groups was expected since participants in both groups were receiving ART medications and were likely to show clinical improvements related to the duration of treatment [15, 37, 38]. However, the intervention group participants showed a higher increase in both CD4 counts and hemoglobin levels compared to the control group. Close follow up of PLH during the *NAMWEZA* intervention could have prompted more clinic visits and greater adherence to ART by exposed participants compared to unexposed group participants. Furthermore, the intervention addressed psychosocial concerns which have been reported to hinder adherence to ART and retention in care [21]. This is similar to what was observed in Zimbabwe and Zambia where a psychosocial intervention known as "mothers2mothers" (m2m) was found to improve retention and adherence to the Option B+ antiretroviral regimens among HIV infected women [39, 40]. Although these studies were based on pregnant and breastfeeding women, the participants were taking a full regimen of ART similar to participants in this study. Better management of psychosocial concerns in the intervention group could also explain the significantly higher weight gain over time for *NAMWEZA* when comparing participants to those in the unexposed group.

Table 5 Factors associated with LTFU among the intervention and comparison group participants

Factor	Intervention				Comparison group			
	Univariate HR (95% CI)	p value	Multivariate HR (95% CI)	p value	Univariate HR (95% CI)	p value	Multivariate HR (95% CI)	p value[1]
CD4		0.01		0.12		<0.001		<0.0001
<200	0.75 (0.54, 0.03)		1.55 (1.11, 2.15)		3.20 (2.52, 4.53)		2.13 (1.63, 2.75)	
200 to <350	0.31 (0.21, 0.45)		0.86 (0.58, 1.27)		2.52 (1.98, 3.21)		1.83 (1.41, 2.36)	
350+	Reference		Reference		Reference		Reference	
Weight WT		0.83		0.65		0.001		0.0200
<45	0.98 (0.99, 1.02)		0.29 (0.02, 0.32)		0.96 (0.68, 1.36)		1.48 (0.95, 2.31)	
45–60	Reference		Reference		Reference		Reference	
60+	0.94 (0.97, 2.03)		0.34 (0.03, 2.01)		1.60 (1.31, 1.96)		2.01 (1.63, 2.49)	
HBG		0.74		0.09		<0.001		<0.000
<8.5	1.11 (0.60, 2.07)		1.93 (0.91, 3.67)		0.40 (0.38, 0.43)		3.24 (2.97, 3.55)	1
8.5 to <10	0.68 (0.47, 0.99)		0.10 (0.06,0.16)		0.44 (0.42, 0.46)		0.48 (0.46, 0.51)	
10 to <12	1.91 (1.32, 2.77)		1.17 (1.11, 0.26)		0.57 (0.55, 0.60)		1.00 (0.95, 1.05)	
12+	Reference		Reference		Reference		Reference	
ART duration		<0.0001		<0.0001		<0.0001		<0.001
<12	Reference		Reference		Reference		Reference	
12+	0.39 (0.27–0.57)		0.42 (0.28–0.63)		2.34 (1.98–0.21)		2.51 (1.84–0.43)	
Gender						<0.000		0.0400
Male	0.02 (0.01–10.47)	0.85			1.49 (1.22–0.82)	1	1.28 (1.01–0.63)	
Female	Reference				Reference			
Age		0.89				0.002		0.0300
<30	3.31 (0.01–0.67)				0.87 (0.64–0.99)		0.73 (0.54–0.99)	
30 to <40	3.23 (0.01–0.23)				0.92 (0.79–0.15)		0.89 (0.69–0.14)	
40 to <50	Reference				Reference		Reference	
50+	5.21 (0.02–0.23)				0.24 (0.06–0.38)		0.14 (0.06–0.35)	

[1] p value was obtained from Chi square test

Table 6 Cumulative attendance of scheduled clinic visits, LTFU, LTFU by sessions at and follow up time the end of the 24 months among the intervention and comparison groups

	Control	Intervention	p value[1]
Average number of scheduled visits in months, n (SD)	16.9 (6.27)	22.8 (2.01)	0.0030
Cumulative lost to follow up by end of 24 months, n (%)	60 (14.7)	20 (4.8)	0.0016
LTFU among those who attended 1–6 sessions, n (%)		12 (60)	0.0330
LTFU among PLH attending 7–10 sessions, n (%)		8 (40)	
Median follow up time (months)	23.3	20.2	0.6800

[1] p value obtained by Chi square test

To our knowledge this is the first intervention study where PLH receiving ART medication were provided a psychosocial intervention that showed improvements in selected ART treatment outcomes. The study took place in an area which has a high HIV prevalence, especially among women, and a significant number of PLH receiving ART medications for varying durations.

There are a number of limitations for this study. The routinely collected clinical data used to select participants for this study had many gaps in information since the purpose of data was for clinical care and not research. We excluded from the analysis of this study (both intervention and control arms), participants who had more than 50% missing information in the 12 months before the study, perhaps limiting the representativeness of the study results. Although the study is observational, major confounders have been controlled for in the study, and selection of participants according to the same eligibility criteria may have reduced potential bias.

Conclusions

The findings suggest that providing additional psychosocial support to PLH receiving ART can reduce LTFU. Such support needs to be formalized and integrated with HIV treatment and care. In addition, working with peer supporters in this context was feasible and is likely generalizable to other resource-limited settings with a significant burden of HIV. Facilitating such interventions could in the long run reduce expenditures due to adverse health outcomes resulting from LTFU in HIV care.

Authors' contributions

HS lead author, lead the development, monitored implementation of the study, data collection, analysis, and interpretation of the results. In addition she revised and incorporated inputs from the rest of the authors on the manuscript. SK contributed on reviewing the proposal, consents development, supervising the implementation of the study, she also participated in the review and editing of the paper. MCSF assisted in development of data collection tools, consent forms the proposal, reviewing and redrafting some of the sections of the paper. EM worked on data cleaning, analysis and interpretation of results. MS worked on reviewing and ensuring consents and study tools are in a clear local language, supervised proper data confidentiality and management at the sites. JK reviewed and advised on the design, analysis and interpretation of findings. FM advised on the methods and participated in the review of the manuscript. JT principle investigator; oversaw the design, data cleaning, and analysis. He advised on the statistical methods, models and tests, and on the interpretation of the results. All authors contributed to the writing of the paper. All authors read and approved the final manuscript.

Author details

[1] Department of Psychiatry and Mental Health, Muhimbili University of Health and Allied Sciences, Dar es Salaam, Tanzania. [2] Management and Development for Health (MDH), Plot number 802, Mwai Kibaki Road, 255 Dar es Salaam, Tanzania. [3] Department of Global Health and Social Medicine, Harvard Medical School, Boston, MA, USA. [4] African Academy for Public Health (AAPH), Dar es Salaam, Tanzania. [5] Department of Epidemiology, Muhimbili University of Health and Allied Sciences, Dar es Salaam, Tanzania. [6] Department of Internal Medicine, Muhimbili University of Health and Allied Sciences, Dar es Salaam, Tanzania. [7] National Institute for Medical Research (NIMR), Mwanza, Tanzania. [8] Department of Epidemiology and Biostatistics, Kilimanjaro Christian Medical University College, Moshi, Tanzania. [9] Population Health Department, London School of Hygiene and Tropical Medicine, London, UK.

Acknowledgements

We would like to acknowledge all our participants, and health facilities' nurses, doctors, managers and all our research assistants who were involved in this study.

Competing interests

All authors declare that they have no competing interests.

Approval to use *NAMWEZA* and CTC2 national data

Approval was sought from the Principle Investigators (PIs) of the main study from which this adjunct study was conducted known as; *NAMWEZA*-change agents study for use of this data. Likewise the use of CTC2 National database from participating sites followed the Tanzanian national guidelines of conducting research through seeking and obtaining approval from the National Institute of Medical Research (NIMR) and the District Medical office of the participating sites before the study rolled out.

Funding

This work was supported by the Tanzania HIV/AIDS and TB Center through International Clinical, Operational, and Health Services Research and Training (ICOHRTA) program at Muhimbili University of Health and Allied Sciences, Dar es Salaam Tanzania, which is funded by the Fogarty funded by Fogarty International Center, National Institutes AQ8 of Health (Grant Number 5U2RTW008258). The funding body did not have any role in the design of the study and collection, analysis, interpretation of data and in writing the manuscript.

References

1. Miller CM, Ketlhapile M, Rybasack-Smith H, Rosen S. Why are antiretroviral treatment patients lost to follow-up? A qualitative study from South Africa. Trop Med Int health. 2010;15(Suppl 1):48–54.
2. Dalal RP, Macphail C, Mqhayi M, Wing J, Feldman C, Chersich MF, et al. Characteristics and outcomes of adult patients lost to follow-up at an antiretroviral treatment clinic in Johannesburg, South Africa. J Acquir Immune Defic Syndr. 2008;47(1):101–7.
3. Rosen S, Fox MP, Gill CJ. Patient retention in antiretroviral therapy programs in sub-Saharan Africa: a systematic review. PLoS Med. 2007;4(10):e298.
4. Krebs DW, Chi BH, Mulenga Y, Morris M, Cantrell RA, Mulenga L, et al. Community-based follow-up for late patients enrolled in a district-wide programme for antiretroviral therapy in Lusaka, Zambia. AIDS Care. 2008;20(3):311–7.
5. Bekolo CE, Webster J, Batenganya M, Sume GE, Kollo B. Trends in mortality and loss to follow-up in HIV care at the Nkongsamba Regional hospital, Cameroon. BMC Res Notes. 2013;6:512.
6. Sibanda EL, Weller IV, Hakim JG, Cowan FM. The magnitude of loss to follow-up of HIV-exposed infants along the prevention of mother-to-child HIV transmission continuum of care: a systematic review and meta-analysis. Aids. 2013;27(17):2787–97.
7. Apisarnthanarak A, Mundy LM. Long-term outcomes of HIV-infected patients with <95% rates of adherence to nonnucleoside reverse-transcriptase inhibitors. Clin Infect Dis. 2010;51(1):115–7.
8. Makunde WH, Francis F, Mmbando BP, Kamugisha ML, Rutta AM, Mandara CI, et al. Lost to follow up and clinical outcomes of HIV adult patients on antiretroviral therapy in care and treatment centres in Tanga City, north-eastern Tanzania. Tanzan Health Res. 2012;14(4):250–6.
9. Brinkhof MW, Pujades-Rodriguez M, Egger M. Mortality of patients lost to follow-up in antiretroviral treatment programmes in resource-limited settings: systematic review and meta-analysis. PloS ONE. 2009;4(6):e5790.
10. Linthicum KJ, Anyamba A, Britch SC, Chretien JP, Erickson RL, Small J, et al. A Rift Valley fever risk surveillance system for Africa using remotely sensed data: potential for use on other continents. Vet Ital. 2007;43(3):663–74.
11. Ceccarelli L, Salpini R, Moudourou S, Cento V, Santoro MM, Fokam J, et al. Characterization of drug resistance mutations in naive and ART-treated patients infected with HIV-1 in Yaounde, Cameroon. J Med Virol. 2012;84(5):721–7.
12. Fox MP, Rosen S. Patient retention in antiretroviral therapy programs up to 3 years on treatment in sub-Saharan Africa, 2007–2009: systematic review. Trop Medicine Int Health. 2010;15(Suppl 1):1–15.
13. PROGRAM T. Community care for people living with HIV/AIDS and orphans/vulnerable children report. 2011.
14. Somi G, Keogh SC, Todd J, Kilama B, Wringe A, van den Hombergh J, et al. Low mortality risk but high loss to follow-up among patients in the Tanzanian national HIV care and treatment programme. Trop Med Int Health. 2012;17(4):497–506.
15. Leroy V, Malateste K, Rabie H, Lumbiganon P, Ayaya S, Dicko F, et al. Outcomes of antiretroviral therapy in children in Asia and Africa: a comparative analysis of the IeDEA pediatric multiregional collaboration. J Acquir Immune Defic Syndr. 2013;62(2):208–19.
16. Somi RG. Attrition from HIV care key operational challenge in implementing HIV care and treatment in Tanzania. Ministry of health and social welfare program (NACP); 2012.
17. Ardura-Garcia C, Feldacker C, Tweya H, Chaweza T, Kalulu M, Phiri S, et al. Implementation and operational research: early tracing of children lost to

follow-up from antiretroviral treatment: true outcomes and future risks. J Acquir Immune Defic Syndr. 2015;70(5):e160–7.

18. Teshome W, Belayneh M, Moges M, Mekonnen E, Endrias M, Ayele S, et al. Do loss to follow-up and death rates from ART care vary across primary health care facilities and hospitals in south Ethiopia? a retrospective follow-up study. Hiv/Aids. 2015;7:167–74.
19. Halkitis PN, Shrem MT, Zade DD, Wilton L. The physical, emotional and interpersonal impact of HAART: exploring the realities of HIV seropositive individuals on combination therapy. J Health Psychol. 2005;10(3):345–58.
20. Tweya H, Gugsa S, Hosseinipour M, Speight C, Ng'ambi W, Bokosi M, et al. Understanding factors, outcomes and reasons for loss to follow-up among women in Option B + PMTCT programme in Lilongwe, Malawi. Trop Med International Health. 2014;19(11):1360–6.
21. Zuniga JA, Yoo-Jeong M, Dai T, Guo Y, Waldrop-Valverde D. The Role of depression in retention in care for persons living with HIV. AIDS Patient Care STDs. 2016;30(1):34–8.
22. WHO. Retention in HIV programmes: defining the challenges and identifying solutions. Geneva: World Health Organization. 2012.
23. Rachlis B, Bakoyannis G, Easterbrook P, Genberg B, Braithwaite RS, Cohen CR, et al. Facility-level factors influencing retention of patients in HIV care in East Africa. PloS ONE. 2016;11(8):e0159994.
24. Kalembo FW, Zgambo M. Loss to followup: a major challenge to successful implementation of prevention of mother-to-child transmission of HIV-1 programs in sub-Saharan Africa. Isrn Aids 2012φ. doi:10.5402/2012/589817.
25. Mugglin C, Estill J, Wandeler G, Bender N, Egger M, Gsponer T, et al. Loss to programme between HIV diagnosis and initiation of antiretroviral therapy in sub-Saharan Africa: systematic review and meta-analysis. Trop Med Int Health. 2012;17(12):1509–20.
26. Gemechu B, Gerbi TH, Tameru B. Psychosocial factors as predictors of HIV/AIDS risky behaviors among people living with HIV/AIDS. J AIDS HIV Res. 2012;1:8–16.
27. Toth M, Messer LC, Quinlivan EB. Barriers to HIV care for women of color living in the Southeastern US are associated with physical symptoms, social environment, and self-determination. AIDS Patient Care STDs. 2013;27(11):613–20.
28. Ribeiro C, Sarmento ECR, Dinis-Ribeiro M, Fernandes L. Effectiveness of psycho-educational intervention in HIV patients' treatment. Front Psychiatr. 2014;5:198.
29. Nakimuli-Mpungu E, Mojtabai R, Alexandre PK, Musisi S, Katabira E, Nachega JB, et al. Lifetime depressive disorders and adherence to antiretroviral therapy in HIV-infected Ugandan adults: a case–control study. J Affect Disord. 2013;145(2):221–6.
30. Tedaldi EM, van den Berg-Wolf M, Richardson J, Patel P, Durham M, Hammer J, et al. Sadness in the SUN: using computerized screening to analyze correlates of depression and adherence in HIV-infected adults in the United States. AIDS Patient Care STDs. 2012;26(12):718–29.
31. Cooperrider DLW. Appreciative Inquiry: a positive revolution in change. In: Holman P, Devane T, editors. The change handbook. Oakland: Berrett-Koehler Publishers, Inc.
32. McCarthy B. Appreciative Inquiry: an alternative to behaviour management. Dementia. 2017;16(2):249–53.
33. Elspeth McAdam AW, Charles Steinberg, Kicki Oljemark, Keith McAdam. Namweza programme overview 2011. http://www.namweza.org/?page_id=145. Accessed 12 Feb 2017.
34. Program Nac. Implementation of HIV/AIDS care and treatment services in Tanzania report. 2013.
35. know TPt. SAS® 9.3 Software 2011 (cited 16 Jun 2016). http://support.sas.com/software/93/. Accessed 19 Jan 2017.
36. Somi G. Attrition from HIV care key operational challenge. 2012. http://slideplayer.com/slide/7083119/. Accessed 10 Mar 2017.
37. Bangsberg DR. Less than 95% adherence to nonnucleoside reverse-transcriptase inhibitor therapy can lead to viral suppression. Clin Infect Dis. 2006;43(7):939–41.
38. Menon S. Early initiation of antiretroviral therapy and universal HIV testing in sub-Saharan Africa: has WHO offered a milestone for HIV prevention? J Public Health Policy. 2010;31(4):385–400.
39. Karfakis EKaJ. Current practices to increase uptake, retention and adherence for option B+ in Malawi. Mothers to mothers Malawi 2014 (cited 2016 August 26). https://www.m2m.org/wp-content/uploads/2014/10/m2m_Malawi-PMTCT-Report.pdf
40. Shroufi A, Mafara E, Saint-Sauveur JF, Taziwa F, Vinoles MC. Mother to mother (M2M) peer support for women in prevention of mother to child transmission (PMTCT) programmes: a qualitative study. PloS ONE. 2013;8(6):e64717.

5

What influences quality of life in older people living with HIV?

Jose Catalan[1*], Veronica Tuffrey[2], Damien Ridge[2], Dana Rosenfeld[3] and On behalf of the HALL (HIV and Later Life) Team

Abstract

Background: People with HIV with access to treatment are growing older and living healthier lives than in the past, and while health improvements and increased survival rates are welcome, the psychological and social consequences and quality of life of ageing are complex for this group. Understanding how ageing, HIV and quality of life intersect is key to developing effective interventions to improve QoL.

Methods: One hundred people with HIV over the age of 50 (range 50–87, mean 58), were recruited through HIV community organizations, and clinics, and included men who have sex with men (MSM), and Black African and White heterosexual men and women. The WHOQOL-HIV BREF was used, as well as the Every Day Memory Questionnaire, and additional questions on anxiety and depression to supplement the WHOQOL.

Results: While most rated their quality of life (QoL) positively, bivariate analysis showed that better QoL (total score and most domains) was strongly associated with being a man; in a relationship; in paid employment; having higher level of income; not on benefits, and to a lesser degree with being MSM, having higher level of education, and diagnosed after the age of 40. Multivariate analysis showed that not being on benefits was the variable most consistently associated with better quality of life, as was being partnered. Concerns about everyday memory difficulties, and anxiety and depression scores were strong predictors of poorer quality of life.

Conclusion: While the cross-sectional nature of the investigation could not establish that the associations were causal, the findings indicate that concerns about memory difficulties, anxiety and depression, as well as gender, ethnicity, financial factors, and relationship status, are important contributors to QoL in this group. These findings point towards the need for further research to clarify the mechanisms through which the factors identified here affect QoL, and to identify possible interventions to improve the QoL of older people living with HIV.

Background

People living with HIV with access to effective antiviral treatments nowadays are growing older and living healthier lives than they were before these treatments became available in the mid-1990s [1, 2], while more people are acquiring HIV at an older age [3, 4]. In the UK there are now more than 25,000 people aged 50 and older living with HIV [4]. Yet, while health improvements and much increased survival rates are to be welcomed, the psychological and social consequences of ageing with HIV are complex. Although the individual impact of getting older with HIV can be positive e.g. [5, 6], the problems faced by older people with HIV include high levels of stigma [7–10]; concerns about dependence on benefits [11], ongoing concerns about disclosure [12], and uncertainty over how ageing, HIV, and its treatment affect health [13]. Gender, ethnicity, sexuality, and social supports play an important role in how older people living with HIV adapt [5, 14–18]. There is evidence for poorer reported quality of life (QoL) in older people living with HIV compared with younger people with the infection [19–21], although this has not been a consistent finding [22, 23]. None of these studies has included a control group without HIV. There is concern about the physical impact of HIV infection in older people, both in terms of non-AIDS related

*Correspondence: J.catalan@nhs.net
[1] CNWL NHS Foundation Trust, South Kensington and Chelsea Mental Health Centre, London, UK
Full list of author information is available at the end of the article

morbidity [24], and cognitive function [25–27]. Understanding how ageing, HIV, and QoL intersect is key to furthering our knowledge and to developing appropriate interventions to improve their QoL.

Aims

This paper is based on analysis of quantitative data gathered for the multi-method HIV and Later Life (HALL) Study [18]. The aims of the study were to uncover self-reported QoL, social supports, and mental health among older people living with HIV in the UK; identify links between them; and identify factors associated with reported mental health and QoL in this population. The study received ethical approval from Keele University and from the NHS-Research Ethics Committee in London.

Methods

Participants

A total of 100 (73 men and 27 women) people over the age of 50 years living with HIV, including 76 interviewees and 24 on line participants, completed the self-administered questionnaires. In terms of ethnicity, 57 were White British, 13 White other, 28 Black African, and 2 Black other. There were 51 MSM, 45 heterosexual, and 4 bisexual participants. Age ranged from 50 to 87 years, median 56 (see Rosenfeld et al. [18] for further details).

Participants were recruited through London-based HIV community organizations and HIV clinics. Staff and volunteers reviewed records to identify patients who met the study inclusion criteria, including having being diagnosed with HIV for at least 12 months, and not suffering acute or severe psychological symptoms. Surveys were completed immediately post-interview, and 24 surveys were completed on-line by non-interviewed participants. There were no differences between participants that completed the surveys post-interview and online in terms of their QoL scores, memory concerns, anxiety, depression, proportions partnered, educational level, on benefits, paid employment, living alone, attending support groups, and time since diagnosis.

Instruments

The WHOQOL- HIV BREF [28], a self-reported 31-item questionnaire, was used. It gives a multidimensional profile across six domains (physical health; psychological health; level of independence; social relationships; environment; and spirituality), as well as an overall rating of QoL.

The Every Day Memory Questionnaire (EMQ), a self-reported 13-item questionnaire was used to establish the subjective perception of cognitive failure [29].

Participants were asked to rate their anxiety and depression on a scale from 0 (not at all) to 10 (extremely) from the Bournemouth Questionnaire, a self-report instrument that has been used in other populations with medical disorders [30].

Analysis

Data were analysed using the statistical package for Social Science Version 18.0 (SPSS, Chicago, Illinois, USA). The independent samples *t* test was used to compare scores for each QoL domain, total QoL, and memory by binary categories of exposure variables. Since the anxiety and depression ratings were derived from single questions, and the shape of their distributions was not normal, a non-parametric test (Mann–Whitney) was used to compare scores by binary categories of exposure variables instead of *t* tests. Two-tailed tests with $p < 0.05$ were considered statistically significant. p values were not adjusted for multiple testing because the objective was simply to identify patterns of associations.

Stepwise linear regression was used to identify the best combination of exposure variable to predict the outcomes of interest. The process repeatedly applies multiple regression, each time searching for the predictor that has the highest correlation with the outcome variable, and removing the weakest correlated variable (the criterion for entry was $p < 0.05$ and for removal $p > 0.10$). The final model includes the variables that best explain the distribution.

It was expected that multicollinearity (correlation between predictor variables) could affect the parameters of the regression models, and lead to poor estimation of the regression coefficients. The variance inflation factor was used to assess whether correlation between independent variables in the multivariate models was of concern.

Results

Response to single questions on overall QoL, anxiety and depression in the last 4 weeks

Over half of the participants (56%) rated their QoL as 'good or very good', 24% as 'neither good nor poor', 9% as 'poor', and 1% as 'very poor'.

For the anxiety and depression scores, on a scale of 1–10 (where 0 is not at all anxious or depressed, and 10 is extremely anxious or depressed), the median scores for both variables were 5, with 26% reporting 0 or 1 for depression, and 22% reporting 0 or 1 for anxiety. For both variables 12% of the participants scored the highest scores of 9 or 10.

Bivariate analysis of WHOQOL-HIV BREF scores versus demographic, socio-economic, social support, and year of diagnosis

Table 1 shows the findings from the bivariate analysis of QoL. Men reported higher QoL, total QoL score

Table 1 Findings from bivariate analysis of quality of life and memory scores v. binary demographic, socio-economic and social support variables (one-way ANOVA)

		WHOQoL-HIV domain scores						Total WHOQoL-HIV score	Everyday memory score	Trends
		Physical health	Psychological health	Independence	Social relations	Environmental health	Spirituality			
Mean (SD)		13.0 (3.8)	12.8 (3.3)	12.9 (3.9)	12.9 (3.4)	14.4 (2.9)	13.7 (3.3)	79.7 (16.6)	1.4 (1.1)	
Gender	*p*	0.008**	0.133	0.001**	0.038*	0.002**	0.052	0.002**	0.137	Men (27) have higher QoL values and lower memory scores than women (73)
Ethnicity	*p*	0.774	0.512	0.051	0.568	0.004**	0.581	0.382	0.481	White group (70) have higher QoL values and lower memory scores than Black group (30)
Partnership	*p*	0.129	0.036*	0.031*	0.001**	0.038*	0.119	0.009**	0.248	Partnered group (33) have higher QoL values and lower memory scores than singles group (67)
Sexual orientation	*p*	0.315	0.496	0.247	0.033*	0.001**	0.723	0.086	0.717	MSM (46) have higher QoL values and lower memory scores than Other group (53)
Age	*p*	0.152	0.340	0.167	0.993	0.242	0.417	0.230	0.386	Those aged 50–55 years (55) have higher QoL values and lower memory scores than those aged ≥56 years (45)
Education	*p*	0.024*	0.471	0.021*	0.722	0.385	0.905	0.151	<0.001***	Those with higher education (57) have higher QoL and lower memory scores than those without HE (43)
Income	*p*	0.004**	0.236	<0.001***	0.040*	<0.001***	0.208	0.001**	0.001**	Those earning ≥£10 K/year (45) have higher QoL and lower memory scores than those earning <£10 K/year (42)
Benefits	*p*	<0.001***	<0.001***	<0.001***	0.002**	<0.001***	0.026*	<0.001***	<0.001***	Those not on benefits (45) have higher QoL values and lower memory scores than those receiving benefits (55)
Children	*p*	0.461	0.759	0.151	0.150	0.073	0.565	0.294	0.522	Those without children (48) have higher QoL values and lower memory scores than those with children (52)

Table 1 continued

		WHOQoL-HIV domain scores						Total WHOQoL-HIV score	Everyday memory score	Trends
		Physical health	Psychological health	Independence	Social relations	Environmental health	Spirituality			
Grand-children	p	0.116	0.180	0.001**	0.066	0.001**	0.316	0.012*	0.051	Those without grandchildren (65) have higher QoL and lower memory scores than those with grandchildren (24)
Working	p	0.004**	0.019*	<0.001***	0.004**	<0.001***	0.026*	<0.001***	<0.001***	Those in paid work (28) have higher QoL values and lower memory scores than those with no paid work (72)
Live alone	p	0.669	0.593	0.797	0.817	0.971	0.342	0.922	0.748	Inconsistent direction of difference between those living alone (59) and those living with someone (41)
Religious	p	0.793	0.483	0.076	0.102	0.001**	0.738	0.113	0.102	Those who rarely or never attend services (52) have higher QoL and lower memory scores than those who attend (48)
Support group	p	0.874	0.164	0.291	0.807	0.074	0.490	0.824	0.603	Inconsistent direction of difference between those who do not attend a support group (45) and those who attend (55)
Year of diagnosis	p	0.149	0.219	0.109	0.427	0.727	0.411	0.184	0.653	Those diagnosed during or after 1997 (77) have higher QoL and similar memory scores to those diagnosed earlier (21)
Age of diagnosis	p	0.030*	0.019*	0.021*	0.213	0.285	0.267	0.031*	0.168	Those diagnosed at age 40 years or younger (23) have lower QoL values and higher memory scores than those diagnosed after the age of 40 (75)

Findings from one-way ANOVA * $0.05 > p \geq 0.01$ ** $0.01 > p \geq 0.001$ *** $p < 0.001$

($p < 0.01$) and in several domains: physical ($p < 0.01$), level of independence ($p < 0.01$), environment ($p < 0.01$), and social relationships ($p < 0.05$). White participants reported higher scores on the environment domain only ($p < 0.01$). Partnered participants reported a higher total QoL score ($p < 0.01$), and for the social relations ($p < 0.01$), psychological, environment, and level of independence domains (all $p < 0.05$). MSM reported higher scores for environment ($p < 0.01$), and social relations ($p < 0.05$).

Participants diagnosed with HIV at 40 or younger had worse QoL than those diagnosed with HIV over the age of 40, with worse total QoL score ($p < 0.05$), and worse physical ($p < 0.05$), psychological health ($p < 0.05$), and level of independence ($p < 0.05$) scores.

Those with higher education reported higher QoL in physical and level of independence (both $p < 0.05$). Participants earning more than £10,000/year reported higher total QoL score ($p < 0.01$), and scored higher for level of independence and environment (both $p < 0.001$), physical ($p < 0.01$), and social relations ($p < 0.05$). Those not receiving state benefits had a higher QoL in total score ($p < 0.001$), and in all domains: physical, psychological, level of independence, and environment (all $p < 0.001$), social relations ($p < 0.01$) and spiritual ($p < 0.05$). Participants in employment reported higher QoL in total score ($p < 0.001$), and in all domains: level of independence and environment (both $p < 0.001$), physical, and social relations (both $p < 0.01$), and psychological and spiritual ($p < 0.05$).

Participants without grandchildren reported better QoL with respect to total score ($p < 0.05$), and to level of independence and environment (both $p < 0.01$). Those who attended religious services had higher QoL for the environment domain ($p < 0.01$).

Multivariate analysis of WHOQOL scores

Stepwise regression was used to identify the best combination of exposure variables to predict the QoL scores. Table 2 shows the findings from stepwise multiple regression analysis of QoL scores by binary demographic, socio-economic and social support variables. Exposure variables with $p < 0.05$ in the bivariate analysis reported above were included for potential selection in the regression models. Findings from the exposure variables gender, income, age of diagnosis, and religious attendance are not included in the table, as these variables were no longer significant when included in models together with the other variables. The findings for those variables finally selected by the stepwise process for inclusion in each regression model are shown in the table (the criterion for entry was $p < 0.05$, and for removal was $p > 0.10$).

Existence of problematic levels of correlation between the independent variables in the multivariate models was checked using the variance inflation factor (VIF) using a threshold of five to indicate high correlation. In the regression models the highest value of VIF was 3.1, and most values were below two, so multicollinearity is unlikely to have adversely affected selection of the best predictors.

The exposure variable benefits remained a strong predictor of total QoL and all QoL domain scores (except social relations) in the final regression models. For the social relations domain, the best combination of predictors was partnership ($p < 0.01$) and paid employment ($p < 0.05$).

After adjusting for the exposure variable of benefits, Black African ethnicity was associated with better QoL in three domains: physical ($p < 0.01$), psychological ($p < 0.01$), and spiritual ($p < 0.05$), in contrast with the bivariate analysis, that showed no differences between ethnic groups in QoL (apart from the environmental domain for which those of white ethnicity had significantly higher scores, $p = 0.004$). The significant association between sexual orientation and QoL was still evident for the environment domain ($p < 0.05$) after adjustment for the exposure variable benefits, but this association did not remain evident for the social relations domain. After adjusting for being on benefits, being partnered was still associated with better scores for total QoL ($p < 0.05$), and for the domains of social relations ($p < 0.01$) and independence ($p < 0.05$).

The exposure variable grandchildren was a significant predictor of QoL on the physical health domain after adjustment for being on benefits, whereby higher QoL scores were observed in those who were not grandparents.

Anxiety, depression, every day memory difficulties, and WHOQOL

Findings from the analysis of the associations between the scores derived from single questions on anxiety and depression, and the binary variables, are similar to the findings from the analysis of the QoL scores for the psychological health domain (results in Table 1), apart from the finding that both anxiety and depression are positively associated with being in the low income group (both $p < 0.05$ with the Mann–Whitney test).

Total score for QoL was highly associated (negatively) with depression score (Spearman's rho −0.62, $p < 0.001$) and anxiety score (Spearman's rho −0.58, $p < 0.001$): the better the QoL, the lower the levels of reported anxiety and depression. Total score for QoL was also strongly negatively correlated with everyday memory score

Table 2 Findings from multivariate analysis of WHOQoL-HIV quality of life and memory scores v. binary demographic, socio-economic and social support variables

	WHOQoL-HIV domain scores												Total WHOQoL-HIV score		Everyday memory score[a]	
	Physical health		Psychological health		Level of independence		Social relations		Environmental health		Spirituality					
	Coeff.	*p*	Coeff.	*p*	Coeff.	*p*	Coeff.	*p*	Coeff.	*p*	Coeff.	*p*	Coeff.	*p*	Coeff.	*p*
Constant	17.83	*<0.001****	15.68	*<0.001****	14.65	*<0.001****	11.68	*<0.001****	15.23	*<0.001****	16.77	*<0.001****	86.54	*<0.001****	0.80	*0.004***
Ethnicity (White)	−3.25	*0.002***	−1.65	*0.044**							−1.83	*0.024**			0.45	*0.046**
Partnership (partnered)					1.78	*0.029**	2.28	*0.008***					8.32	*0.027**		
Sexual orientation (MSM)									1.47	*0.012**						
Education (with higher education)															−0.47	*0.023**
Benefits (on benefits)	−3.38	*<0.001****	−2.62	*0.001**	−3.73	*<0.001****			−2.48	*<0.001****	−2.63	*0.001***	−14.54	*<0.001****	0.74	*0.001***
Grand-children (grandparent)	−2.10	*0.048**														
Working (paid work)							2.00	*0.018**								
Adjusted R^2	0.23	*<0.001****	0.14	*0.002***	0.33	*<0.001****	0.16	*0.001***	0.29	*<0.001****	0.15	*0.001***	0.27	*<0.001****	0.22	*<0.001****
N	89[b]		100		100		100		99		100		100		100	

* $0.05 > p \geq 0.01$ ** $0.01 > p \geq 0.001$ *** $p < 0.001$

Exposures with p < 0.05 in the bivariate analysis (Table 1) were included for potential selection in regression models, applying the stepwise linear regression process. The table shows significance values and unstandardized coefficients for those variables selected for inclusion in models, having applied criteria p to enter <0.05 and p to remove <0.10

[a] Higher scores for everyday memory score indicate greater memory difficulties, so the coefficients for memory have opposite signs to those for QoL scores

[b] The sample size included in the analysis is lower for this outcome variable because only 89 of the 100 participants responded to the question about being grandparents

(Spearman's rho −0.61, $p < 0.001$) (higher scores for this variable indicated more memory difficulties).

In the bivariate analysis, lower everyday memory scores were associated with higher education ($p < 0.001$), and with higher income ($p = 0.001$), not being on benefits ($p < 0.001$), and with being in paid employment ($p < 0.001$) (see Table 1). However, multivariate analysis, adjusting for exposure to other variables, showed a change in the direction of the association between everyday memory scores and ethnicity, so that participants of Black African ethnicity reported lower memory scores (indicating fewer memory difficulties).

A key finding was the association between reported memory difficulties and QoL. When the variable everyday memory score was included as a potential predictor variable in stepwise regression analysis, together with the same demographic, socio-economic, and social support exposure variables that had been included in the analysis reported above, score on the memory difficulties questionnaire was the strongest predictor of total QoL score ($p < 0.001$). Again, statistical criterion for entry was $p < 0.05$, and for removal was $p > 0.10$. The best combination of exposure variables to predict the total QoL score were Everyday Memory Questionnaire score (negative effect $p < 0.001$); being on benefits (negative effect $p < 0.01$); being partnered (positive effect $p < 0.05$); and having higher education (negative effect $p < 0.05$). The unexpected direction of effect of higher education is due to having adjusted for the very high correlation between higher education and memory score (see Table 1). This residual negative correlation of higher education with QoL suggests that in addition to the strong positive effect of higher education on QoL via improved cognitive functioning, there may exist an additional weak adverse effect, and while it may be spurious, this finding should be borne in mind for future investigations.

Discussion

Most study participants reported their QoL to be 'good' or 'very good' and reported low levels of depressive or anxious self-ratings. Bivariate analysis showed that better QoL was strongly associated with male gender, being in a relationship, in employment and not on state benefits, and having higher level of income; and to a lesser extent with being MSM, having higher education, and having being diagnosed after the age of 40. Multivariate analysis demonstrated that not being on state benefits was most consistently associated with better quality of life, as was being partnered. Concerns about everyday memory difficulties, and anxiety and depression scores were strong predictors of poor quality of life.

These results were comparable to those of Owen and Catalan [5] and Ribeiro Nobre and colleagues [6], whose participants, all older people living with HIV, reported finding meaning in life and having a positive attitude towards the future. In contrast, in a study comparing younger and older people living with HIV and using the same QoL instrument used in our study, Monteiro and colleagues [21] found older people living with HIV to have lower QoL in a number of domains (physical, level of independence, and social relationships), as well as more depressive symptoms. Differences in the heterogeneity of the populations and transmission categories in the studies, and the use of different instruments to measure depressive symptoms, as well as differences in the medical and social context of the participants may explain the discrepancies between these two studies.

Interestingly, two other studies using the same instrument to measure QoL as Monteiro and colleagues [21] and ourselves also gave contrasting results, Skevington and colleagues [23] not finding older people with HIV to have poorer quality of life than younger ones, while the WHOQoL HIV group [19] found older people to have worse quality of life than younger ones. The use of the same instrument suggests that the discrepant results are related to sampling and population differences: the former study [23] carried out their investigation in samples from 23 areas, including developing and developed ones, while the latter [19] included samples from six areas, most of them developing countries. Socio-economic factors and the context of medical services are likely have influenced the participants' reported quality of life. These inconsistent findings in relation to age and QoL in the population of people living and ageing with HIV requires further research.

Reported memory difficulties, and depressive and anxious feelings, were strongly associated with lower QoL. Although neurocognitive disorders in older people with HIV are more common than in younger people [25–27], subjective reports of memory problems do not always indicate the presence of cognitive impairment. Rather, these problems may reflect wider concerns over the ways in which age and HIV intersect to shape physical and mental health, which our analysis of qualitative data also revealed [13], and it is important to ensure appropriate cognitive screening [31].

Better economic indicators were shown to be strongly associated with better QoL, as reported by Monteiro and colleagues [21]. While not surprising, it highlights the risks that as people living with HIV continue ageing, financial independence is frequently further compromised [11].

Male gender was a strong predictor of better QoL, in contrast with the findings of the WHOQOL-HIV field test (WHOQOL-HIV Group, 2004). In agreement with our findings, Miners and colleagues [32] in a large study with a general population control group also found male gender to be associated with better quality of life. Male participants in our study were mostly MSM, and thus belonged to a group with a relatively lower intra-group stigmatisation of HIV [18]. This might also explain another of our findings, that being an MSM was associated with better QoL. In the qualitative part of the study, MSM participants described greater sense of belonging to a community of people living with HIV [18].

Being in a partnership was also found to be a strong predictor of QoL for total score, as well as several domains (social relations, psychological, level of independence, and environment). Grov and colleagues [15] identified loneliness as an important factor in terms of depressive feelings in older people living with HIV, and not being in a partnership may similarly contribute to lower QoL associated with isolation.

Not having grandchildren was associated with better QoL in some domains. Although our qualitative data indicate that having grandchildren was a source of comfort for some [18]. The quantitative data, however, suggest that being free from the demands of looking after grandchildren was a positive factor with respect to QoL.

Findings in relation to ethnicity are more complex. Multivariate analysis, after adjusting for being on benefits, showed that Black Ethnicity was associated with significantly better QoL in several domains, and when adjusted for the effect of being on benefits, being in the White ethnic group appeared to be a risk factor for low QoL rather than protective against it. More research with a larger sample size is needed to clarify the relationship between ethnicity and QoL.

There were some limitations to our investigation. Our sample was largely London-based, and included few participants from rural environments who might have experienced greater levels of isolation and thus lower quality of life. Also under-represented were non-White and non-Black ethnic groups (e.g. South Asians), and people of Black ethnicity who were not from African countries (e.g. Black Caribbean). Finally, our participants were recruited through HIV clinics and community organizations, thus excluding potential participants who were not engaged with services and support groups, and perhaps experiencing lower quality of life. Further research should aim at expanding the sample of participants, so as to strengthen and widen its findings.

Studies comparing people living with HIV with the general population have shown the former group to have worse quality of life [32], but we are not aware of research comparing PLWH with people with other chronic diseases. As HIV becomes a more manageable condition as a result of new therapies and more people are ageing with HIV, the question of similarities and differences with other chronic disorders is becoming an important one, but complicated by the continued stigmatisation of the virus and of those living with it, and by the increased likelihood that people ageing with HIV will also be living with other chronic disorders, and thus comparison populations should be included in further research.

Conclusions

Despite growing research into the psycho-social dimensions of ageing with HIV, our understanding of QoL among people living and ageing with HIV remains limited. Our analysis shows that while, overall, older people with HIV reported high levels of QoL and low levels of anxious or depressive feelings, specific variables were associated with QoL, suggesting areas of further intervention and research.

Although, in our sample, ethnicity in relation to QoL did not show clear-cut results, suggesting a complex association needing further research, other associations were more easily identifiable. Unfavourable economic factors were associated with lower QoL, and further research is required to understand the impact of financial concerns linked to ageing in older people living with HIV (e.g. changes to disability benefits). Gender was shown to be a predictor of QoL, with men reporting higher levels. The mechanisms explaining this finding are likely to include differential levels of stigma and feelings of isolation in heterosexual women with HIV, and further research is needed to elucidate the relevant factors. Finally, being in a partnership had a positive effect on QoL, and, surprisingly, not having grandchildren appeared to have a positive impact on some domains of QoL, another finding that requires further investigation, especially given the ageing of the population of people with HIV, and the increased proportion of heterosexuals with children within this population.

These findings, while requiring further exploration, suggest specific policy responses on the part of service providers and policy makers working with this population. We have listed elsewhere several recommendations for policy and practice (see Rosenfeld et al. [18]), but of these, the following are the most relevant given the findings reported here.

First, service providers should be aware of the low QoL and high levels of depressive and anxious feelings among specific groups in older people with HIV (such as those on low income or state benefits, women, those without partners, and those reporting memory concerns), and to be prepared to provide them with the appropriate help and support. Second, older people with HIV should be screened for depressive or anxious feelings, neurocognitive function, and QoL, as part of the regular monitoring of their health. Finally, service providers caring for older people with HIV should not assume that the medical care they receive is necessarily sufficient to identify or manage the psychological and social stressors that can lower their QoL.

Authors' contributions

JC participated in the design of the study and took responsibility for writing the manuscript. VT carried out the statistical analysis and helped to draft the manuscript. DR participated in the design of the study and helped to draft the manuscript. DR conceived and oversaw the study and helped to draft the manuscript. All authors read and approved the final manuscript.

Author details

[1] CNWL NHS Foundation Trust, South Kensington and Chelsea Mental Health Centre, London, UK. [2] Faculty of Science and Technology, University of Westminster, London, UK. [3] School of Social Science and Public Policy, Keele University, London, UK.

Acknowledgements

We thank the other members of the HALL (HIV AND Later Life) Team: Jane Anderson, David Asboe, Simon Collins, and Valerie Delpech. We are very grateful to the older people living with HIV who participated in the study, and to the clinics and HIV organizations who helped us to recruit participants for the research. We also thank the MRC Lifelong Health and Wellbeing (LLHW) Phase 3 Pilot Studies Programme for supporting the research. Dominic Lopez-Welsch provided invaluable assistance in the preparation of the manuscript.

Competing interests

The authors declare that they have no competing interests.

Funding

The study was funded by the UK's Medical Research Council's Life-Long Health and Wellbeing Phase 3 Pilot Studies Programmes, G1001817.

References

1. May M, Gompels M, Sabin C. Life expectancy of HIV-1-positive individuals approaches normal conditional on response to antiretroviral therapy: UK Collaborative HIV Cohort Study. J Int AIDS Soc. 2012;15:18078.
2. Nakagawa F, May M, Phillips A. Life expectancy living with HIV: recent estimates and future implications. Curr Opin Infect Dis. 2013;26:17–25.
3. Cresswell F, Fisher M. HIV and the ageing patient. Medicine. 2013;41:456–60.
4. Yin Z, Brown A, Hughes G, Nardone A, Gill O, Delpech V. HIV in the United Kingdom 2014 report: data to end 2013. London: Public Health England; 2014.
5. Owen G, Catalan J. 'We never expected this to happen': narratives of ageing with HIV among gay men living in London, UK. Cult Health Sex. 2012;14:59–72.
6. Ribeiro Nobre N, Kylma J, Kirsi T. I Live Quite a Good Balanced Life: a pilot study on the life experiences of ageing individuals living with HIV. Nurs Res Prac. 2012;2012:128108.
7. Emlet CA. You're awfully old to have this disease: experiences of stigma and ageism in adults 50 years and older living with HIV/AIDS. Gerontologist. 2006;46:781–90.
8. Emlet CA, Brennan DJ, Brennenstuhl S, Rueda S, Hart TA, Rourke SB. The impact of HIV-related stigma on older and younger adults living with HIV disease: does age matter? AIDS Care. 2015;27:520–8.
9. Hudson A, Mbewe R, Delpech V. Stigma index study: a continued issue in the UK. In: British HIV association (BHIVA) autumn conference 12–13 November 2015, London; 2015.
10. Grodensky CA, Golin CE, Jones C, Mamo M, Dennis AC, Abernethy MG, et al. I Should Know Better: the roles of relationships, spirituality, disclosure, stigma, and shame for older women living with HIV seeking support in the south. J Assoc Nurses AIDS Care. 2015;26:12–23.
11. Power L, Bell M, Freemantle I. A national study of people over 50 living with HIV. York: Joseph Rowntree Foundation; 2010.
12. Rosenfeld D, Ridge D, Catalan J, Delpech V. Age and life course location as interpretive resources for decisions regarding disclosure of HIV to parents and children: findings from the HIV and later life study. J Aging Stud. 2016;38:81–91.
13. Rosenfeld D, Ridge D, Von Lob G. Vital scientific puzzle or lived uncertainty? Professional and lived approaches to the uncertainties of ageing with HIV. Health Sociol Rev. 2014;23:20–32.
14. Chesney MA, Chambers DB, Taylor JM, Johnson LM. Social support, distress, and well-being in older men living with HIV infection. J Acquir Immune Defic Syndr. 2003;33:S185–93.
15. Grov C, Golub SA, Parsons JT, Brennan M, Karpiak SE. Loneliness and HIV-related stigma explain depression among older HIV-positive adults. AIDS Care. 2010;22:630–9.
16. Lyons A, Pitts M, Grierson J, Thorpe R, Power J. Ageing with HIV: health and psychosocial well-being of older gay men. AIDS Care. 2010;22:1236–44.
17. Sankar A, Nevedal A, Neufeld S, Berry R, Luborsky M. What do we know about older adults and HIV? A review of social and behavioral literature. AIDS Care. 2011;23:1187–207.
18. Rosenfeld D, Anderson J, Ridge D, Asboe D, Catalan J, Collins S, et al. Social support, mental health, and quality of life among older people living with HIV: findings from the HIV and Later Life (HALL) project. Newcastle: Keele University; 2015.
19. WHO QoL HIV Group. WHOQOL-HIV for quality of life assessment among people living with HIV and AIDS: results from the field test. AIDS Care. 2004;16:882–9.
20. McGowan J, Sherr L, Rodger A, Fisher M, Miners A, Johnson M, et al. Effects of age on symptom burden, mental health and quality of life amongst people with HIV in the UK. J Int AIDS Soc. 2014;17:19511.
21. Monteiro F, Canavarro MC, Pereira M. Factors associated with quality of life in middle-aged and older patients living with HIV. AIDS Care. 2016;28:92–8.
22. Nokes KM, Coleman CL, Hamilton MJ, Corless IB, Sefcik E, Kirksey KM, et al. Age-related effects on symptom status and health-related quality of life in persons with HIV/AIDS. Appl Nurs Res. 2011;24:10–6.
23. Skevington SM. Is quality of life poorer for older adults with HIV/AIDS? International evidence using the WHOQOL-HIV. AIDS Care. 2012;24:1219–25.
24. Deeks SG, Phillips AN. Clinical review: HIV infection, antiretroviral treatment, ageing, and non-AIDS related morbidity. BMJ. 2009;338:288–92.
25. Malaspina L, Woods SP, Moore DJ, Depp C, Letendre SL, Jeste D, et al. Successful cognitive aging in persons living with HIV infection. J Neurovirol. 2011;17:110–9.
26. Valcour V. HIV, aging, and cognition: emerging issues. Top Antivir Med. 2013;21:119–23.
27. Heikinheimo T, Poutiainen E, Salonen O, Elovaara I, Ristola M. Three-decade neurological and neurocognitive follow-up of HIV-1-infected patients on best-available antiretroviral therapy in Finland. BMJ Open. 2015;5:e007986.
28. O'Connell KA, Skevington SM. An international quality of life instrument to assess wellbeing in adults who are HIV-positive: a short form of the WHOQOL-HIV (31 items). AIDS Behav. 2012;16:452–60.
29. Royle J, Lincoln NB. The Everyday Memory Questionnaire–revised: development of a 13-item scale. Disabil Rehabil. 2008;30:114–21.
30. Bolton JE, Breen AC. The Bournemouth Questionnaire: a short-form comprehensive outcome measure. I. Psychometric properties in back pain patients. J Manip Physiol Ther. 1999;22:503–10.
31. Barber T, Bansi L, Pozniak A, Asboe D, Nelson M, Moyle G, et al. Low levels of neurocognitive impairment detected in screening HIV-infected men who have sex with men: the MSM Neurocog Study. Int J STD AIDS. 2016;11:e0159286.

6

Late presentation increases risk and costs of non-infectious comorbidities in people with HIV

Giovanni Guaraldi[1*], Stefano Zona[1], Marianna Menozzi[1], Thomas D. Brothers[2], Federica Carli[1], Chiara Stentarelli[1], Giovanni Dolci[1], Antonella Santoro[1], Ana Rita Domingues Da Silva[4], Elisa Rossi[5], Julian Falutz[3] and Cristina Mussini[1]

Abstract

Background: Late presentation (LP) at the time of HIV diagnosis is defined as presentation with AIDS whatever the CD4 cell count or with CD4 <350 cells/mm. The objective of our study was to assess the prevalence of non-infectious comorbidities (NICM) and multimorbidity among HIV-positive individuals with and without a history of LP (HIV + LP and HIV + EP, respectively), and compare them to matched HIV-negative control participants from a community-based cohort. The secondary objective was to provide estimates and determinants of direct cost of medical care in HIV patients.

Methods: We performed a matched cohort study including HIV + LP and HIV + EP among people attending the Modena HIV Metabolic Clinic (MHMC) in 2014. HIV-positive participants were matched in a 1:3 ratio with HIV-negative participants from the CINECA ARNO database. Multimorbidity was defined as the concurrent presence of ≥2 NICM. Logistic regression models were constructed to evaluate associated predictors of NICM and multimorbidity.

Results: We analyzed 452 HIV + LP and 73 HIV + EP participants in comparison to 1575 HIV-negative controls. The mean age was 46 ± 9 years, 27.5% were women. Prevalence of NICM and multimorbidity were fourfold higher in the HIV + LP compared to the general population ($p < 0.001$), while HIV + EP present an intermediate risk. LP was associated with increased total costs in all age strata, but appear particularly relevant in patients above 50 years of age, after adjusting for age, multimorbidity, and antiretroviral costs.

Conclusions: LP with HIV infection is still very frequent in Italy, is associated with higher prevalence of NICM and multimorbidity, and contributes to higher total care costs. Encouraging early testing and access to care is still urgently needed.

Keywords: HIV, Late presentation, Comorbidities, Costs

Background

The World Health Organization defines "late presentation" (LP) as a new HIV diagnosis with concurrent acquired immunodeficiency syndrome (AIDS) defining events, whatever the CD4+ T cell count, or else a new human immunodeficiency virus (HIV) diagnosis with CD4+ count less than 350 cells/mm^3 [1, 2]. LP is associated with adverse outcomes, including shorter life expectancy [3–5], and may also impair the efficacy and tolerability of combined antiretroviral therapy (cART) [4, 6]. Although most HIV-positive individuals who begin therapy with a CD4+ count above 200 cells/mm^3 eventually achieve a CD4+ count >500 cells/mm^3, those with LP are far less likely to ever experience a robust CD4+ cell gain [7]. LP has also been associated with enhanced risk for drug toxicities including anemia [8] and immune reconstitution inflammatory syndrome (IRIS) [9].

*Correspondence: giovanni.guaraldi@unimore.it
[1] Department of Medical and Surgical Sciences for Adults and Children, Clinic of Infectious Diseases, University of Modena and Reggio Emilia, Emilia-Romagna, Modena, Italy
Full list of author information is available at the end of the article

Approximately 40–60% of new HIV diagnoses in Italy are made in the context of LP [10]. The Collaboration of Observational HIV Epidemiological Research Europe (COHERE) study observed a small decrease in LP across Europe from 57.3% in 2000 to 51.7% in 2010/11, suggesting that the prevalence of LP remains stubbornly high over time [5].

Older age represents a consistent risk factor for LP [11–14], as a result of barriers to HIV testing among older adults at the individual, medical and public health policy levels [15, 16]. With an increasing number of people being diagnosed with HIV at an older age, the association between older age and LP is becoming even more significant and it is important to understand how LP might affect the health of people aging with HIV.

Nevertheless, it is still unknown whether there is an association between LP and age-related non-infectious co-morbidities (NICM) among people living with HIV, including cardiovascular disease (CVD), hypertension, type 2 diabetes mellitus (T2DM), chronic kidney disease (CKD), and osteopenia/osteoporosis. These heterogeneous comorbidities recognize age and HIV disease as independent risk factors, and tend to aggregate into complex multimorbidity (MM) patterns (usually defined as two or more NICM being present in the same individual at the same assessment).

The objective of our study was to assess the prevalence of NICM and MM among HIV-positive individuals with and without a history of LP, and compare them to matched HIV-negative control participants from a community-based cohort. The secondary objective was to provide estimates and determinants of direct cost of medical care in LP HIV patients.

Methods

The study took place at the multidisciplinary Modena HIV Metabolic Clinic (MHMC), which was initiated in 2004 to assess longitudinal metabolic changes among people with HIV. As previously described [17, 18], patients undergo annual comprehensive assessments in multiple domains, including metabolic and endocrinological variables, bone mineral density (BMD), organ function, and social factors.

In the past 10 years a gradual decline in LP was observed in people attending MHMC, similar to that found in other European countries [5, 14, 19]. In 2004 LP prevalence in our cohort was 87%, while in 2012 it was 65% of the new patients.

The current cross-sectional study was performed using data from two groups of individuals with visits to the MHMC in 2014. One group were all patients identified with a history of LP at the time of HIV diagnosis (HIV + LP). The other were all patients without a history of LP, and were therefore early presenters (HIV + EP). LP was defined according to the WHO definition, as a new HIV diagnosis with concurrent AIDS defining events, whatever the CD4+ T-cell count, or else a new HIV diagnosis with CD4+ count less than 350 cells/mm^3 [1, 2].

HIV + LP and HIV + EP participants were each matched in a 1:3 ratio, on age, sex, and race (all Caucasian) and geographical area of origin, to participants in a community-based cohort of the general population, the CINECA ARNO database [18]. The ARNO Observatory is an online, multi-centre observational database in which population-based data is collected and epidemiological methods [20] are used to combine and aggregate large volumes of health and healthcare-related data for each individual patient. These data include primary care provider-generated medication prescriptions, inpatient hospital records and discharge, summaries, diagnostic laboratory tests and radiographic examinations. This information is linked to other sources of patient data (including vital statistics and patient demographics) in order to provide comprehensive tracking of clinical diagnoses and healthcare use trends throughout Italy. Lifestyle, anthropometric and metabolic data are not collected in the CINECA ARNO database. All CINECA ARNO participants included in this study did not have a diagnosis of HIV infection, and were therefore assumed to be HIV negative.

Outcomes

NICM diagnoses were based according the following criteria previously used in our studies [18]. The category of CVD included the following diagnoses: myocardial infarction, coronary artery disease, peripheral vascular disease, stroke, angina pectoris, coronary artery bypass grafting, and angioplasty. Among MHMC participants, diagnostic criteria for hypertension, T2DM, and CKD included, respectively, blood pressure measurements >140/90 mmHg over two consecutive measurements, fasting serum glucose levels >126 mg/dL and eGFR <60 ml/min using the modification of diet in renal disease (MDRD) estimating equation [21]. Drug tracing criteria used to establish hypertension and T2DM diagnoses in both cohorts included current use of antihypertensive and hypoglycemic drugs. In the HIV-positive groups only we analyzed low bone mineral density (t-score <−2SD) using dual-energy X-ray absorptiometry (DXA).

Direct healthcare cost assessments

The cost of care analysis is referred to the economic point of view of the Italian public healthcare system, which offers drugs and health assistance free of charge to any HIV-positive patients. Direct healthcare costs were retrospectively analyzed in the calendar year 2013, as previously described [22] using the following indicators:

1. Hospital costs
   Hospitalization costs were calculated by collecting International Classification of Diseases, ninth edition (ICD9) codes in both cohorts. All hospitalization with a primary or secondary ICD-9 diagnosis codes including CVD, hypertension, T2DM, bone fractures, and renal failure diagnosis were selected [23] (Additional file 1: Table S1).
2. Outpatient HIV medical care cost
   With the movement of HIV care into the outpatient setting, it is not possible to evaluate the total cost of medical care using ICD9 codes. For outpatient cares we attributed a mean patient care cost obtained by the most recent reference value, which was able to better define HIV related care cost in patient with cART. This estimate is adjusted for current CD4 count strata, accounting 1381 USD/year for patients with CD4 <75 cell/mmc, 1241 USD/year for 76 < CD4 < 200 cell/mmc and 190 USD/year for CD4 > 201 cell/mmc [24] (Additional file 1: Table S1).
3. NICM medication costs
   NICM medication costs were calculated using pharmaceutical tracing by average wholesale prices obtained by National Pharmaceutical Prontuary of Agenzia Italiana del Farmaco (AIFA) [25].
4. cART medication costs
   cART medication cost were calculated using pharmaceutical tracing, by average hospital-sale price.

We converted hospital cost and outpatient HIV medical care cost from USDs to euros using conversion rate at the 31th of December, 2014 [26]. Total cost was defined as the sum of mean of NICM-costs plus mean of HIV-hospitalization costs plus mean of drug costs.

Statistical analysis

Comparisons among groups were performed using χ^2 test for categorical variables with Bonferroni adjusted post hoc analyses (significance level fixed at $p < 0.017$) and T-test or Mann–Whitney U-test for normally and non-normally distributed continuous variables, respectively. The probability of MM was drawn in the three comparative groups across age distribution using a logistic model. Univariate and multivariable logistic regression models were constructed to determine factors associated with LP using general population as reference after correction for sex and age (in years).

Considering the non-normal distribution of total costs, generalized linear models were constructed to evaluate independent factors associated with total cost in the whole population and in the subgroup of HIV-infected patients, using inverse Gaussian family distribution.

The variables for regression analyses were chosen on the basis of their clinical relevance.

Statistical analyses were performed STATA Software package, Intercooled version 13 for Mac (StataCorp ltd, Collage Station, TX, USA).

Results

525 individuals presented to the MHMC with new HIV diagnosis in 2014: 452 (85%) were HIV + LP and 73 (15%) were HIV + EP. These HIV-positive MHMC participants were matched to 1575 HIV-negative CINECA ARNO participants. Overall mean age was 46 ± 9 years and 27.5% were women, being the same across study groups per matching criteria.

With regards to HIV patients all the HIV + LP were on ART regimen, while 30.3% of HIV + EP had not yet started ARV.

Table 1 shows descriptive characteristics of the sample and their association with HIV + LP in comparison to HIV + EP.

NICM prevalence are reported in Fig. 1. A trend in higher prevalence of any NICM was observed in HIV + LP participants. With regard to MM the difference in prevalence reached significant levels when comparing HIV- and HIV + EP with HIV + LP (respectively $p < 0.001$ and $p < 0.001$), being present in 11% in HIV + LP, 4% in HIV + EP and 3% in HIV-negative controls, respectively.

According to our study hypothesis we explored the probability of NICM and MM across age distribution using a logistic model in the three comparative groups. CVD, T2DM and MM were significantly higher in HIV + LP when compared to both HIV + EP and HIV-negative participants ($p < 0.01$ for all comparisons) (Fig. 2).

No difference was found in hypertension risk across age distribution in the three groups.

CKD and low BMD data were not available for comparison in the HIV-negative group, but a non-significant trend in higher prevalence was observed in HIV + LP when compared to HIV + EP, respectively 7.52 vs. 4.11%, $p = 0.291$ and 20.13 vs. 12.33%, $p = 0.147$.

In multivariable models including age and sex, we observed fourfold increased odds of MM in HIV + LP participants compared to HIV-negative individuals (OR 4.3, 95% CI 2.8–6.7, $p < 0.001$). On the contrary, HIV + EP was not a risk factor for MM when compared to HIV-negative (OR 1.5, 95% CI 0.4–5.5, $p = 0.503$) (Fig. 3).

With regards to our secondary objective we estimated NICM related costs, HIV outpatient costs and cART costs in the 3 patient groups. Additional file 1: Figure S1 describes total costs across age strata and Fig. 4 also stratify HIV patients in EP and LP.

Table 1 Demographic, anthropometric and metabolic characteristics associated with late presentation

	All HIV + Patients (n = 525)	HIV + LP (n = 452)	HIV + EP (n = 73)	OR (95% CI)	p value
Men (n)	381 (72.5%)	319 (71.2%)	60 (82.2%)	0.59 (0.28–1.00)	0.050
Age (mean, SD)	46 (±9)	46 (±8)	43 (±10)	1.03 (1.01–1.08)	0.010
Current CD4 (n/microL) (median, IQR)	590 (441–756)	570 (423–729)	750 (589–981)	0.997 (0.996–0.998)	<0.001
Smoke					
None	318 (60.6%)	282 (62.4%)	36 (49.3%)	1 (ref.)	–
<10 cigs (moderate)	76 (14.4%)	63 (14.0%)	13 (17.8%)	0.61 (0.31–1.23)	0.173
>10 cigs (intense)	99 (18.9%)	84 (18.6%)	15 (20.6%)	0.71 (0.37–1.37)	0.311
Missing	32 (6.1%)	23 (5.1%)	9 (12.3%)	Not included	
BMI (kg/m^2) (SD)	24.7 (±4.7)	24.7 (±4.7)	24.8 (±4.7)	0.99 (0.94–1.05)	0.891
Waist circompherence (cm) (SD)	89.1 (±12)	89.2 (±12)	88.6 (±12)	1.08 (0.98–1.03)	0.467
Lipodystrophy					
No lipodystrophy	184 (35.0%)	144 (31.9%)	40 (54.8%)	1 (ref.)	–
Lipoatrophy	129 (24.6%)	112 (25.0%)	16 (21.9%)	1.96 (1.04–3.68)	0.036
Fat accumulation	212 (40.4%)	195 (43.1%)	17 (23.3%)	3.18 (1.73–5.84)	<0.001
Cardiovascular and metabolic					
Triglycerides (mg/dL) (medican, IQR)	142 (95–207)	143 (96–209)	127 (93–185)	1.00 (0.99–1.00)	0.494
Total cholesterol (mg/dL) (mean, SD)	198 (±45)	197 (±45)	197 (±43)	1.00 (0.99–1.00)	0.929
HDL (mg/dL) (mean, SD)	46 (±14)	46 (±14)	47 (±16)	0.99 (0.98–1.00)	0.645
LDL (mg/dL) (mean, SD)	117 (±33)	117 (±33)	119 (±33)	0.99 (0.99–1.00)	0.710
Glucose (mg/dL) (mean, SD)	94 (±19)	95 (±21)	90 (±10)	1.03 (1.01–1.05)	0.011
HOMA (median, IQR)	2.4 (1.4–3.8)	1.9 (1.2–2.9)	1.9 (1.2–3.0)	1.29 (1.09–1.54)	0.003

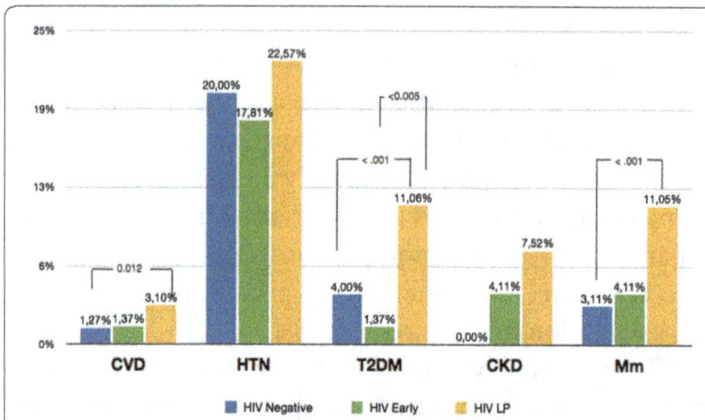

Fig. 1 NICM and MM prevalence distribution across study groups

A multivariable logistic regression was built to predict total cost in the whole population including clinically significant covariates (Table 2).

A second linear regression model was built to identify independent predictors of total cost in HIV-infected patients only. Predictors of total cost in cases were: LP (β, 2994; CI 1561–4427, $p < 0.001$); MM (β, 7818; CI 5653–9985, $p < 0.001$); age (β, 150; CI 87–212, $p < 0.001$); current CD4 count < 200 (β, 2723; CI −270 to 5716, $p = 0.075$); male sex (β, 281; CI −865 to 1427, $p = 0.630$); protease inhibitors (PIs) exposure in months (β, 33; CI 6–60, $p = 0.015$).

Discussion

Data from MHMC cohort study show that individuals with late presentation for HIV diagnosis (HIV + LP) exhibit an increased risk for age-related NICM and MM compared to individuals with early presentation for HIV diagnosis (HIV + EP) and matched HIV-negative individuals sampled from the general population. This difference translates into increased total costs of medical care in all age strata, but appear particularly relevant in patients above the age of 50. Therefore, LP influences both clinical and economical outcomes.

At any age, the risk for individual NICM as well as MM was fourfold higher in HIV + LP compared to people without HIV, while HIV + EP had an intermediate risk.

Our results should be interpreted with caution, in particular with regard to reproducibility of our results in different HIV settings. It could be argued that the tertiary referral setting of the MHMC may concentrate patients with higher prevalence of NICM and MM, however the prevalence of these conditions has previously been demonstrated to be similar between local MHMC attendees and those referred from other centers [18]. In Italy,

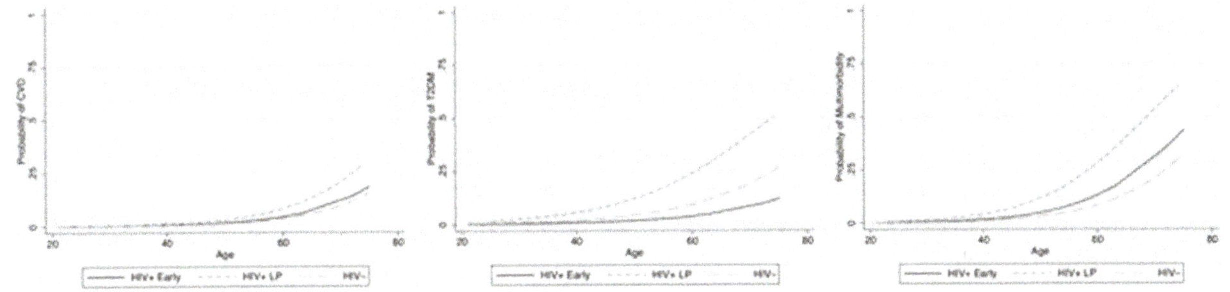

Fig. 2 Age-related risk probability for CVD, T2DM and MM

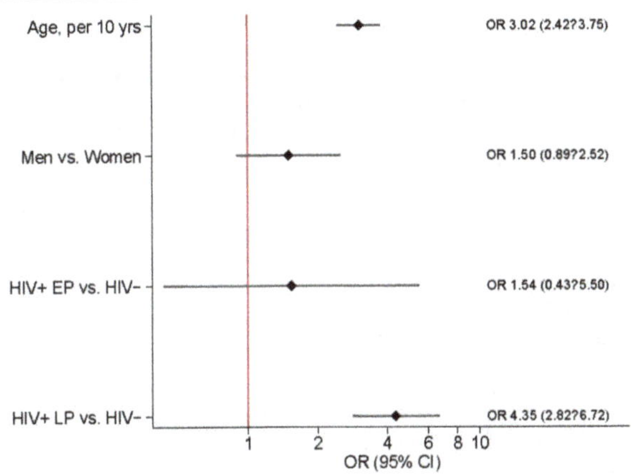

Fig. 3 Multivariable logistic regression model to detect independent predictors of MM in the cohort

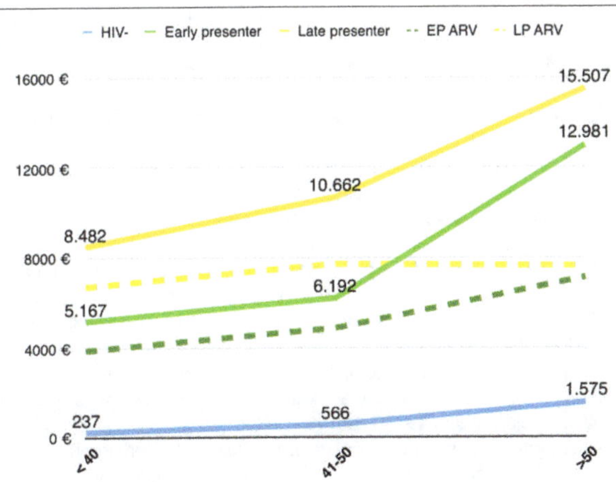

Fig. 4 Total and cART costs of medical care in HIV negative, HIV + EP and HIV + LP across age strata (mean)

people with HIV have full free access not only to cART but also to clinical care including diagnostic procedures with no co-pay. This might result in a selection bias as screening activities are offered relatively more frequently to individuals with HIV than the general population, which might result in higher rates of incidentally identified asymptomatic disease. The information available in the CINECA-ARNO administrative database limited further comparisons in rates of NICM diagnoses, as not all major risk factors for NICM are collected and clinical assessments are not provided. Moreover, with regard to CKD, the number of clinical events was very limited and BMD measurements were not available in CINECA cohort. Furthermore, the HIV + EP group is relatively small. Finally, the cross-sectional design of our study cannot prove causality regarding the impact of LP on NICM or MM risk, nor we were able to collect biomarkers of systemic and tissue inflammation to argue a pathogenic link between LP and these outcomes.

Table 2 Independent predictors of total cost in the whole population

	β-coeff	95% CI	p value
HIV + EP vs. HIV−	1400	422–2380	0.005
HIV + LP vs. HIV−	3246	2233–4260	<0.001
Multimorbidity	6578	6049–7107	<0.001
Age	53	41–64	<0.001
Sex			
Women	0 (Ref)	-	-
Men	114	−106 to 334	0.309
ART	5606	4602–6610	<0.001

The total cost of medical care was higher in HIV-positive participants than in the general population in any age strata. Higher costs was, as expected, mainly attributable to antiretroviral drugs costs, especially PIs [27–29]. Of interest, total and ART costs for the HIV + EP group aged less than 40 years is much lower than the other HIV + EP strata. This can be explained with the fact that 30.3% of these patients were not on ART, following WHO 2013 guidelines [30].

Notably NICM-related care costs contributed significantly to the higher cost burden of HIV-infected patients in the context of LP.

These findings reinforce what has already been suggested by Krentz and Gill, that early initiation of ART may result in a cost-saving intervention [24]. Conversely, increasing age and concurrent MM represent a good indicator of increased total cost.

We believe that, in a demographic setting, particularly in a resource-rich setting, in which the majority of HIV-infected patients are older than 50 years, total care cost will continue to increase [28, 31, 32].

These results suggest that, in the absence of targeted HIV prevention and diagnostic campaigns, the proportion of HIV+/LP will continue to increase, which will increase the burden of higher MM-related clinical and economic costs. In light of the unmistakable message recently provided by the strategic timing of antiretroviral therapy (START) study [33], which demonstrated a beneficial effect of immediate antiretroviral therapy for both serious AIDS-related and serious non–AIDS-related events, we can hope a reduction of the proportion of HIV + LP with a reduction in the burden and cost of comorbidities.

In conclusion, LP with HIV infection remains very common today in Italy and is associated with higher NICM and MM which is associated with higher total care costs. Promoting early testing and access to care is still urgently needed.

Abbreviations

AIDS: acquired immuno deficiency syndrome; AIFA: Agenzia Italiana del Farmaco; BMD: bone mineral density; cART: combined anti retroviral therapy; CKD: chronic kidney disease; COHERE: collaboration of observational HIV epidemiological research Europe; CVD: cardio vascular disease; DXA: dual-energy X-ray absorptiometry; EP: early presentation; HIV: human immunodeficiency virus; HIV + EP: HIV-positive patients with early presentation; HIV + LP: HIV-positive patients with late presentation; ICD-9: international classification of diseases, ninth edition; IRIS: immune reconstitution inflammatory syndrome; LP: late presentation; MDRD: modification of diet in renal disease; MHMC: Modena HIV metabolic clinic; MM: multi morbidity; NICM: non infectious comorbidities; START: strategic timing of antiretroviral therapy; T2DM: type 2 diabetes mellitus.

Authors' contributions

GG, SZ, FC, CS carried out the field work. SZ, MM carried out the statistical analysis. GG, SZ, GD prepared the manuscript. GG, SZ, FC, CS, MM prepared the study design. CM was guarantor of the study. All authors read and approved the final manuscript.

Author details

[1] Department of Medical and Surgical Sciences for Adults and Children, Clinic of Infectious Diseases, University of Modena and Reggio Emilia, Emilia-Romagna, Modena, Italy. [2] Faculty of Medicine, Dalhousie University, Halifax, NS, Canada. [3] McGill University Health Center, Montreal, QC, Canada. [4] Infectious Disease Department, Hospital Beatriz Ângelo, Regiao de Lisboa, Loures, Portugal. [5] Health Care Department, Cineca-Interuniversity Consortium, Casalecchio di Reno, Emilia-Romagna, Bologna, Italy.

Acknowledgements

The authors would like to thank all the patients who attend the Metabolic Clinic. Without them this publication would not be possible.

Competing interests

The authors declare that they have no competing interests.

Funding

This study is supported by 'Co-morbidity in relation to AIDS' Grant agreement (305522), European Union Seventh Framework. Thomas Brothers was supported by Canadian Institutes of Health Research Summer Research Studentship.

References

1. Antinori A, Coenen T, Costagiola D, Dedes N, Ellefson M, Gatell J, et al. Late presentation of HIV infection: a consensus definition. HIV Med. 2011;12:61–4.
2. World Health Organization. Anti retroviral therapy for HIV infection in adults and adolescents. Recommendations for a public health approach: 2010 revision. http://www.who.int/hiv/pub/arv/adult2010/en/ 13 Dec 2015.
3. Antiretroviral Therapy Cohort Collaboration. Life expectancy of individuals on combination antiretroviral therapy in high-income countries: a collaborative analysis of 14 cohort studies. Lancet. 2008;372:293–9.
4. Sterne JAC, May M, Costagliola D, de Wolf F, Phillips AN, Harris R. Timing of initiation of antiretroviral therapy in AIDS-free HIV-1-infected patients: a collaborative analysis of 18 HIV cohort studies. Lancet. 2009;373:1352–63.
5. Mocroft A, Lundgren JD, Sabin ML, d'Arminio MA, Brockmeyer N, Casabona J. Risk factors and outcomes for late presentation for HIV-positive persons in Europe: results from the collaboration of observational HIV epidemiological research Europe study (COHERE). PLoS Med. 2013;10:1001510.
6. Op de Coul EL, van Sighem A, Brinkman K, van Benthem BH, van der Ende ME, Geerlings S. Factors associated with presenting late or with advanced HIV disease in the Netherlands, 1996–2014: results from a national observational cohort. BMJ Open. 2016;6:e009688.
7. Kelley CF, Armstrong WS. Update on immune reconstitution inflammatory syndrome: progress and unanswered questions. Curr Infect Dis Rep. 2009;11:486–93. http://www.ncbi.nlm.nih.gov/pubmed/19857389.
8. Sullivan PS, Hanson DL, Chu SY, Jones JL, Ward JW. Epidemiology of anemia in human immunodeficiency virus (HIV)-infected persons: results from the multistate adult and adolescent spectrum of HIV disease surveillance project. Blood. 1998;91:301–8.
9. Shelburne SA, Visnegarwala F, Darcourt J, Graviss EA, Giordano TP, White ACJ, et al. Incidence and risk factors for immune reconstitution inflammatory syndrome during highly active antiretroviral therapy. AIDS. 2005;19:399–406.
10. Girardi E, Aloisi MS, Arici C, Pezzotti P, Serraino D, Balzano R. Delayed presentation and late testing for HIV: demographic and behavioral risk factors in a multicenter study in Italy. J Acquir Immune Defic Syndr. 2004;36:951–9.
11. Zoufaly A, van der Heiden M, Marcus U, Hoffmann C, Stellbrink H, Voss L, et al. Late presentation for HIV diagnosis and care in Germany. HIV Med. 2012;13:172–81.

12. Bai F, Tincati C, Merlini E, Pacioni C, Sinigaglia E, Carpani G. Reduced central memory CD4+ T cells and increased T-cell activation characterise treatment-naive patients newly diagnosed at late stage of HIV infection. AIDS Res Treat. 2012;2012:314849.
13. de Olalla PG, Manzardo C, Sambeat MA, Ocana I, Knobel H, Humet V, et al. Epidemiological characteristics and predictors of late presentation of HIV infection in Barcelona (Spain) during the period 2001–2009. AIDS Res Ther. 2011;8:22.
14. d'Arminio Monforte A, Cozzi-Lepri A, Girardi E, Castagna A, Mussini C, Di Giambenedetto S, et al. Late presenters in new HIV diagnoses from an Italian cohort of HIV-infected patients: prevalence and clinical outcome. Antivir Ther. 2011;16:1103–12.
15. Deblonde J, De Koker P, Hamers FF, Fontaine J, Luchters S, Temmerman M. Barriers to HIV testing in Europe: a systematic review. Eur J Public Health. 2010;20:422–32.
16. Mensforth S, Goodall L, Bodasing N, Coultas J. Late diagnosis among our ageing HIV population: a cohort study. J Int AIDS Soc. 2014;17:19692.
17. Guaraldi G, Orlando G, Murri R, Vandelli M, De Paola M, Beghetto B, et al. Quality of life and body image in the assessment of psychological impact of lipodystrophy: validation of the Italian version of assessment of body change and distress questionnaire. Qual Life Res. 2006;15:173–8.
18. Guaraldi G, Orlando G, Zona S, Menozzi M, Carli F, Garlassi E, et al. Premature age-related comorbidities among HIV-infected persons compared with the general population. Clin Infect Dis. 2011;53:1120–6.
19. Vives N, Carnicer-Pont D, Garcia de Olalla P, Camps N, Esteve A, Casabona J. Factors associated with late presentation of HIV infection in Catalonia Spain. Int J STD AIDS. 2012;23:475–80.
20. CINECA ARNO observational database. https://osservatorioarno.cineca.org 9 Aug 2014.
21. Levey AS, Bosch JP, Lewis JB, Greene T, Rogers N, Roth D. A more accurate method to estimate glomerular filtration rate from serum creatinine: a new prediction equation modification of diet in renal disease study group. Ann Intern Med. 1999;130:461–70.
22. Guaraldi G, Zona S, Menozzi M, Carli F, Bagni P, Berti A, et al. Cost of non-infectious comorbidities in patients with HIV Clinicoecon. Outcomes Res. 2013;5:481–8.
23. International classification of diseases (ICD): 9th revision, basic tabulation list with alphabetic index. Geneva: World Health Organization;1978. http://www.cdc.gov/nchs/icd/icd9.htm.
24. Krentz HB, Gill MJ. Cost of medical care for HIV-infected patients within a regional population from 1997 to 2006. HIV Med. 2008;9:721–30.
25. Agenzia Italiana del Farmaco (AIFA)]. http://www.agenziafarmaco.gov.it/5 Mar 2015.
26. Banca d'Italia—Cambi di riferimento del 31 dicembre 2014. https://www.bancaditalia.it/compiti/operazioni-cambi/cambio/cambi_rif_20141231.
27. Bozzette SA, Joyce G, McCaffrey DF, Leibowitz AA, Morton SC, Berry SH, et al. Expenditures for the care of HIV-infected patients in the era of highly active antiretroviral therapy. N Engl J Med. 2001;344:817–23.
28. Gebo KA, Fleishman JA, Conviser R, Hellinger J, Hellinger FJ, Josephs JS, et al. Contemporary costs of HIV healthcare in the HAART era. AIDS. 2010;24:2705–15.
29. Magoni M, Scarcella C, Vassallo F, Lonati F, Carosi G, Castelnuovo F, et al. The evolving burden of HIV infection compared with other chronic diseases in northern Italy. HIV Med. 2011;12:129–37.
30. WHO. Consolidated ARV guidelines. 7.1.1 When to start ART in adults and adolescents. 2013. http://www.who.int/hiv/pub/guidelines/arv2013/art/statartadolescents/en/.
31. Luther VP, Wilkin AM. HIV infection in older adults. Clin Geriatr Med. 2007;23:567–83.
32. Mandalia S, Mandalia R, Looo G, Chadborn T, Sharott P, Youle M, et al. Rising population cost for treating people living with HIV in the UK, 1997–2013. PLoS ONE. 2010;5:15677.
33. INSIGHT START study group. Initiation of antiretroviral therapy in early asymptomatic HIV infection. N Engl J Med. 2015;373:1–13.

7

The therapeutic landscape of HIV-1 via genome editing

Alexander Kwarteng[1,2*], Samuel Terkper Ahuno[1] and Godwin Kwakye-Nuako[3]

Abstract

Current treatment for HIV-1 largely relies on chemotherapy through the administration of antiretroviral drugs. While the search for anti-HIV-1 vaccine remain elusive, the use of highly active antiretroviral therapies (HAART) have been far-reaching and has changed HIV-1 into a manageable chronic infection. There is compelling evidence, including several side-effects of ARTs, suggesting that eradication of HIV-1 cannot depend solely on antiretrovirals. Gene therapy, an expanding treatment strategy, using RNA interference (RNAi) and programmable nucleases such as meganuclease, zinc finger nuclease (ZFN), transcription activator-like effector nuclease (TALEN), and clustered regularly interspaced short palindromic repeats/CRISPR-associated proteins (CRISPR–Cas9) are transforming the therapeutic landscape of HIV-1. TALENS and ZFNS are structurally similar modular systems, which consist of a *FokI* endonuclease fused to custom-designed effector proteins but have been largely limited, particularly ZFNs, due to their complexity and cost of protein engineering. However, the newly developed CRISPR–Cas9 system, consists of a single guide RNA (sgRNA), which directs a Cas9 endonuclease to complementary target sites, and serves as a superior alternative to the previous protein-based systems. The techniques have been successfully applied to the development of better HIV-1 models, generation of protective mutations in endogenous/host cells, disruption of HIV-1 genomes and even reactivating latent viruses for better detection and clearance by host immune response. Here, we focus on gene editing-based HIV-1 treatment and research in addition to providing perspectives for refining these techniques.

Background

Human immunodeficiency virus-1 (HIV-1) infection is still a major contributor to global disease burden. The brunt of the infection is borne mostly by resource-limited populations [1]. Despite much effort by regional and international public health organizations, sub-Saharan Africa accounts for approximately 70% of all 36.73 million people living with HIV-1 world-wide [2]. On the other hand, the availability of early treatment therapies are changing the epidemiology of the disease, contributing to decreasing HIV-1 incidence as a result of drastic reductions of the risk of transmission of the infection [1].

One of the key challenges to the effective treatment and management of HIV-1 infection is the persistence of transcriptionally silent but replication competent integrated viral DNA (provirus) in long-lived memory CD4+ T cells, naïve CD4+ T cells, myeloid cells in the CNS, tissue-based macrophages and other sanctuary sites [3]. A larger proportion of latent HIV-1 is housed by resting CD4+ T cells in the periphery. Resting CD4+ T cells are less endowed with key transcriptional factors such as NF-kB, positive transcription elongation factor b (P-TEFb) and CDK11, all of which are important for HIV-1 replication [4, 5]. Ideally, one clinical important role of latent HIV-1 with regards to the pathogenesis of the disease is by functioning as a repertoire of the HIV-1 viruses for sustained infection, tropism or disease progression.

In many instances, latent viral reservoirs evade host immune response, therefore remain refractory to standard treatment strategies, such as antiretroviral therapies [6]. Several studies have reported viral recrudescence upon interruption or cessation of antiretroviral therapy. However, this scenario is correlated with increased risk of morbidity and definitely mortality among such patients with history of treatment interruption [7, 8].

*Correspondence: akwarteng@knust.edu.gh
[1] Department of Biochemistry and Biotechnology, Kwame Nkrumah University of Science and Technology (KNUST), PMB, Kumasi, Ghana
Full list of author information is available at the end of the article

The exact mechanisms mediating viral latency remains elusive. Previous studies propose that HIV-1 quiescence is predominantly driven by complex epigenetic mechanisms/pathways as well as transcriptional interferences by both viral and host factors [9]. Overcoming the barriers posed by latent HIV-1 will be key to the eradication of the infection. Several approaches have been proposed, some of which are under early stages of development, to target latent HIV-1. These strategies are predominantly based on the "shock and kill" strategy. The shock and kill strategy is a hypothetical term in which viral reservoirs are awaken, thereby making them susceptible to clearance by host immune defences and or therapeutic agents such as ARTs. Conversely, rather than awakening latent HIV-1 reservoirs, these viral reservoirs could be silenced by targeting key signaling pathways or molecules important for cytokine activation. Existing evidence shows that reduction of T cell activation is correlated with decrease HIV-1 associated inflammation in HIV-1+ individuals [10]. Moreover, murine studies using JAK and STAT inhibitors such as ruxolitinib and tofacitinib have demonstrated suppression of T cell activation. This suggests their high potential of being translated into clinical studies [11, 12].

Conversely, there are a number of pre-existing techniques/tools for "brute-force" activation of latent viral cells given that the chances of effectively clearing these cells are greatly increased by several folds after activation. Latent reversing agents (LRAs) such as histone deacetylase inhibitors (HDACis) promote acetylation and remodelling of the chromatin, therefore support enhanced expression of cell-associated HIV-1 RNA from latent viral reservoirs. However, there are a number of challenging results that report low coverage of all intended latent cells, thus only a small subset of latent cells were targeted by HDACi interventions [13–16]. This sheds lights on the complex signaling networks in vivo that are intricately fashioned to maintain memory cells (and for this matter HIV-1 infected memory cells) in a resting stage. The stochastic nature of latency reversal is a huge impediment to the study of LRAs activity over protracted periods and therefore supports the development of animal models, especially non-human primates, for in vivo studies [17].

Another class of LRAs, capable of reactivating HIV-1 in cell line models of latency are the BET bromodomain inhibitors (BETis) such as JQI [18]. Unfortunately, BETis are ineffective HIV-1 reactivating agents in human primary resting infected T cells primarily due to the inability of these humanized cells to express sufficient levels of essential transcription factors (TFs) [19, 20].

However, protein kinase C (PKC) agonists [21, 22] (such as prostratin, bryostatin and ingenols) [23–25] and MAPK agonists (including procyanidin) [26, 27] can reactivate HIV-1 in primary CD4+ T cells and almost all other cell line models. The success of PKC and MAPK agonists is based on their ability to increase cellular concentrations of required TFs needed for reactivation of primary CD4+ T cells in human cells [23]. The use of PKC and MAPK agonists are not without side effects. For instance, respiratory distress, muscle pain and toxicity even at therapeutic levels with prostratin and bryostatin use have been documented. Another cause for alarm, is the high cost of producing bryostatina, natural product derived from marine sources, warranting the need for the development of novel and cost-effective MAPK and PKC agonists such as synthetic bryostatin or igenol analogues with superior or comparable therapeutic efficacy with no or few side-effects [28, 29].

In contrast, HDACis and BETis mono-therapies have enormous therapeutic potential. Combined with other therapeutic agents, such as powerful immune stimulating agents, appear promising to effectively purge all latent viral reservoirs [29, 30]. Powerful immune activating agents, such as interleukin-2 (IL-2) [31] and anti-CD3 antibody [32] in combination with antiretroviral drugs has demonstrated enhanced HIV-1 expression from latent viral reservoirs and increased clearance of infected resting memory CD4+ T cells [33]. More specifically, LRAs in combination with powerful immune boosters may be used to induce viral proteins or processed antigens on cell surfaces that can be sufficiently recognized by the host immune cells such as cytotoxic T lymphocytes (CTLs) and NK cells for killing infected cells [34]. Similarly, activation of broadly neutralizing antibodies (bNAbs) with capabilities of recognizing several clades of HIV-1 together with even escape mutants represents another dimension being harnessed to kill HIV-1 latent/infected cells by host defences [35, 36]. Recently, chimeric antigen receptors (CARs), which can be engineered to recognize specific viral proteins have been developed to enhance T cell receptor avidity and activation. However, concerns over the longevity of CARs-bound cells as well as substantial off-target effects are limitations of the widespread application of CARs [37] for therapeutic purposes.

At a glance, the expanding promise of the various anti-HIV-1 "shock and kill" strategies leaves little room for reservations. Given that some latent HIV-1 activating agents are also capable of dampening CTL functions, there is the need for a more careful investigation into the mechanisms underlying these 'shock" agents [37] in order to fine-tune these strategies where needed. Furthermore, continuous expansion of the already vast body of knowledge surrounding viral infection and molecular evolution is still needed. Studies relating to the regulatory mechanisms of HIV-1 gene expression during latency, in addition to the molecular underpinning underlying key viral processes such as HIV-1 nuclear mRNA export, splicing and translation will not only lead to more understanding of the virus but also promote the development of novel therapeutic strategies [3]. Moreover, a thorough understanding of the pathophysiology of infected cells at the various sanctuary sites, the effects of tissue microenvironment on viral latency, in addition to the canonical cell types involved in latency are urgently need to garner efforts towards targeting HIV-1 latent reservoirs. Taken together, it will be almost impossible to effectively purge all HIV-1 latent reservoirs without a deeper understanding of replication capacity and extent of viral expression at the various sanctuary sites [38].

HIV-1 therapeutic landscape

The call to end the global pandemic might be achieved through two therapeutic approaches. Firstly, the sterilizing approach, which theoretically implies purging all HIV-1 latent reservoirs (as described above). Secondly, the functional cure approach, which seeks to empower the host immune defences to fight the infection and other opportunistic infections that arise as the disease progresses. Generally, both approaches are effective and heavily depend on HAART. Research into anti-HIV-1 gene therapy has intensified following the so called "Berlin-patient" where scientists eradicated HIV from his body after receiving a bone marrow transplant. Therefore, gene and nucleic acid based therapies including gene editing with programmable nucleases, RNA decoy, DNA/RNA aptamers, ribozymes, antisense, inhibitory proteins, fusion inhibitors and sh/siRNA have also been developed of which some are candidates for ongoing clinical trials (Table 1) [39–48].

Chemotherapy (drugs)

Treatment with HAART, the primary treatment strategy, has greatly impacted the epidemiology of HIV-1 infection changing the previously life-threatening disease into a chronic disease. The move by world leaders to make these drugs available to endemic regions, particularly developing nations, led to significant reduction in the number of AIDS-related deaths as well as an increase in the quality of life of infected individuals [49, 50]. However, HAART is intensive and life-long, usually leading to treatment fatigue, with considerable side effects [50]. Moreover, poor pharmacokinetics of these drugs and tissue toxicity, on top of viral resistance after prolonged treatment, have also been widely documented throughout the volumes of scientific literature and clinical practice [51]. Added to these are the huge economic and logistical challenges borne by developing countries in order to make treatment sustainable. The constellation of drawbacks warrants the development of robust and effective treatment regimens to supplant HAART, which will result in better treatment and management as well as the possible eradication of the virus. The advancement of biomedical research and engineering, nano-delivery of drugs to specific and key anatomical barriers hold the promise of increasing the efficiency of HIV-1 chemotherapy [52–54].

Nano-medicine

Anti-HIV-1 nanomedicine involves the administration of minute (on the nano-scale, 10^{-9} m) anti-HIV-1 therapeutic agents to allow precise delivery to virtually any therapeutic target sites particularly HIV-1 sanctuary sites such as the central nervous system. The development of biocompatible, biodegradable, non-toxic nanoparticles are feasible depending on the material of manufacturing and are therefore a keen research focus in biomedical engineering [55]. Nanotechnology-based anti-HIV-1 therapeutic agents could range from various drug formulations to gene therapy toolkits (such as RNA interference and anti-HIV-1 ribozymes), which could either be bound to or encapsulated in nano-carriers [56]. Anti-HIV-1 nano-based therapeutic agents have been upheld for their ability to facilitate stable and prolonged drug circulation coupled with the ability to specifically target intended cells/tissues with improved toxicity profiles and low side effects [53]. These ground-breaking techniques facilitate the permeation of the blood–brain barrier of the CNS with remarkable precision and accuracy [57]. However, a move to translate nanotechnology-based anti-HIV-1 agents into clinical practice would require a critical review of existing delivery routes as well as the development of novel delivery routes for nano-formulations. This precaution has now become necessary given that both the pharmacodynamics and pharmacokinetics (absorption, distribution, metabolism and elimination) of nano-formulations are at times affected by the mode of delivery [58]. Such assessments would deepen our knowledge of the efficacy and safety of this treatment approach while opening up new frontiers for HIV-1 research and treatment. A critical assessment of the cost-to-benefit ratio is of equal importance, particularly to ensure wider coverage of middle and lower income individuals as well as resource-limited countries in the upcoming years.

Anti-HIV-1 RNA interference (RNAi)-based therapeutic landscape

RNA interference is a widely used technique in endogenous cells and biomedical research for regulating gene expression and cellular defense against viral infections [59]. The technique has served as the bedrock for the

Table 1 Anti-HIV-1 gene therapy landscape

Therapeutic approach	Gene therapy	Interventions	Targets	Identifier	Stage/status	Company/Institute
Drug shRNA peptide	Dual anti-HIV gene Transfer construct, LVsh5/C46 (Cal)	CCR5 shRNA; C46 peptide Busulfan	Host co-receptor; viral Env; transplant conditioning	NCT01734850	Phase I/II recruiting	Calimmune/CalTech/UCLA
shRNA	Long term follow up of delayed adverse events in Cal-1 recipients	Blood test for general health, complete blood count and Cal-1 specific analyses		NCT02390297	Recruiting by invitation	Calimmune/CalTech/UCLA
Endoribonuclease	Redirected MazF-CD4 autologous T-cells	CCR5 MazF	Host co-receptor	NCT01787994	Phase I ongoing	University of Pennsylvania
Ribozyme	Autologous CD34+ HSCs transduced with anti-HIV-1 ribozyme (OZ1)	Tat-vpr anti-HIV ribozyme	tat-vpr mRNA	NCT00074997	Phase II completed	Janssen-Cilag Pty Ltd, UCLA
Ribozyme	Long term follow up of OZ1 Gene therapy	Blood test for quantitative marking of the gene transfer product in PBMCs overtime		NCT01177059	Phase II Recruiting by invitation	Janssen-Cilag Pty Ltd, UCLA
Antisense	Tolerability and therapeutic effects of repeated doses of autologous T cells with VRX496	VRX496 antisense RNA	Env mRNA	NCT00295477	Phase I/II Ongoing/ not recruiting	University of Pennslyvernia/NIAID
Antisense	Safety and efficacy of T-cell genetic immunotherapy	VRX496 antisense RNA	Env mRNA	NCT00131560	Phase II Ongoing	VIRxSYS Corporation
Ribozyme	L-TR/Tat-neo in HIV+ Patients with Non-Hodgkin's Lymphoma	Tat ribozyme	Tat-rev mRNA	NCT00002221	Phase II completed	Ribozyome/City of Hope
Inhibitory peptides	M87o autologous HSCs for HIV+ patients with malignant disease	C46 peptide	Viral Env	NCT00858793	Phase I/II suspended	University Medical Center Hamburg-Eppendorf
Ribozyme, inhibitory peptide	C46/CCR5/P140K modified autologous HSCs in patients with lymphoma	C46 peptide, CCR5 ribozyme, MGMTP140 K mutant	Viral Env, CCR5 mRNA, Alkylating agent resistance	NCT02343666	Phase I, recruiting	Fred Hutchinson Cancer Research Center/NCI/NHLBI
shRNA,peptide	Autologous transplantation of HSCs with LVsh5/C46 (Cal-1) for treatment of HIV-related lymphoma	CCR5 shRNA, C46 peptide	Host co-receptor, viral Env	NCT02378922	Phase I recruiting	Fred Hutchinson Cancer Research Center/NCI
shRNA, ribozyme,RNA decoy, drugs	rHIV7-shI-TAR-CCR5RZ-transduced HSC in patient with AIDS-related Non-Hodgkin Lymphoma	tat/rev shRNA, TAR decoy, CCR5 ribozyme, Prednisone, Rituximab, Etoposide, Doxorubicin Hydrochloride, Vincristine Sulfate, Cyclophosphamide	Viral mRNA, Viral tat proteinm, CCR5 mRNA, Transplant conditioning	NCT02337985	Pilot recruiting	City of Hope Medical Center/NCI
shRNA, ribozyme,RNA decoy, drugs	rHIV7-shI-TAR-CCR5RZ-transduced HSC in patient with AIDS-related Non-Hodgkin Lymphoma	tat/rev shRNA, TAR decoy, CCR5 ribozyme, Busulfan	Viral mRNA, Viral tat proteinm, CCR5 mRNA	NCT01961063	Pilot recruiting	City of Hope Medical Center/NCI
shRNA, ribozyme,RNA decoy, drugs	rHIV7-shI-TAR-CCR5RZ-transduced HSC in patient undergoing stem cell transplant for AIDS-related lymphoma	tat/rev shRNA, TAR decoy, CCR5 ribozyme, carmustine, cyclophosphamide, etoposide	viral mRNA, viral tat protein, CCR5 mRNA, transplant conditioning	NCT00569985	Pilot ongoing, not recruiting	City of Hope Medical Center/NCI
shRNA, RNA decoy	shRNA/TRIM5alpha/TAR decoy-transduced Autologous HSC in patient with HIV-Related Lymphoma	CCR5 shRNA, RNF88,TAR decoy	Host co-receptor, Gag p24, Viral tat protein	NCT02797470	Phase I/II	City of Hope Medical Center/NCI

Table 1 continued

Therapeutic approach	Gene therapy	Interventions	Targets	Identifier	Stage/status	Company/Institute
RNA decoy	RNA decoy (ex vivo retroviral modified CD34+ HPC)	Rev reponse element decoy	Rev Protein	NCT00001535	Phase 0-pilot	Children's Hospital
	Redirected high affinity gag-specific autologous T cells	WT-gag-TCR or alpha/6-gag-TCR	CD8 TCR	NCT00991224	Phase I completed	University of Pennslyvernia/Adaptimmune
ZFN	T-cells modified at CCR5 gene by ZFN SB-728mR	CCR5 ZFN	CCR5 DNA	NCT02388594	Phase 1 recruiting	University of Pennsylvania/NIAID
	Repeated doses of SB-728mR-T after cyclophosphamide conditioning in HIV+ on HAART	CCR5 ZFN (SB-728mR-T)	CCR5 DNA	NCT02225665	PHASE I/II ongoing	Sangamo biosciences
	Autologous T cells modified at CCR5 gene by ZFN SB-728	CCR5 ZFN	CCR5 DNA	NCT00842634	Phase 1 completed	Sangamo biosciences/ Uni. Of Pennsylvania
	Autologous T-cells genetically modified at the CCR5 gene by zinc finger nucleases (SB-728-T) in HIV-infected patients	CCR5 ZFN	CCR5 DNA	NCT01044654	Phase I completed	Sangamo Therapeutics
	Safety of ZFN CCR5-modified HPS/progenitor cells in HIV+	SB-728mR-HSPC infusion after busulfan conditioning	CCR5 DNA	NCT02500849	Phase 1	City of Hope Medical Center|Sangamo Therapeutics
	Autologous T-cells genetically modified at the CCR5 Gene by zinc finger nucleases in HIV-infected subjects	CCR5 ZFN (SB-728-T)	CCR5 DNA	NCT01252641	Phase I/II completed	Sangamo Therapeutics

elucidation of complex signaling pathways in biological systems, functional genomics and gene therapy. RNA interference has been extensively applied to the elucidation of HIV-1 pathogenesis as well as identification of novel therapeutic targets for controlling HIV-1 infections.

microRNAs (miRNAs) and small interference or short hairpin RNAi (si/shRNA) are the two RNAi toolkits used for RNAi mediated gene silencing studies. miRNAs are short endogenous single-stranded oligonucleotides (~22 bp) that specifically binds to and suppresses mRNA expression. They are therefore capable of modulating key cellular processes, such as developmental processes and even influencing the pathogenesis of diseases [60]. In contrast, sh/siRNAs are double stranded RNA molecules (21–23 bp) generated by the cleavage of either an endogenous or exogenous RNA. Dicer is a ribonuclease, which functions primarily by cleaving RNA to generate sh/siRNAs for targeted gene silencing. Following cleavage, siRNA forms a large complex, RNA-induced silencing complex, (RISC) with helicase (in the case of plants and drosophila cells) and other nucleases such as Argonaute (Argo) proteins. The complex facilitates uncoiling of the siRNA thus promoting precise RNA binding to targeted transcripts, which could lead to sequence-directed gene silencing by mRNA repression [61], translational repression [62], or heterochromatin formation [63]. In humans, the transactivation response RNA-binding proteins (TRBP) is an addition to the RNA-induced silencing complex.

There are two main pathways for targeted gene silencing by RNAi, namely, post transcriptional gene silencing (PTGS) [64] and transcriptional gene silencing (TGS) [65]. PTGS occurs mostly in the cytoplasm where complementary base-pairing of siRNA with target mRNA leads to the degradation of the targeted mRNA. TGS occurs predominantly in the nucleus but unlike PTGS, the target sequences for TGS are usually gene promoter sequences. Therefore, binding of the siRNA to these sequences induces epigenetic silencing of the targeted gene. Although, TGS has been least explored for gene silencing by RNAi, both pathways have been the heart for the development of powerful RNAi therapeutic agents [66, 67]. RNAi can be achieved by targeting conserved viral mRNAs, particularly the ones involved in viral entry, reverse transcription and integration as well as genes that encode structural and enzymatic proteins needed for viral assembly and infection (Table 2). In principle, cutting or editing small pieces of nucleotides in the coding region may give rise to critical mutations that will disrupt the activities or viability of the virus [68]. Host cellular co-factors such as the CD4, CCR5, and CXCR4 receptors essential for viral infection have thus been the center of RNAi based HIV-1 therapy. Moreover, other host co-factors such chaperonin, LEDGF/p75, and importin-7 involved in HIV-1 integration are veritable RNAi as well as other gene therapy targets for anti-HIV-1 treatment.

Table 2 Potential gene therapy targets for HIV-1 therapy

HIV-1 gene targets	Function	Reference
Gag	Proteolytic processing of the HIV-1 genome	[135, 136]
Pol	Transcription	[137]
env	Receptor binding and fusion	[138, 139]
tat	Transcription or RNAi modulation	[140]
rev	Reverse transcription, integration	[141]
nef	Immune modulation	[124, 142–145]
pol (integrase)	Integration	[146, 147]
pol (reverse transcriptase)	Reverse transcription	[148]
Promoter	Transcription	[149]
Long terminal repeats	Genome expression	[145, 150]
P17	Assembly and budding of HIV-1	[68]
Cellular targets		
CCR5	Receptor binding and fusion	[151]
CD4	Receptor binding and fusion	
CXCR4	Receptor binding and fusion	[152, 153]
Chaperonin	Integration	[154]
LEDGF/p75	Integration	[155]
Importin-7	Integration	[156]
Cyclin T1	Transcription	[157]
P-TEFb	Transcription	[158]
Tat-SF1	Transcription	[159]
SPT5	Transcription	[160]
DDX3	Export	[161]
SOCS1	Trafficking or immune modulation	[162]
TRBP	Immune modulation or RNAi pathway	[163, 164]
TNPO3	Nuclear entry of viral pre-integration complex	[141, 165]

Challenges with RNAi

Conversely, despite the popularity of RNAi mediated anti-HIV-1 treatment and research, some trade-offs exist. Of particular importance, is the high likelihood of generating viral escape mutants also known as siRNA escape mutants. This is due to the high error rate of the viral reverse transcriptase (1 in 1000 nucleotides per replication cycle) hence a change in even 1 bp could lead to mutations in the targeted sequences therefore limiting the regulatory effects of siRNAs [69]. However, one of the surest ways of offsetting this challenge is by deploying multiple anti-HIV-1 siRNAs. Another is the combination of other anti-HIV-1 therapeutics, in particular antiretroviral drugs.

Some inherent factors of siRNA, such as anionic charge and large molecular weight, makes it difficult for successful migration across the cell membrane by simple diffusion, thereby preventing its full utilization in certain jurisdictions [56]. In addition, siRNAs are susceptible to degradation by RNAses making it imperative for the development of novel delivery methods. RNA nanotechnology and hydrodynamic cell transfection are making it more practical to delivery RNAi toolkits to targeted cells for research and therapeutic purposes. Furthermore, plasmids and lentiviral vectors that encode siRNA have been useful in delivering RNAi therapeutic agents to targeted cells or tissues for gene therapy.

Anti-HIV-1 gene editing therapeutic landscape

The arrival of gene editing tools such as zinc finger nucleases (ZFNs), transcription activator-like effector nucleases (TALENs), and clustered regularly interspaced short palindromic repeats/CRISPR-associated proteins (CRISPR–Cas9) has revolutionized biomedical research. Similar to other seminal scientific breakthroughs, the adoption of these reagents by modern research have increased exponentially since their invention—and undoubtedly proves promising as arsenals for eradicating HIV-1 infections as well as other viral infections (such as Hepatitis B and C virus, human papilloma virus and herpes simplex virus) even in resource-limited populations.

Previous and ongoing applications of these proof-of-concept technologies may not be limited to programming cells to be permanently resistant to HIV-1 infection and interfering with HIV-1 replication by targeting viral proteins such as Tat, Env, and Gag. HIV-1 resistant cells can be generated by editing genes that encode important cellular factors needed for viral invasion such as CCR5 or CXCR4 co-receptor (Table 2). Ideally, conferring resistance to HIV-1 susceptible or infected cells would require highly efficient, precise, accurate in vivo strategies. However, in vivo delivery approaches are imperfect and cannot produce precise, distributed and sustained delivery of therapeutic agents to targeted cells. Current delivery methods rely on ex vivo manipulation of autologous cells reintroduced into the host after treatment to observe the intended therapeutic effect.

Zinc-finger nucleases (ZFNs)

The structure of ZFNs is basically the combination of 2 domains: the nonspecific *FokI* restriction endonuclease for cleavage of targeted sequences and the custom-designed Cys_2-His_2 zinc-finger proteins (ZFPs) for specific DNA-binding (Fig. 1). The domains are stabilized by zinc ions. Unlike other DNA binding proteins, which depends on the twofold symmetry of the double helix, ZFNs have the advantage of being linked linearly in tandem to recognize nucleic acids of varying lengths, allowing unprecedented combinatorial possibilities for specific gene targeting and manipulations [70]. Ideally, ZFN subunits recognize target sequences in a head-to-tail conformation. After recognition and binding of ZFNs to specific genomic loci, there is the dimerization of the two nuclease domains which leads to a double-stranded break (DSB) of the targeted DNA [70].

ZFNs have been widely used as intervention in several gene therapy clinical trials. Out of the six ZFN anti-HIV-1 clinical trials, three studies have been completed with promising results (NCT00842634, NCT01044654, and NCT01252641). The studies involved the removal of white blood cells that contain CD4+ T cells from consented HIV-1+ patients. The extracted cells were genetically modified by ZFNs, which lead to mutations in the CCR5 gene encoding proteins that function as co-receptors on the surfaces of CD4+ T cells needed for HIV-1 entry. The genetically modified cells were then re-infused back into the individuals with the expectations that these new cells will remain resistant to HIV-1 and possibly produce several generations of HIV-1 resistant cells eventually. Furthermore, another ongoing clinical trial (NCT02500849) that is being sponsored by Sangamo Therapeutics and the City of Hope Medical Center applies CCR5-targeted ZFNs to Hematopoietic Stem/Progenitor cells in HIV-1 infected patients. One of the primary outcomes of the study was to evaluate the safety of SB-728-mR-HSPC (CCR5-targeted HSPCs using ZFNs) after bulsulfan dose in HIV-1 infected individuals. Indeed, this particular study is timely due to the associated risk of developing tumours when HSPCs are genetically manipulated [71].

On the other hand, there are credible reasons to explore other gene editing techniques other than ZFNs. Despite being the forerunner of all gene editing techniques, challenges with engineering customized proteins needed for precise DNA-protein interaction by ZFN are hampering further exploitation [72]. In addition, the development of off-target effects are anecdotes, which needs careful consideration when using ZFNs.

Transcription activator-like effector nucleases (TALENs)

TALENs are structurally similar to ZFNs comprising of a TALE DNA-binding region and a *FokI* restriction endonuclease domain (Fig. 2) [73]. Transcription activator-like effectors (TALEs) are naturally occurring DNA

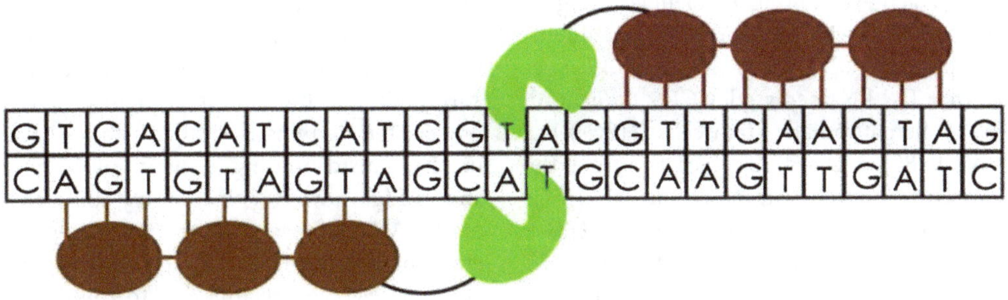

Fig. 1 Zinc finger nucleases

binding proteins from the plant bacterial pathogen, Xanthomonas [74]. In contrast to ZFNs where each finger module recognizes three target DNA nucleotides, TALE proteins contain a highly conserved, central domain, usually consisting of 33–35 amino acid TALE repeats for which each protein monomer is capable of recognizing single base pairs of the target DNA [75]. However, the specificity of these DNA-protein interactions are dictated by two hypervariable residues as shown by studies, which investigated the crystal structure of TALEs bound to DNA. The results from these studies show that each TALEN repeat forms a two-helix structure connected by a loop which presents the hypervariable residues into the major groove as the protein wraps around the DNA in a super-helical structure [76, 77]. The flexibility of joining these modular TALE repeats to form long arrays with custom DNA-binding specificities has proved useful in targeted gene editing of a variety of cells for therapeutic purposes [78–80]. Although TALENs are cost effective when compared to ZFNs, they are difficult to generate. The bulkiness of both ZFNs and TALENs makes it more difficult to deliver these reagents to several targeted cell types [81]. It has been shown that the presence of multiple sequence repeats in TALEN genes renders them unsuitable cargos for lentiviral vector repeats [81]. However, the single-nucleotide precision give rise to superior editing efficiency with minimal off-target and cytotoxicity effects when compared to ZFNs thereby making TALENs good candidates for sequence-specific genome modification [82].

TALENs have not yet been applied for HIV-1 treatment in clinical studies. However, several experimental studies have shown promising results with potential for optimization for large scale anti-HIV-1 treatment. Shi and colleagues recently generated 28 CCR5-TALEN screens to target several domains on the CCR5 of CD4+ T cells [82]. CCR5-ZFNs similar to the anti-HIV-1 ZFNs currently being applied for ongoing clinical trials were used as controls in this study for comparative studies. The results were remarkable and showed increased editing efficiency and minimal cytotoxicity activity compared to the CCR5-ZFN currently undergoing clinical trials [83]. Furthermore, cleavage of HIV-1 matrix protein P17 gene sequences with custom designed TALENs delivered by lentiviral vectors to Jurkat-HIV-1 cell lines has been reported with editing efficiency of ~43% [68]. HIV-1 P17 helps in the assembly and budding of HIV-1, and shows relatively little sequence diversity, therefore serves as a suitable candidate for clinical applications. TALENS have been used to target a highly conserved sequence in the transcription response element of the HIV-1 proviral DNA [84]. The HIV-1 TALEN constructs

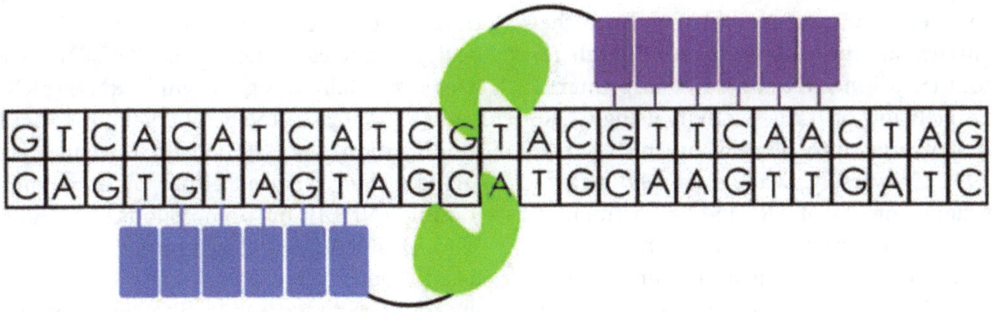

Fig. 2 TALENS

used were able to achieve editing efficiencies ranging between 30 and 60%. Elsewhere capsid modified adenovirus (helper dependent adenovirus, HD-Ad5/35) vectors for ZFN and TALEN-mediated CCR5 truncation of human CD34+ hematopoietic stem cells (HSCs) has been documented [85]. HD-Ad5/35 vectors target the CD46 receptor constitutively expressed on all HSCs [86] and are effective transducers of human CD34+ HSCs in vitro with minimal effects of cytotoxicity [87]. HD-Ad5/35 have a large carrying capacity with capabilities to efficiently transduce primitive subsets of HSCs [88]. Moreover, Ru and colleagues [89] used a cell-penetrating peptide (TAT peptide, YGRKKRRQRRR) bound to ZFN and TALEN to disrupt genes encoding the CCR5 co-receptors of human induced pluripotent stem cells (hiPSCs). Cell-penetrating peptides (CPPs) such as TAT, are promising therapeutic delivery systems that have been used for the treatment of several diseases [90]. Their versatility is based on the fact that CPPs are applicable to all cell types with high transduction efficiency under controlled administration [91]. CPPs have been used for delivery of large cargos including biomolecules (such as nucleic acids and large proteins with low transmembrane permeability) [91–94] and drugs [95, 96]. A dose-dependent TAT-TALEN activity was observed under hypothermic conditions with disruption efficiency of 3 and 5% with HeLa and hiPSCs respectively. There was a lack of certainty of the factors that contributed to the differences in the editing efficiencies in the different cell types. Perhaps the differences in cell membrane composition and endocytosis capabilities were contributing factors that affected the varying CCR5-edting efficiency of HeLa and hiPSCs. The limited use of TAT-ZFN is due to its low protein expression and low binding affinity which largely contributed to challenges in purifying TAT-ZFN proteins for analysis in cell culture. Interestingly, an earlier study has reported considerable success with TAT-ZFNs for cell transduction and gene editing [97]. Additional studies are required in light of these contrasting results to support the conclusion that TAT-TALENs are superior to TAT-ZFNs for anti-HIV-1 therapeutic purposes.

On anti-HIV-1 experimental studies with huge therapeutic potentials, another study reported high-rate CCR5 knockout (>90% in PM1 and >50% in primary T cells) with relatively low off-target activity using CCR5-Uco-TALENs delivered into T cells by mRNA electroporation [98]. Conversely, Wang et al. [99] attained an editing efficiency of 40% of TRIM5α (tripartite motif containing 5) genes of rhesus macaques using TALENs. TRIM5α, among other HIV-1 capsid-binding proteins such as Fv1 and TRIMCypA are well characterized anti-HIV-1 proteins, which restricts early HIV-1 replication in non-human primate cells [100]. TRIM5α consists of RING, B-box 2, coiled-coil and B30.2 (SPRY), the major determinant of anti-HIV-1 potency [101, 102]. Although the human orthologues (TRIM5αhu) does not confer significant viral resistance, point mutations in the capsid-binding domain of human TRIM5αhu shows high anti-HIV-1 activity [103]. The exploitation of TRIM5α transgenes as candidates for anti-HIV-1 gene therapy is currently ongoing [104, 105]. The emergence of escape variants due to the fast evolution rate of HIV-1 are major potential challenges that may hamper the development and scalability of this therapeutic strategy.

Conversely, the lens epithelium-derived growth factor (LEDGF/p75) is a cellular co-factor needed for tethering and proper integration of HIV-1 genome into the host genome and thus remains an attractive therapeutic target. Gene therapy techniques such as RNAi and ribozymes have shown minimal success in knocking-out *PSIP1*, the gene which encodes LEDGF/p75, needed to confer HIV-1 resistance to cells. This is due to the fact that even a small residual of the tightly chromatin-bound protein is just enough to promote integration function [106]. Recently, Fadel and colleagues [107] provided the proof-of-concept by demonstrating that TALENs could effectively knockout *PSIP1* genes thereby blocking HIV-1 propagation in human cell lines.

Taken together, although there are currently no clinical studies applying TALENs as interventions for HIV-1 treatment, the existing pool of evidence from experimental studies indicates that TALENs are potential candidates for future anti-HIV-1 therapeutic agents.

Clustered regularly interspaced short palindromic repeats/CRISPR-associated proteins (CRISPR–Cas9)

The emergence of CRISPR–Cas9, a proof-of-principle technique based on the adaptive immune systems of bacteria and archae [108] has transformed the therapeutic landscape of HIV-1. CRISPR–Cas9, has gained so much popularity in the research community due to the preciseness, cost-effectiveness and simplicity with its design thus allowing superior genetic manipulations of targeted sequences [109]. Unlike the former designer nucleases (ZFN and TALENs) CRISPR–Cas9 uses a specially designed guide RNA (gRNA) to direct a nuclease (Cas9) to specific genomic loci for genomic modification (Fig. 3) [110]. The disrupted genomic DNA is then repaired either by non-homologous end joining (NHEJ) or homologous recombination (HR) (Fig. 4). DNA repair via non-homologous end joining usually leads to mutations that interrupt the open reading frame, which could lead to gene inactivation when a template is provided.

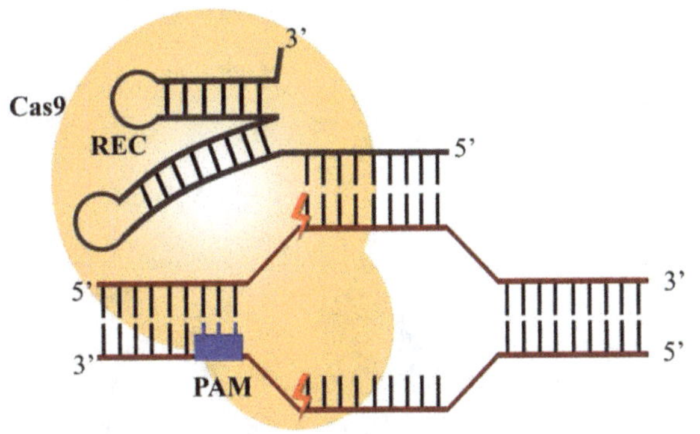

Fig. 3 CRISPR–Cas9

Currently there are no ongoing clinical trials using CRISPR–Cas9 as anti HIV-1 therapeutic intervention. This is not surprising given the labyrinthine process and regulatory network surrounding approval for running a clinical trial. However, preclinical studies have demonstrated the importance of this approach as a golden tool for anti-HIV-1 therapeutic intervention. For example, Wang et al, used lentivirus vectors to express CCR5-sgRNA and Cas9 to knockout CCR5 co-receptors of CD4+ T cells thereby conferring HIV-1 resistance to these cells [111]. In addition, no mutations were reported at potential off-target sites that were homologous to the CCR5-sgRNA, even several days (85 days) after transduction. Furthermore, CRISPR–Cas9 system was recently used to remove the entire HIV-1 genome, spanning the full length 5′ and 3′ LTRs, of integrated HIV-1 proviral DNA from latently infected human CD4+ T-cells with no off-target effects [112]. The CRISPR–Cas9 mediated proviral DNA excision had no significant deleterious effect on several cell health indices such as cell viability, cell cycle progression and apoptosis. Moreover, continuous expression of sgRNA and Cas9 nuclease by T cells where HIV-1 was eliminated, showed protection from new HIV-1 infection as compared to T-cells expressing Cas9 or sgRNA alone. CRISPR–Cas9 has also been successfully used to activate latently infected cells to promote better detection and clearance of these latent cells by effector immune cells [109].

Natronobacterium gregoryi Argonaute (NgAgo): the next golden editor?

Another valuable addition to the gene editing toolbox has been NgAgo, a DNA-guided endonuclease [113] with possibilities of generating site-specific modification

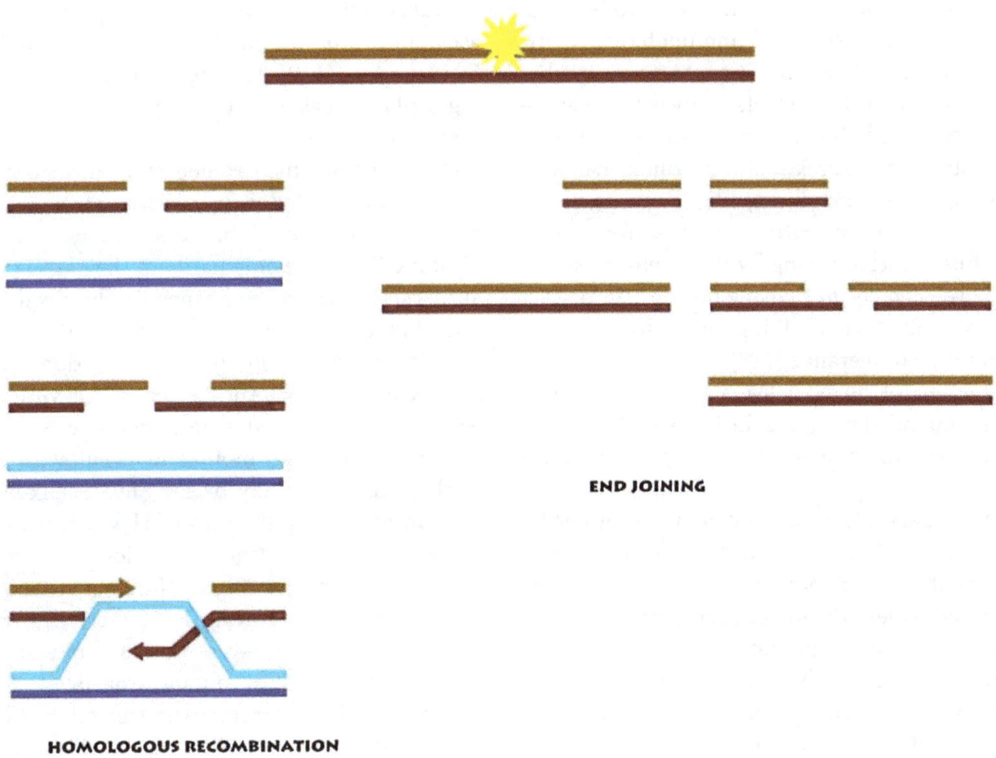

Fig. 4 DNA repair mechanism

of human cells. Unlike CRISPR–Cas9, NgAgo-gDNA system operates without a protospacer-adjacent motif (PAM) with remarkable low tolerance to guide-target mismatches as well as high efficiency in editing (G+C)-rich genomic loci. Although promising, the reproducibility of the original protocols could prolong the huge benefits such a tool could offer biomedical researchers with profound interest in gene modifications [114]. There are no reported studies using this latest addition to the genome editing toolbox for HIV-1 treatment and research, suggesting the need for future research to explore the potentials of NgAgo for HIV-1 research.

Challenges and perspective

Programmable nucleases could be exploited to deepen current knowledge of host-viral interaction and to create improved animal models that mimics HIV-1 infections in humans. As a result our current knowledge of the molecular pathogenesis of the infection would be enhanced. However, genetic manipulations using non-human primates can be problematic due to several factors such as slow sexual maturity, possibility of generating mosaic mutations, off-targets, and low quality of publicly available non-human primate gene sequences, in particular monkey, as well as expensive embryos [72, 115]. The arrival of CRISPR–Cas9 [116] and TALENs [117] are breakthroughs of the century, which have facilitated the successful generation of transgenic HIV-1 non-human primate models to elucidate the key components in HIV-1 susceptibility, infection and immunobiology. Furthermore, programmable nucleases could boost studies with particular focus on the interplay between the adaptive immune system and HIV-1 in mice models after successful substitution and expression of murine genes with human homolog (such as cytokines) [72].

HIV-1 researchers have battled with some crucial challenges while experimenting with recent designer nucleases. These include editing inefficiency, imperfect delivery systems, off-targets editing and cytotoxicity in addition to immune intolerance [118].

The development of novel delivery systems that can target precisely intended cells with little possibility of not being tolerated by immune defences are crucial in moving forward.

Gene therapy interventions can be achieved either by in vivo or ex vivo methods. In vivo delivery approaches relies on packaging into nanoparticles and administering directly to the patient through intravenous infusions. Ex vivo approaches involve sampling of host cells, culturing and treatment of target cells, such as CD4+ T-cells or CD34+ HSCs with biological interventions after which treated cells are infused back into the patient (Fig. 5). Transduction of targeted cells could be achieved either by nanodelivery or with biological vectors, such as adenovirus and lentivirus vectors. Adenovirus and lentivirus vectors are the two main biological delivery systems for targeted gene editing by programmable nucleases. However, the two viral vectors demonstrate differential integrity profiles. Adenovirus vectors are superior in transducing targeted cells with programmable nucleases and promote high site-specific double-stranded DNA breaks [119]. Scaling-up production and processing for large scale anti-HIV-1 gene therapy needs further investigation.

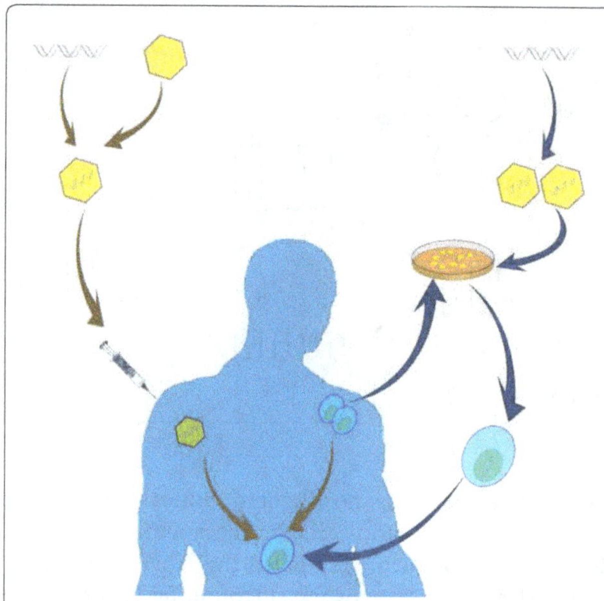

Fig. 5 In vivo and ex vivo delivery methods

Until recently, the detailed mechanisms of viral escape (or resistance) following treatment with anti-retrovirals, small molecule inhibitors, and gene editors such as CRISPR/Ca9 were enigmatic. In the case of gene-editing antiviral therapies, resistance could result due to the introduction of target site mutations that would usually permit viral replication but inhibit endonuclease binding and cleavage [120]. Another cause for viral resistance is when a defective viral gene target is restored to its wild-type state by a recombination event with a functional viral genome. A study by De Silva Feelixge et al. [121] supported existing theories of HIV-1 resistance by demonstrating that insertional mutations introduced into the HIV-1 provirus following ZFN therapy enabled virus replication and ZFN cleavage resistance. The study showed similar replication levels of mutant and wild-type viruses and the persistence of mutant progeny even in activated primary T cells. Their findings stressed the need for combination therapy that would target multiple regions of the viral genome to avert the emergence of viral resistance.

Similarly, recent studies have supported previous theories of the mechanisms of HIV-1 resistance following treatment with CRISPR–Cas9 [122, 123]. The former used HIV-1 evolution experiments with CRISPR–Cas9, and revealed rapid and consistent viral escape even when conserved HIV-1 sequences were attacked by CRISPR–Cas9 [123]. This was done by sequencing the entire HIV-1 escape variants, which provided evidences of nucleotide insertions, deletions, and substitutions around the Cas9/gRNA cleavage site as a result of an imperfect non-homologous end-joining pathway of DNA repair pathway [123]. Conversely, the latter study supported these findings by showing mutations at HIV-1 pol, env, and LTR target sites which contributed to viral resistance [122].

Insight into the detailed mechanisms of Cas9/sgRNA HIV-1 resistance would be invaluable to the development of novel strategies to mitigate several viral escape. Nevertheless, some precautionary measures could be put in place to avoid incidence of escape mutants. CRISPR–Cas9 multiplex system could be fully exploited using multiple sgRNA to target conserved regions of the viral genomes [124]. Alternatively, customised or modified Cas9 proteins (such as Cpf1) [125, 126] or SpCas9 with novel PAM specificities [127] could be programmed to target sequences outside the targeted regions. This strategy would ensure that mutations arising from NHEJ repair will not prevent Cas9/sgRNA binding and DNA cleavage which previously were the cause of viral resistance.

Despite the discovery of smaller, yet effective Cas9 nucleases and improved strategies for transducing both CD4+ T cells and CD34 hematopoietic stem cells via lentiviral vectors [128, 129], there are substantial challenges with in vivo delivery of CRISPR–Cas9-encoding genes to certain cell types. Of most importance is the risk of insertional oncogenesis associated with integrating lentiviral vectors for successful gene transfer into cells and tissues. However, the use of highly efficient virus-like particles (such as the newly developed Lent-One Trans Vectors) that effectively packages the transcription activator joined with the Cas9 and single guide RNA, (Vpr-Cas9/sgRNA) are recommended for transient delivery into target cells. This could save HIV-1 researchers who are often trapped in the limbo of finding suitable delivery systems for CRSIPR-Cas9 [130].

In an attempt to combat insertional mutagenesis at antiviral therapeutic sites, the use of small molecule inhibitors [131], RNAi-based suppressors [132] and other chemotherapeutic agents, [133, 134] which silence specific enzymes involved in the NHEJ pathway while promoting homology-directed repair (HDR) could be adopted. Additionally, given the drawbacks of HAART as well as the limitation of current genome editing tools, exploring the synergistic power of combinatorial therapy (such as CRISPR–Cas9 with HAART) in actively suppressing HIV-1 replication could advance current efforts in finding a functional cure to HIV-1 in resource-limited countries.

Conclusion

In this review, we have highlighted some of the mechanisms underlying the application of genome editing as a major control to augment existing strategies against HIV-1 infection. It will be interesting to investigate the efficacy of clearing HIV-1 proviral DNA while shedding more light on the outcome of such strategies on the health and safety of individuals.

While the research community is still keen on finding an anti-HIV-1 vaccine, gene therapy a budding therapeutic approach has seen many developments with promising potential for perpetually eliminating the disease.

Single gRNA has been shown to mediate suppression of HIV-1 replication following treatment. In addition to T cells we anticipate that genome editing approaches could be further explored to target other immune cell populations such as monocytes, macrophages and dendritic cells to harness functional treatment of HIV-1 infections. While most research focus on either the application of CRISPR–Cas9 in vitro or in vivo, there is the need for novel genome editing protocols, which are capable of transmigrating the blood-brain barrier (BBB) to target HIV-1-infected and latently-infected HIV-1 brain reservoirs to overcome the incidence of neuro-acquired immunodeficiency syndrome (neuroAIDS) in the brain [57]. Despite the fast pace of current research to end HIV-1, there is compelling evidence, as highlighted throughout this communication, that fighting HIV-1 cannot be achieved using a single therapeutic strategy but by a combinational approach of existing and new strategies yet to be developed. Given that the brunt of these infections are borne largely by developing countries, such as sub-Saharan Africa there is the need for careful consideration of the scalability and cost of promising gene therapy in order to make such treatments deliverable to the world's bottom billion. Nevertheless, given the current hurdles with CRISPR–Cas9 and other recent genome editors, it is imperative for intensive and collaborative research across various biomedical disciplines to develop better strategies for optimization of these tools while opening up new avenues for the treatment of HIV-1.

Abbreviations

CRISPR–Cas9: clustered regularly interspaced short palindromic repeats/CRISPR-associated protein 9; HAART: highly active antiretroviral therapy; HDR: homology-directed repair; NHEJ: non-homologous end joining; NgAgo:

Natronobacterium gregoryi Argonaute; sgRNA: single guide RNA; TALENS: transcription activator-like effector nucleases; ZFNS: zinc finger nucleases.

Authors' contributions

AK conceived the idea. AK, STA and GKN equally wrote and critically edited the paper. All authors read and approved the final manuscript.

Author details

[1] Department of Biochemistry and Biotechnology, Kwame Nkrumah University of Science and Technology (KNUST), PMB, Kumasi, Ghana. [2] Kumasi Centre for Collaborative Research in Tropical Medicine (KCCR), Kumasi, Ghana. [3] Department of Biomedical Sciences, School of Allied Health Sciences, College of Health and Allied Sciences, University of Cape Coast, Cape Coast, Ghana.

Acknowledgements

We would like to thank Emmanuel Kobla Atsu Amewu, Biochemistry and Biotechnology Department, KNUST, for the illustrations in the manuscript.

Competing interests

The authors declare that they have no competing interests.

Funding

The authors received no funding towards this study.

References

1. Maartens G, Celum C, Lewin SR. HIV infection: epidemiology, pathogenesis, treatment, and prevention. Lancet. 2014;384(9939):258–71.
2. United Nations Programme on HIV/AIDS. AIDS by the numbers. Geneva: Joint United Nations Programme on HIV/AIDS (UNAIDS); 2016.
3. Deeks SG, Lewin SR, Ross AL, Ananworanich J, Benkirane M, Cannon P, Chomont N, Douek D, Lifson JD, Lo YR, et al. International AIDS Society global scientific strategy: towards an HIV cure 2016. Nat Med. 2016;22(8):839–50.
4. Bartholomeeusen K, Xiang Y, Fujinaga K, Peterlin BM. Bromodomain and extra-terminal (BET) bromodomain inhibition activate transcription via transient release of positive transcription elongation factor b (P-TEFb) from 7SK small nuclear ribonucleoprotein. J Biol Chem. 2012;287(43):36609–16.
5. Yu W, Ramakrishnan R, Wang Y, Chiang K, Sung TL, Rice AP. Cyclin T1-dependent genes in activated CD4 T and macrophage cell lines appear enriched in HIV-1 co-factors. PLoS ONE. 2008;3(9):e3146.
6. Margolis DM. Mechanisms of HIV latency: an emerging picture of complexity. Curr HIV/AIDS Rep. 2010;7(1):37–43.
7. Chun TW, Justement JS, Moir S, Hallahan CW, Maenza J, Mullins JI, Collier AC, Corey L, Fauci AS. Decay of the HIV reservoir in patients receiving antiretroviral therapy for extended periods: implications for eradication of virus. J Infect Dis. 2007;195(12):1762–4.
8. Wong JK, Hezareh M, Gunthard HF, Havlir DV, Ignacio CC, Spina CA, Richman DD. Recovery of replication-competent HIV despite prolonged suppression of plasma viremia. Science. 1997;278(5341):1291–5.
9. Cary DC, Fujinaga K, Peterlin BM. Molecular mechanisms of HIV latency. J Clin Investig. 2016;126(2):448–54.
10. Marin B, Thiebaut R, Bucher HC, Rondeau V, Costagliola D, Dorrucci M, Hamouda O, Prins M, Walker S, Porter K, et al. Non-AIDS-defining deaths and immunodeficiency in the era of combination antiretroviral therapy. AIDS. 2009;23(13):1743–53.
11. Gavegnano C, Detorio M, Montero C, Bosque A, Planelles V, Schinazi RF. Ruxolitinib and tofacitinib are potent and selective inhibitors of HIV-1 replication and virus reactivation in vitro. Antimicrob Agents Chemother. 2014;58(4):1977–86.
12. Haile WB, Gavegnano C, Tao S, Jiang Y, Schinazi RF, Tyor WR. The Janus kinase inhibitor ruxolitinib reduces HIV replication in human macrophages and ameliorates HIV encephalitis in a murine model. Neurobiol Dis. 2016;92(Pt B):137–43.
13. Archin NM, Liberty AL, Kashuba AD, Choudhary SK, Kuruc JD, Crooks AM, Parker DC, Anderson EM, Kearney MF, Strain MC, et al. Administration of vorinostat disrupts HIV-1 latency in patients on antiretroviral therapy. Nature. 2012;487(7408):482–5.
14. Sogaard OS, Graversen ME, Leth S, Olesen R, Brinkmann CR, Nissen SK, Kjaer AS, Schleimann MH, Denton PW, Hey-Cunningham WJ, et al. The depsipeptide romidepsin reverses HIV-1 latency in vivo. PLoS Pathog. 2015;11(9):e1005142.
15. Elliott JH, McMahon JH, Chang CC, Lee SA, Hartogensis W, Bumpus N, Savic R, Roney J, Hoh R, Solomon A, et al. Short-term administration of disulfiram for reversal of latent HIV infection: a phase 2 dose-escalation study. Lancet HIV. 2015;2(12):e520–9.
16. Rasmussen TA, Tolstrup M, Brinkmann CR, Olesen R, Erikstrup C, Solomon A, Winckelmann A, Palmer S, Dinarello C, Buzon M, et al. Panobinostat, a histone deacetylase inhibitor, for latent-virus reactivation in HIV-infected patients on suppressive antiretroviral therapy: a phase 1/2, single group, clinical trial. Lancet HIV. 2014;1(1):e13–21.
17. Ho YC, Shan L, Hosmane NN, Wang J, Laskey SB, Rosenbloom DI, Lai J, Blankson JN, Siliciano JD, Siliciano RF. Replication-competent noninduced proviruses in the latent reservoir increase barrier to HIV-1 cure. Cell. 2013;155(3):540–51.
18. Boehm D, Calvanese V, Dar RD, Xing S, Schroeder S, Martins L, Aull K, Li PC, Planelles V, Bradner JE, et al. BET bromodomain-targeting compounds reactivate HIV from latency via a Tat-independent mechanism. Cell Cycle. 2013;12(3):452–62.
19. Spina CA, Anderson J, Archin NM, Bosque A, Chan J, Famiglietti M, Greene WC, Kashuba A, Lewin SR, Margolis DM, et al. An in-depth comparison of latent HIV-1 reactivation in multiple cell model systems and resting CD4+ T cells from aviremic patients. PLoS Pathog. 2013;9(12):e1003834.
20. Blazkova J, Chun TW, Belay BW, Murray D, Justement JS, Funk EK, Nelson A, Hallahan CW, Moir S, Wender PA, et al. Effect of histone deacetylase inhibitors on HIV production in latently infected, resting CD4(+) T cells from infected individuals receiving effective antiretroviral therapy. J Infect Dis. 2012;206(5):765–9.
21. Korin YD, Brooks DG, Brown S, Korotzer A, Zack JA. Effects of prostratin on T-cell activation and human immunodeficiency virus latency. J Virol. 2002;76(16):8118–23.
22. Perez M, de Vinuesa AG, Sanchez-Duffhues G, Marquez N, Bellido ML, Munoz-Fernandez MA, Moreno S, Castor TP, Calzado MA, Munoz E. Bryostatin-1 synergizes with histone deacetylase inhibitors to reactivate HIV-1 from latency. Curr HIV Res. 2010;8(6):418–29.
23. Pandelo Jose D, Bartholomeeusen K, da Cunha RD, Abreu CM, Glinski J, da Costa TB, Bacchi Rabay AF, Pianowski Filho LF, Dudycz LW, Ranga U, et al. Reactivation of latent HIV-1 by new semi-synthetic ingenol esters. Virology. 2014;462–463:328–39.
24. Jiang G, Mendes EA, Kaiser P, Sankaran-Walters S, Tang Y, Weber MG, Melcher GP, Thompson GR 3rd, Tanuri A, Pianowski LF, et al. Reactivation of HIV latency by a newly modified Ingenol derivative via protein kinase Cdelta-NF-kappaB signaling. AIDS. 2014;28(11):1555–66.
25. Abreu CM, Price SL, Shirk EN, Cunha RD, Pianowski LF, Clements JE, Tanuri A, Gama L. Dual role of novel ingenol derivatives from *Euphorbia tirucalli* in HIV replication: inhibition of de novo infection and activation of viral LTR. PLoS ONE. 2014;9(5):e97257.
26. Hori T, Barnor J, Huu TN, Morinaga O, Hamano A, Ndzinu J, Frimpong A, Minta-Asare K, Amoa-Bosompem M, Brandful J, et al. Procyanidin trimer C1 derived from *Theobroma cacao* reactivates latent human immunodeficiency virus type 1 provirus. Biochem Biophys Res Commun. 2015;459(2):288–93.
27. Wang C, Yang S, Lu H, You H, Ni M, Shan W, Lin T, Gao X, Chen H, Zhou Q, et al. A natural product from *Polygonum cuspidatum* Sieb. Et Zucc. Promotes Tat-dependent HIV latency reversal through triggering P-TEFb's release from 7SK snRNP. PLoS ONE. 2015;10(11):e0142739.
28. DeChristopher BA, Loy BA, Marsden MD, Schrier AJ, Zack JA, Wender PA. Designed, synthetically accessible bryostatin analogues potently induce activation of latent HIV reservoirs in vitro. Nat Chem. 2012;4(9):705–10.

29. Wender PA, Nakagawa Y, Near KE, Staveness D. Computer-guided design, synthesis, and protein kinase C affinity of a new salicylate-based class of bryostatin analogs. Org Lett. 2014;16(19):5136–9.
30. Darcis G, Kula A, Bouchat S, Fujinaga K, Corazza F, Ait-Ammar A, Delacourt N, Melard A, Kabeya K, Vanhulle C, et al. An in-depth comparison of latency-reversing agent combinations in various in vitro and ex vivo HIV-1 latency models identified bryostatin-1+JQ1 and ingenol-B+JQ1 to potently reactivate viral gene expression. PLoS Pathog. 2015;11(7):e1005063.
31. Chun TW, Engel D, Mizell SB, Hallahan CW, Fischette M, Park S, Davey RT Jr, Dybul M, Kovacs JA, Metcalf JA, et al. Effect of interleukin-2 on the pool of latently infected, resting CD4+ T cells in HIV-1-infected patients receiving highly active anti-retroviral therapy. Nat Med. 1999;5(6):651–5.
32. Prins JM, Jurriaans S, van Praag RM, Blaak H, van Rij R, Schellekens PT, ten Berge IJ, Yong SL, Fox CH, Roos MT, et al. Immuno-activation with anti-CD3 and recombinant human IL-2 in HIV-1-infected patients on potent antiretroviral therapy. AIDS. 1999;13(17):2405–10.
33. Perelson AS, Essunger P, Cao Y, Vesanen M, Hurley A, Saksela K, Markowitz M, Ho DD. Decay characteristics of HIV-1-infected compartments during combination therapy. Nature. 1997;387(6629):188–91.
34. Shan L, Deng K, Shroff NS, Durand CM, Rabi SA, Yang HC, Zhang H, Margolick JB, Blankson JN, Siliciano RF. Stimulation of HIV-1-specific cytolytic T lymphocytes facilitates elimination of latent viral reservoir after virus reactivation. Immunity. 2012;36(3):491–501.
35. Halper-Stromberg A, Nussenzweig MC. Towards HIV-1 remission: potential roles for broadly neutralizing antibodies. J Clin Investig. 2016;126(2):415–23.
36. Chun TW, Murray D, Justement JS, Blazkova J, Hallahan CW, Fankuchen O, Gittens K, Benko E, Kovacs C, Moir S, et al. Broadly neutralizing antibodies suppress HIV in the persistent viral reservoir. Proc Natl Acad Sci USA. 2014;111(36):13151–6.
37. Cary DC, Peterlin BM. Targeting the latent reservoir to achieve functional HIV cure. F1000Research. 2016;5.
38. Chun TW, Moir S, Fauci AS. HIV reservoirs as obstacles and opportunities for an HIV cure. Nat Immunol. 2015;16(6):584–9.
39. Zeller SJ, Kumar P. RNA-based gene therapy for the treatment and prevention of HIV: from bench to bedside. Yale J Biol Med. 2011;84(3):301–9.
40. Zhou J, Rossi JJ. Current progress in the development of RNAi-based therapeutics for HIV-1. Gene Ther. 2011;18(12):1134–8.
41. Subramanya S, Kim SS, Manjunath N, Shankar P. RNA interference-based therapeutics for human immunodeficiency virus HIV-1 treatment: synthetic siRNA or vector-based shRNA? Expert Opin Biol Ther. 2010;10(2):201–13.
42. Rossi JJ. RNAi as a treatment for HIV-1 infection. BioTechniques. 2006;40:25–9.
43. Manjunath N, Yi G, Dang Y, Shankar P. Newer gene editing technologies toward HIV gene therapy. Viruses. 2013;5(11):2748–66.
44. Cullen BR. Does RNA interference have a future as a treatment for HIV-1 induced disease? AIDS Rev. 2005;7(1):22–5.
45. Blake SJ, Bokhari FF, McMillan NA. RNA interference for viral infections. Curr Drug Targets. 2012;13(11):1411–20.
46. Ban HS, Lee SK, Kumar P. Delivering antiviral siRNA into human T-cells: new approaches in RNAi-based HIV therapy. IDrugs: Investig Drugs J. 2009;12(12):774–8.
47. Chong H, Xue J, Xiong S, Cong Z, Ding X, Zhu Y, Liu Z, Chen T, Feng Y, He L, et al. A lipopeptide HIV-1/2 fusion inhibitor with highly potent in vitro, ex vivo and in vivo antiviral activity. J Virol. 2017;91:e00288.
48. Bobbin ML, Burnett JC, Rossi JJ. RNA interference approaches for treatment of HIV-1 infection. Genome Med. 2015;7(1):50.
49. Lessells RJ, Mutevedzi PC, Iwuji CC, Newell ML. Reduction in early mortality on antiretroviral therapy for adults in rural South Africa since change in CD4+ cell count eligibility criteria. J Acquir Immune Defic Syndr. 2014;65(1):e17–24.
50. Deeks SG, Lewin SR, Havlir DV. The end of AIDS: hIV infection as a chronic disease. Lancet. 2013;382(9903):1525–33.
51. Volberding PA, Deeks SG. Antiretroviral therapy and management of HIV infection. Lancet. 2010;376:49–62.
52. Otieno MO. Why novel nanoparticle-based delivery platforms hold key for HIV/AIDS treatment and prevention? HIV/AIDS Res Treat Open J. 2015;2(3):81–5.
53. Gomes MJ, Neves J, Sarmento B. Nanoparticle-based drug delivery to improve the efficacy of antiretroviral therapy in the central nervous system. Int J Nanomed. 2014;9:1757–69.
54. Edagwa BJ, Zhou T, McMillan JM, Liu XM, Gendelman HE. Development of HIV reservoir targeted long acting nanoformulated antiretroviral therapies. Curr Med Chem. 2014;21(36):4186–98.
55. Bhaskar S, Tian F. Stoeger Tea: multifunctional nanocarriers for diagnostics, drug delivery and targeted treatment across blood-brain barrier: perspectives on tracking and neuroimaging. Part Fibre Toxicol. 2010;7:3.
56. Adesina SK, Akala EO. Nanotechnology approaches for the delivery of exogenous siRNA for HIV therapy. Mol Pharm. 2015;12(12):4175–87.
57. Kaushik A, Jayant RD, Nair M. Advancements in nano-enabled therapeutics for neuroHIV management. Int J Nanomed. 2016;11:4317–25.
58. Moss DM, Siccardi M. Optimizing nanomedicine pharmacokinetics using physiologically based pharmacokinetics modelling. Br J Pharmacol. 2014;171(17):3963–79.
59. Kitabwalla M, Ruprecht RM. RNA interference—a new weapon against HIV and beyond. N Engl J Med. 2002;347(17):1364–7.
60. Lemons D, Maurya MR, Subramaniam S, Mercola M. Developing microRNA screening as a functional genomics tool for disease research. Front Physiol. 2013;4:223.
61. Hammond SM, Bernstein E, Beach D, Hannon GJ. An RNA-directed nuclease mediates post-transcriptional gene silencing in Drosophila cells. Nature. 2000;404(6775):293–6.
62. Huntzinger E, Izaurralde E. Gene silencing by microRNAs: contributions of translational repression and mRNA decay. Nat Rev Genet. 2011;12(2):99–110.
63. Djupedal I, Ekwall K. Epigenetics: heterochromatin meets RNAi. Cell Res. 2009;19(3):282–95.
64. Hoffer P, Ivashuta S, Pontes O, Vitins A, Pikaard C, Mroczka A, Wagner N, Voelker T. Posttranscriptional gene silencing in nuclei. Proc Natl Acad Sci. 2011;108(1):409–14.
65. Weinberg MS, Morris KV. Transcriptional gene silencing in humans. Nucleic Acids Res. 2016;44(14):6505–17.
66. Ruigrok MJ, Frijlink HW, Hinrichs WL. Pulmonary administration of small interfering RNA: the route to go? J Controll Release. 2016;235:14–23.
67. Balakrishna Pillai A, Nagarajan U, Mitra A, Krishnan U, Rajendran S, Hoti SL, Mishra RK. RNA interference in mosquito: understanding immune responses, double-stranded RNA delivery systems and potential applications in vector control. Insect Mol Biol. 2017;26(2):127–39.
68. Kishida T, Ejima A, Mazda O. Specific destruction of HIV proviral p17 gene in T lymphoid cells achieved by the genome editing technology. Front in Microbiol. 1001;2016:7.
69. Jacque JM, Triques K, Stevenson M. Modulation of HIV-1 replication by RNA interference. Nature. 2002;418(6896):435–8.
70. Klug A. The discovery of zinc fingers and their applications in gene regulation and genome manipulation. Annu Rev Biochem. 2010;79:213–31.
71. Liang C, Wainberg MA, Das AT, Berkhout B. CRISPR/Cas9: a double-edged sword when used to combat HIV infection. Retrovirology. 2016;13(1):37.
72. Drake MJ, Bates P. Application of gene-editing technologies to HIV-1. Curr Opin HIV AIDS. 2015;10(2):123–7.
73. Zhao J, Sun W, Liang J, Jiang J, Wu Z. A one-step system for convenient and flexible assembly of transcription activator-like effector nucleases (TALENs). Mol Cells. 2016;39(9):687–91.
74. Bogdanove AJ, Schornack S, Lahaye T. TAL effectors: finding plant genes for disease and defense. Curr Opin Plant Biol. 2010;13(4):394–401.
75. Joung JK, Sander JD. TALENs: a widely applicable technology for targeted genome editing. Nat Rev Mol Cell Biol. 2013;14(1):49–55.
76. Cong L, Ran FA, Cox D, Lin S, Barretto R, Habib N, Hsu PD, Wu X, Jiang W, Marraffini LA, et al. Multiplex genome engineering using CRISPR/Cas systems. Science. 2013;339(6121):819–23.
77. Jinek M, East A, Cheng A, Lin S, Ma E, Doudna J. RNA-programmed genome editing in human cells. eLife. 2013;2:E00471.
78. Miller JC, Tan S, Qiao G, Barlow KA, Wang J, Xia DF, Meng X, Paschon DE, Leung E, Hinkley SJ, et al. A TALE nuclease architecture for efficient genome editing. Nat Biotechnol. 2011;29(2):143–8.

79. Cermak T, Doyle EL, Christian M, Wang L, Zhang Y, Schmidt C, Baller JA, Somia NV, Bogdanove AJ, Voytas DF. Efficient design and assembly of custom TALEN and other TAL effector-based constructs for DNA targeting. Nucleic Acids Res. 2011;39(12):e82.
80. Hockemeyer D, Wang H, Kiani S, Lai CS, Gao Q, Cassady JP, Cost GJ, Zhang L, Santiago Y, Miller JC, et al. Genetic engineering of human pluripotent cells using TALE nucleases. Nat Biotechnol. 2011;29(8):731–4.
81. Mock U, Riecken K, Berdien B, Qasim W, Chan E, Cathomen T, Fehse B. Novel lentiviral vectors with mutated reverse transcriptase for mRNA delivery of TALE nucleases. Sci Rep. 2014;4:6409.
82. Shi B, Li J, Shi X, Jia W, Wen Y, Hu X, Zhuang F, Xi J, Zhang L. TALEN-mediated knockout of CCR5 confers protection against infection of human immunodeficiency virus. J Acquir Immune Defic Syndr. 2017;74(2):229–41.
83. Perez EE, Wang J, Miller JC, Jouvenot Y, Kim KA, Liu O, Wang N, Lee G, Bartsevich VV, Lee Y-L, et al. Establishment of HIV-1 resistance in CD4+ T cells by genome editing using zinc-finger nucleases. Nat Biotechnol. 2008;26(7):808–16.
84. Strong CL, Guerra HP, Mathew KR, Roy N, Simpson LR, Schiller MR. Damaging the integrated HIV proviral DNA with TALENs. PLoS ONE. 2015;10(5):e0125652.
85. Saydaminova K, Ye X, Wang H, Richter M, Ho M, Chen H, Xu N, Kim JS, Papapetrou E, Holmes MC, et al. Efficient genome editing in hematopoietic stem cells with helper-dependent Ad5/35 vectors expressing site-specific endonucleases under microRNA regulation. Mol Ther Methods Clin Dev. 2015;1:14057.
86. Li L, Krymskaya L, Wang J, Henley J, Rao A, Cao LF, Tran CA, Torres-Coronado M, Gardner A, Gonzalez N, et al. Genomic editing of the HIV-1 coreceptor CCR5 in adult hematopoietic stem and progenitor cells using zinc finger nucleases. Mol Ther. 2013;21(6):1259–69.
87. Wang H, Cao H, Wohlfahrt M, Kiem H-P, Lieber A. Tightly regulated gene expression in human hematopoietic stem cells after transduction with helper-dependent Ad5/35 vectors. Exp Hematol. 2008;36(7):823–31.
88. Wang H, Shayakhmetov DM, Leege T, Harkey M, Li Q, Papayannopoulou T, Stamatoyannopolous G, Lieber A. A capsid-modified helper-dependent adenovirus vector containing the β-globin locus control region displays a nonrandom integration pattern and allows stable erythroid-specific gene expression. J Virol. 2005;79(17):10999–1013.
89. Ru R, Yao Y, Yu S, Yin B, Xu W, Zhao S, Qin L, Chen X. Targeted genome engineering in human induced pluripotent stem cells by penetrating TALENs. Cell Regen. 2013;2(1):5.
90. Guidotti G, Brambilla L, Rossi D. Cell-penetrating peptides: from basic research to clinics. Trends Pharmacol Sci. 2017;38(4):406–24.
91. Tashima T. Intelligent substance delivery into cells using cell-penetrating peptides. Bioorg Med Chem Lett. 2017;27(2):121–30.
92. Cerrato CP, Kunnapuu K, Langel U. Cell-penetrating peptides with intracellular organelle targeting. Expert Opin Drug Deliv. 2017;14(2):245–55.
93. Bolhassani A, Jafarzade BS, Mardani G. In vitro and in vivo delivery of therapeutic proteins using cell penetrating peptides. Peptides. 2017;87:50–63.
94. Juks C, Lorents A, Arukuusk P, Langel U, Pooga M. Cell-penetrating peptides recruit type A scavenger receptors to the plasma membrane for cellular delivery of nucleic acids. FASEB J. 2017;31(3):975–88.
95. Boisguérin P, Deshayes S, Gait MJ, O'Donovan L, Godfrey C, Betts CA, Wood MJA, Lebleu B. Delivery of therapeutic oligonucleotides with cell penetrating peptides. Adv Drug Deliv Rev. 2015;87:52–67.
96. Dissanayake S, Denny WA, Gamage S, Sarojini V. Recent developments in anticancer drug delivery using cell penetrating and tumor targeting peptides. J Controll Release. 2017;250:62–76.
97. Gaj T, Guo J, Kato Y, Sirk SJ, Barbas CF. Targeted gene knockout by direct delivery of zinc-finger nuclease proteins. Nat Methods. 2012;9(8):805–7.
98. Mock U, Machowicz R, Hauber I, Horn S, Abramowski P, Berdien B, Hauber J, Fehse B. mRNA transfection of a novel TAL effector nuclease (TALEN) facilitates efficient knockout of HIV co-receptor CCR5. Nucleic Acids Res. 2015;43(11):5560–71.
99. Wang X, Yu Q, Yuan Y, Teng Z, Li D, Zeng Y. Targeting the rhesus macaque TRIM5alpha gene to enhance the susceptibility of CD4+ T cells to HIV-1 infection. Arch Virol. 2017;162(3):793–8.
100. Sanz-Ramos M, Stoye JP. Capsid-binding retrovirus restriction factors: discovery, restriction specificity and implications for the development of novel therapeutics. J Gen Virol. 2013;94(Pt 12):2587–98.
101. Stremlau M, Perron M, Welikala S, Sodroski J. Species-specific variation in the B30.2(SPRY) domain of TRIM5alpha determines the potency of human immunodeficiency virus restriction. J Virol. 2005;79(5):3139–45.
102. Kovalskyy DB, Ivanov DN. Recognition of the HIV capsid by the TRIM5alpha restriction factor is mediated by a subset of pre-existing conformations of the TRIM5alpha SPRY domain. Biochemistry. 2014;53(9):1466–76.
103. Jung U, Urak K, Veillette M, Nepveu-Traversy ME, Pham QT, Hamel S, Rossi JJ, Berthoux L. Preclinical assessment of mutant human TRIM5alpha as an anti-HIV-1 transgene. Hum Gene Ther. 2015;26(10):664–79.
104. Richardson MW, Guo L, Xin F, Yang X, Riley JL. Stabilized human TRIM5alpha protects human T cells from HIV-1 infection. Mol Ther. 2014;22(6):1084–95.
105. Neagu MR, Ziegler P, Pertel T, Strambio-De-Castillia C, Grutter C, Martinetti G, Mazzucchelli L, Grutter M, Manz MG, Luban J. Potent inhibition of HIV-1 by TRIM5-cyclophilin fusion proteins engineered from human components. J Clin Investig. 2009;119(10):3035–47.
106. Llano M, Vanegas M, Hutchins N, Thompson D, Delgado S, Poeschla EM. Identification and characterization of the chromatin-binding domains of the HIV-1 integrase interactor LEDGF/p75. J Mol Biol. 2006;360(4):760–73.
107. Fadel HJ, Morrison JH, Saenz DT, Fuchs JR, Kvaratskhelia M, Ekker SC, Poeschla EM. TALEN knockout of the PSIP1 gene in human cells: analyses of HIV-1 replication and allosteric integrase inhibitor mechanism. J Virol. 2014;88(17):9704–17.
108. Sorek R, Kunin V, Hugenholtz P. CRISPR–a widespread system that provides acquired resistance against phages in bacteria and archaea. Nat Rev Microbiol. 2008;6(3):181–6.
109. Doudna JA, Charpentier E. Genome editing. The new frontier of genome engineering with CRISPR-Cas9. Science. 2014;346(6213):1258096.
110. Sternberg SH, Doudna JA. Expanding the biologist's toolkit with CRISPR-Cas9. Mol Cell. 2015;58(4):568–74.
111. Wang W, Ye C, Liu J, Zhang D, Kimata JT, Zhou P. CCR5 gene disruption via lentiviral vectors expressing Cas9 and single guided RNA renders cells resistant to HIV-1 infection. PLoS ONE. 2014;9(12):e115987.
112. Kaminski R, Chen Y, Fischer T, Tedaldi E, Napoli A, Zhang Y, Karn J, Hu W, Khalili K. Elimination of HIV-1 genomes from human T-lymphoid cells by CRISPR/Cas9 gene editing. Sci Rep. 2016;6:22555.
113. Gao F, Shen XZ, Jiang F, Wu Y, Han C. DNA-guided genome editing using the *Natronobacterium gregoryi Argonaute*. Nat Biotechnol. 2016;34(7):768–73.
114. Cyranoski D. Replications, ridicule and a recluse: the controversy over NgAgo gene-editing intensifies. Nature. 2016;536(7615):136–7.
115. Guo X, Li X-J. Targeted genome editing in primate embryos. Cell Res. 2015;25(7):767–8.
116. Niu Y, Shen B, Cui Y, Chen Y, Wang J, Wang L, Kang Y, Zhao X, Si W, Li W, et al. Generation of gene-modified cynomolgus monkey via Cas9/RNA-mediated gene targeting in one-cell embryos. Cell. 2014;156(4):836–43.
117. Liu H, Chen Y, Niu Y, Zhang K, Kang Y, Ge W, Liu X, Zhao E, Wang C, Lin S, et al. TALEN-mediated gene mutagenesis in rhesus and cynomolgus monkeys. Cell Stem Cell. 2014;14(3):323–8.
118. Han Y, Li Q. Application progress of CRISPR/Cas9 genome editing technology in the treatment of HIV-1 infection. Yi chuan=Hereditas/Zhongguo yi chuan xue hui bian ji. 2016;38(1):9–16.
119. Holkers M, Maggio I, Liu J, Janssen JM, Miselli F, Mussolino C, Recchia A, Cathomen T, Goncalves MA. Differential integrity of TALE nuclease genes following adenoviral and lentiviral vector gene transfer into human cells. Nucleic Acids Res. 2013;41(5):e63.
120. Stone D, Niyonzima N, Jerome KR. Genome editing and the next generation of antiviral therapy. Hum Genet. 2016;135(9):1071–82.
121. De Silva Feelixge HS, Stone D, Pietz HL, Roychoudhury P, Greninger AL, Schiffer JT, Aubert M, Jerome KR. Detection of treatment-resistant infectious HIV after genome-directed antiviral endonuclease therapy. Antivir Res. 2016;126:90–8.
122. Wang Z, Pan Q, Gendron P, Zhu W, Guo F, Cen S, Wainberg MA, Liang C. CRISPR/Cas9-derived mutations both inhibit HIV-1 replication and accelerate viral escape. Cell Rep. 2016;15(3):481–9.
123. Wang G, Zhao N, Berkhout B, Das AT. CRISPR-Cas9 can inhibit HIV-1 replication but NHEJ repair facilitates virus escape. Mol Ther. 2016;24(3):522–6.

124. ter Brake O, Konstantinova P, Ceylan M, Berkhout B. Silencing of HIV-1 with RNA interference: a multiple shRNA approach. Mol Ther. 2006;14:883–92.
125. Yamano T, Nishimasu H, Zetsche B, Hirano H, Slaymaker IM, Li Y, Fedorova I, Nakane T, Makarova KS, Koonin EV, et al. Crystal structure of Cpf1 in complex with guide RNA and target DNA. Cell. 2016;165(4):949–62.
126. Zetsche B, Gootenberg JS, Abudayyeh OO, Slaymaker IM, Makarova KS, Essletzbichler P, Volz SE, Joung J, van der Oost J, Regev A, et al. Cpf1 is a single RNA-guided endonuclease of a class 2 CRISPR-Cas system. Cell. 2015;163(3):759–71.
127. Kleinstiver BP, Prew MS, Tsai SQ, Topkar VV, Nguyen NT, Zheng Z, Gonzales AP, Li Z, Peterson RT, Yeh JR, et al. Engineered CRISPR-Cas9 nucleases with altered PAM specificities. Nature. 2015;523(7561):481–5.
128. Bilal MY, Vacaflores A, Houtman JC. Optimization of methods for the genetic modification of human T cells. Immunol Cell Biol. 2015;93(10):896–908.
129. Walker JE, Chen RX, McGee J, Nacey C, Pollard RB, Abedi M, Bauer G, Nolta JA, Anderson JS. Generation of an HIV-1-resistant immune system with CD34(+) hematopoietic stem cells transduced with a triple-combination anti-HIV lentiviral vector. J Virol. 2012;86(10):5719–29.
130. Choi JG, Dang Y, Abraham S, Ma H, Zhang J, Guo H, Cai Y, Mikkelsen JG, Wu H, Shankar P, et al. Lentivirus pre-packed with Cas9 protein for safer gene editing. Gene Ther. 2016;23(7):627–33.
131. Robert F, Barbeau M, Ethier S, Dostie J, Pelletier J. Pharmacological inhibition of DNA-PK stimulates Cas9-mediated genome editing. Genome Med. 2015;7:93.
132. Basu S, Aryan A, Overcash JM, Samuel GH, Anderson MA, Dahlem TJ, Myles KM, Adelman ZN. Silencing of end-joining repair for efficient site-specific gene insertion after TALEN/CRISPR mutagenesis in Aedes aegypti. Proc Natl Acad Sci USA. 2015;112(13):4038–43.
133. Vartak SV, Raghavan SC. Inhibition of nonhomologous end joining to increase the specificity of CRISPR/Cas9 genome editing. FEBS J. 2015;282(22):4289–94.
134. Jekimovs C, Bolderson E, Suraweera A, Adams M, O'Byrne KJ, Richard DJ. Chemotherapeutic compounds targeting the DNA double-strand break repair pathways: the good, the bad, and the promising. Front Oncol. 2014;4:86.
135. Morris KV, Chung CH, Witke W, Looney DJ. Inhibition of HIV-1 replication by siRNA targeting conserved regions of gag/pol. RNA Biol. 2005;2:17–20.
136. Scarborough RJ, Levesque MV, Boudrias-Dalle E, Chute IC, Daniels SM, Ouellette RJ. A conserved target site in HIV-1 Gag RNA is accessible to inhibition by both an HDV ribozyme and a short hairpin RNA. Mol Ther Nucleic Acids. 2014;3:e178.
137. Cave E, Weinberg MS, Cilliers T, Carmona S, Morris L, Arbuthnot P. Silencing of HIV-1 subtype C primary isolates by expressed small hairpin RNAs targeted to gag. AIDS Res Hum Retrovir. 2006;22:401–10.
138. Park WS, Hayafune M, Miyano-Kurosaki N, Takaku H. Specific HIV-1 env gene silencing by small interfering RNAs in human peripheral blood mononuclear cells. Gene Ther. 2003;10:2046.
139. Flynn NM, Forthal DN, Harro CD, Judson FN, Mayer KH, Para MF. Placebo-controlled phase 3 trial of a recombinant glycoprotein 120 vaccine to prevent HIV-1 infection. J Infect Dis. 2005;191:654–65.
140. DiGiusto DL, Stan R, Krishnan A, Li H, Rossi JJ, Zaia JA. Development of hematopoietic stem cell based gene therapy for HIV-1 infection: considerations for proof of concept studies and translation to standard medical practice. Viruses. 2013;5:2898–919.
141. Zhou J, Neff CP, Liu X, Zhang J, Li H, Smith DD. Systemic administration of combinatorial dsiRNAs via nanoparticles efficiently suppresses HIV-1 infection in humanized mice. Mol Ther. 2011;19:2228–38.
142. Westerhout EM, Ooms M, Vink M, Das AT, Berkhout B. HIV-1 can escape from RNA interference by evolving an alternative structure in its RNA genome. Nucleic Acids Res. 2005;33:796–804.
143. Brake O, Legrand N, Eije KJ, Centlivre M, Spits H, Weijer K. Evaluation of safety and efficacy of RNAi against HIV-1 in the human immune system (Rag-2(−/−)gammac(−/−)) mouse model. Gene Ther. 2009;16:48.
144. Omoto S, Ito M, Tsutsumi Y, Ichikawa Y, Okuyama H, Brisibe EA. HIV-1 nef suppression by virally encoded microRNA. Retrovirology. 2004;1:44.
145. Yamamoto T, Miyoshi H, Yamamoto N, Yamamoto N, Inoue J, Tsunetsugu-Yokota Y. Lentivirus vectors expressing short hairpin RNAs against the U3-overlapping region of HIV nef inhibit HIV replication and infectivity in primary macrophages. Blood. 2006;108:3305–12.
146. Lau TS, Li Y, Kameoka M, Ng TB, Wan DC. Suppression of HIV replication using RNA interference against HIV-1 integrase. FEBS Lett. 2007;581:3253–9.
147. Nishitsuji H, Kohara M, Kannagi M, Masuda T. Effective suppression of human immunodeficiency virus type 1 through a combination of short- or long-hairpin RNAs targeting essential sequences for retroviral integration. J Virol. 2006;80:7658–66.
148. Jacque JM, Triques K, Stevenson M. Modulation of HIV-1 replication by RNA interference. Nature. 2002;418:435.
149. Suzuki K, Ishida T, Yamagishi M, Ahlenstiel C, Swaminathan S, Marks K. Transcriptional gene silencing of HIV-1 through promoter targeted RNA is highly specific. RNA Biol. 2011;8:1035–46.
150. Singh A, Palanichamy JK, Ramalingam P, Kassab MA, Bhagat M, Andrabi R. Long-term suppression of HIV-1C virus production in human peripheral blood mononuclear cells by LTR heterochromatization with a short double-stranded RNA. J Antimicrob Chemother. 2014;69:404–15.
151. Krebs MD, Alsberg E. Localized, targeted, and sustained siRNA delivery. Chemistry. 2011;17:3054–62.
152. Anderson J, Banerjea A, Akkina R. Bispecific short hairpin siRNA constructs targeted to CD4, CXCR4, and CCR5 confer HIV-1 resistance. Oligonucleotides. 2003;13:303–12.
153. Martinez MA, Gutierrez A, Armand-Ugon M, Blanco J, Parera M, Gomez J. Suppression of chemokine receptor expression by RNA interference allows for inhibition of HIV-1 replication. AIDS. 2002;16:2385–90.
154. Al-Mawsawi LQ, Neamati N. Blocking interactions between HIV-1 integrase and cellular cofactors: an emerging anti-retroviral strategy. Trends Pharmacol Sci. 2007;28:526–35.
155. Christ F, Debyser Z. The LEDGF/p75 integrase interaction, a novel target for anti-HIV therapy. Virology. 2013;435:102–9.
156. Zaitseva L, Cherepanov P, Leyens L, Wilson SJ, Rasaiyaah J, Fassati A. HIV-1 exploits importin 7 to maximize nuclear import of its DNA genome. Retrovirology. 2009;6:11.
157. Li MJ, Kim J, Li S, Zaia J, Yee JK, Anderson J. Long-term inhibition of HIV-1 infection in primary hematopoietic cells by lentiviral vector delivery of a triple combination of anti-HIV shRNA, anti-CCR5 ribozyme, and a nucleolar-localizing TAR decoy. Mol Ther. 2005;12:900–9.
158. Chiu YL, Cao H, Jacque JM, Stevenson M, Rana TM. Inhibition of human immunodeficiency virus type 1 replication by RNA interference directed against human transcription elongation factor P-TEFb (CDK9/CyclinT1). J Virol. 2004;78:2517–29.
159. Green VA, Arbuthnot P, Weinberg MS. Impact of sustained RNAi-mediated suppression of cellular cofactor Tat-SF1 on HIV-1 replication in CD4+ T cells. Virol J. 2012;9:272.
160. Ping YH, Chu CY, Cao H, Jacque JM, Stevenson M, Rana TM. Modulating HIV-1 replication by RNA interference directed against human transcription elongation factor SPT5. Retrovirology. 2004;1:46.
161. Ishaq M, Hu J, Wu X, Fu Q, Yang Y, Liu Q, Guo D. Knockdown of cellular RNA helicase DDX3 by short hairpin RNAs suppresses HIV-1 viral replication without inducing apoptosis. Mol Biotechnol. 2008;39:231–8.
162. Subramanya S, Armant M, Salkowitz JR, Nyakeriga AM, Haridas V, Hasan M. Enhanced induction of HIV-specific cytotoxic T lymphocytes by dendritic cell-targeted delivery of SOCS-1 siRNA. Mol Ther. 2010;18:2028–37.
163. Christensen HS, Daher A, Soye KJ, Frankel LB, Alexander MR, Laine S. Small interfering RNAs against the TAR RNA binding protein, TRBP, a Dicer cofactor, inhibit human immunodeficiency virus type 1 long terminal repeat expression and viral production. J Virol. 2007;81:5121–31.
164. Eekels JJ, Geerts D, Jeeninga RE, Berkhout B. Long-term inhibition of HIV-1 replication with RNA interference against cellular co-factors. Antivir Res. 2011;89:43–53.
165. Zhou J, Neff CP, Swiderski P, Li H, Smith DD, Aboellail T. Functional in vivo delivery of multiplexed anti-HIV-1 siRNAs via a chemically synthesized aptamer with a sticky bridge. Mol Ther. 2013;21:192–200.

8

Validity assessment of the PROMIS fatigue domain among people living with HIV

L. E. Gibbons[1,10*], R. Fredericksen[1], D. S. Batey[2], L. Dant[3], T. C. Edwards[4], K. H. Mayer[3,5], W. C. Mathews[6], L. S. Morales[7], M. J. Mugavero[8], F. M. Yang[9], E. Paez[6], M. M. Kitahata[1], D. L. Patrick[4], H. M. Crane[1], P. K. Crane[1] and for the Centers for AIDS Research Network of Integrated Clinical Systems (CNICS)

Abstract

Purpose: To evaluate psychometric characteristics and cross-sectional and longitudinal validity of the 7-item PROMIS® Fatigue Short Form and additional fatigue items among people living with HIV (PLWH) in a nationally distributed network of clinics collecting patient reported data at the time of routine clinical care.

Methods: Cross-sectional and longitudinal fatigue data were collected from September 2012 through April 2013 across clinics participating in the Centers for AIDS Research Network of Integrated Clinical Systems (CNICS). We analyzed data regarding psychometric characteristics including simulated computerized adaptive testing and differential item functioning, and regarding associations with clinical characteristics.

Results: We analyzed data from 1597 PLWH. Fatigue was common in this cohort. Scores from the PROMIS® Fatigue Short Form and from the item bank had acceptable psychometric characteristics and strong evidence for validity, but neither performed better than shorter instruments already integrated in CNICS.

Conclusions: The PROMIS® Fatigue Item Bank is a valid approach to measuring fatigue in clinical care settings among PLWH, but in our analyses did not perform better than instruments associated with less respondent burden.

Keywords: Fatigue, HIV, PROMIS, Validity, Psychometrics, Measurement, Patient burden

Background

Fatigue is a common clinical symptom and adversely impacts health-related quality of life. Fatigue is highly prevalent among persons living with HIV (PLWH) [1, 2]. It is a common side-effect of antiretroviral medications [3], and it is associated with several adverse clinical outcomes, including longer time until depression remission [4], poorer physical functioning [5, 6], poorer adherence to antiretroviral medications [7], and virologic failure [8]. Patients rank fatigue as an important domain for providers to know about in order to provide good care [9].

In many cases fatigue is not systematically assessed as part of clinical care. Challenges that impede fatigue assessment for research in PLWH have been outlined previously, including lack of consistent measurement, lack of longitudinal measurement, and lack of comprehensive clinical data to examine potential predictors of fatigue [10]. Measuring fatigue for clinical care further compounds these issues as there are substantial time constraints and logistical hurdles that must be addressed to minimize impact of assessment on clinical flow.

One option for assessing fatigue among PLWH is the HIV-Related Fatigue Scale [10–12]. This is a well-designed measure with 56 items including subscales addressing concepts such as intensity and impact. Unfortunately, it is too long to be useful in most routine clinical care settings. At the opposite end of the spectrum are very brief assessments such as the single item included in the HIV symptoms index [13].

The Patient Reported Outcomes Measurement and Information System (PROMIS®, http://www.nihpromis.org) is a National Institutes of Health Roadmap initiative to develop item banks to measure patient-reported

*Correspondence: gibbonsl@u.washington.edu
[10] Harborview Medical Center, University of Washington, 325 9th Ave, Box MS 35978, Seattle, WA 98104, USA
Full list of author information is available at the end of the article

symptoms. PROMIS investigators developed a fatigue item bank [14]. Items from the bank can be used as either a fixed-length short-form or as a computerized adaptive test (CAT) [15]. The PROMIS® Fatigue Item Bank was developed for people in general rather than specific patient groups such as PLWH, which facilitates comparisons with the general population and across patient groups [16]. Well-developed and calibrated universal fatigue measures could enhance comparability of findings and serve as a common metric of fatigue across conditions [15]. Yet, previous analyses of the PROMIS® fatigue domain were not conducted among PLWH, and were not carried out in the context of routine clinical care. We conducted this study to better understand the properties of the PROMIS® fatigue instrument as part of routine clinical care for PLWH.

Methods

Study cohort

This study was conducted in the Centers for AIDS Research Network of Integrated Clinical Systems (CNICS) cohort [17], which integrates comprehensive inpatient and outpatient clinical data on PLWH in the cohort [17]. PLWH complete the CNICS clinical assessment of patient reported measures, symptoms, and outcomes (PROs) every 4–6 months as part of routine clinic visits [18, 19]. They use touch screen tablets or personal computers using web-based survey software developed specifically for PROs [18, 20] to complete the clinical assessment which includes a variety of measures such as the HIV Symptoms Index [13], the Patient Health Questionnaire (PHQ-9) [21, 22] for depression, and the modified Alcohol, Smoking, and Substance Involvement Screening Test [23, 24] for illicit drug use. The assessment was integrated into clinical care for regularly scheduled clinic visits at each site. No exclusions were made on the basis of severe fatigue.

Study participants

PLWH 18 years old or older who spoke English or Spanish at four clinics (University of Washington Madison HIV Clinic, Seattle; University of Alabama at Birmingham 1917 Clinic, Birmingham; University of California San Diego HIV Clinic, San Diego; and Fenway Health, Boston) were eligible to participate in this study. Data were collected from 1597 PLWH from September 2012 to April 2013.

Qualitative analyses

We conducted in-depth interviews in English and Spanish with 42 patients endorsing fatigue to elicit concepts regarding the experience of living with fatigue and HIV, as described elsewhere [25]. We excerpted and coded transcribed interview content using codes adapted from PROMIS® Fatigue Item Bank content. We matched coded interview content to bank items. The team assessed unmatched content for possible new item development. We reviewed all proposed items using PROMIS® Qualitative Item Review criteria [26], for readability using the Lexile Analyzer, and for translatability into English or Spanish. We held focus groups with 68 patients and asked them to rank-order the prospective item list in order of importance for their provider to know. We retained the most important items and conducted cognitive interviews with 21 patients to assess item comprehensibility, modifying items as needed [25]. We developed four new items in addition to those already in the PROMIS® Fatigue Item Bank [25].

Item administration

We administered the 7-item PROMIS® Fatigue Short Form [27], an additional 13 items selected from the PROMIS® Fatigue Item Bank (including four items excluded from the final bank and, thus, without PROMIS® item parameters), and our four new items (see Table 1). We modified response options for five existing PROMIS® items because of qualitative feedback. We used PROMIS® item parameters for all of the other PROMIS® items but calibrated the five items with new response options anew.

Quantitative analyses

We used Stata [28] for all analyses unless otherwise noted.

Dimensionality

We used structural equation modeling to determine whether the items were sufficiently unidimensional to use item response theory (IRT) in our sample. All structural equation models were fit in Mplus [29]. We applied the following thresholds for acceptable model fit: confirmatory fit index (CFI) > 0.95, Tucker–Lewis index (TLI) > 0.95, and root mean squared error of approximation (RMSEA) < 0.08 [30].

PROMIS® item parameters

We performed additional analyses to determine whether it was appropriate to use PROMIS® item parameters in our population of PLWH. We initially fixed all seven items from the fatigue short form to their PROMIS® values and used modification indices to identify the item for which constraining parameters to PROMIS® values had the greatest impact on model fit. We then removed those constraints and freely estimated parameters for that item and identified the next item that had the greatest impact on model fit. We repeated this procedure until

Table 1 Fatigue items administered, with a priori subdomains

Item description	Subdomain
PROMIS 7-item Fatigue Short Form	
How often did you feel tired?	Experience
How often did you run out of energy?	Experience
How often were you too tired to take a bath or shower?	Impact
How often did you experience extreme exhaustion?	Experience
How often did your fatigue limit you at work (including work at home)?	Impact
How often were you too tired to think clearly?	Impact
How often did you have enough energy to exercise strenuously?	Impact
Other calibrated PROMIS items	
How often were you physically drained?	Experience
To what degree did you have to force yourself to get up and do things because of your fatigue?	Impact
How run-down did you feel on average?	Experience
How fatigued were you on average?	Experience
Items calibrated in PROMIS but administered with different response options[a]	
How fatigued were you when your fatigue was at its worst?	Experience
To what degree did your fatigue interfere with your physical functioning?	Impact
I felt fatigued	Experience
I had trouble starting things because I was tired	Impact
How much were you bothered by your fatigue on average?	Experience
Uncalibrated PROMIS items	
How often did you wake up feeling exhausted?	Experience
How often did you feel so exhausted that you stayed in bed all day?	Impact
How often were you too exhausted to take your medication?	Impact
How often were you so exhausted that you missed appointments?	Impact
New items from qualitative interviews	
How often were you too exhausted to carry out your daily responsibilities?	Impact
How often did your body feel exhausted?	Experience
How often were you too exhausted to chew and swallow food?	Impact
How often were you too exhausted to concentrate?	Impact

[a] Because different response options were offered in this study, we did not use the PROMIS item parameters for these items

we were left with two anchor items. We extracted factor scores from the PROMIS®-fixed model and from a model with the final two anchor items and five freely estimated items and calculated correlations between these scores. We plotted agreement between scores using a variant of a Bland–Altman plot, with the difference between the scores on the y-axis and the PROMIS®-fixed model scores on the x-axis. We superimposed the standard error of measurement (SEM) curve on this graph and examined whether the differences were smaller than the SEM at each level of fatigue.

Comparison of measurement properties of scores

We computed an IRT score for all 24 items. We fixed item parameters for the 11 PROMIS® items with PROMIS® response options to their PROMIS® values, so scores are on the PROMIS® metric. We freely estimated parameters for the other 13 items. We compared the SEM for the PROMIS®-7a short form to that from all 24 items.

Simulated CAT

We used Firestar [31] to simulate CAT from the 24-item bank we administered. We categorized PLWH into groups based on PROMIS® fatigue scores: <40, 40–50, >50–60, and >60. We set the minimum number of items administered by the simulated CAT at 7 and the default stopping rule of SEM < 0.3 (equivalent: T-metric SEM < 3). We determined the proportion of times each item was administered to people in each fatigue level group. We used seven items as a minimum to determine the extent of overlap between items selected by CAT and items included in the 7-item PROMIS® Fatigue Short Form. As a sensitivity analysis, we performed a second CAT simulation with no minimum number of items and used a 0.3 SEM or seven items maximum stopping rule. We compared patient burden based on the average completion times per item for patients from one site (University of Washington) who completed both instruments, based on the 7-item short form and the number of items in the 2 CAT simulations.

Differential item functioning (DIF)

We used the Stata command—difwithpar—[32] to evaluate items for DIF with respect to age, sex, race, and nadir CD4 count. We used a *P* value criterion of 0.05 for uniform and for non-uniform DIF. The—difwithpar—algorithm uses demographic-specific item parameters for items identified with DIF and generates new scores that account for DIF. We evaluated DIF impact by comparing naïve scores that ignored DIF to those that accounted for DIF. We use differences of score larger than 0.3 points on the theta metric (larger than 3 points on the T metric) as the primary threshold to indicate salient DIF impact and the median SEM as a more stringent threshold.

Associations with clinical characteristics

We used Spearman correlations to compare cross-sectional associations between clinical characteristics and the HIV Symptoms Index fatigue item [13], the "tired" item from the PHQ-9 [21, 22], the PROMIS®-7a score, and the score derived from the entire 24 items we administered. The clinical characteristics included: hepatitis C virus co-infection; nadir and current CD4 count; the number of symptoms endorsed on the HIV Symptoms Index; specific symptoms endorsed on the HIV Symptoms Index; quality of life estimated using EQ-5D responses [33–36]; and the total PHQ-9 score. Among PLWH taking antiretroviral medications for HIV, we also determined associations between fatigue scores and medication adherence based on the last time the person stated they had missed medications, their self-reported ability to take medications, and the proportion of medications they were estimated to have taken [37–42].

Test–retest reliability

We had 51 people return to clinic on a second occasion from 6–14 days following their initial assessment to repeat the assessment. Since this involved an extra visit outside the context of clinical care, we provided an incentive of $15 for this activity. We used intraclass correlation coefficients (ICCs) to measure test–retest reliability.

Longitudinal evaluation

A subset of 249 PLWH had repeat assessment on a second routine clinical care visit from 79–203 days following their initial assessment [median 119 days, interquartile range (IQR) 105–134 days]. Given the episodic nature of HIV symptoms [43], we were interested first in describing changes in fatigue. We also sought to compare changes in fatigue measures in two situations where change might be expected: concurrent with a change in depression symptoms or a change in methamphetamine use on the clinical assessment.

Results

Demographic and clinical characteristics from the cross-sectional quantitative data

English questionnaires were completed by 1597 PLWH (Table 2); we included Spanish speakers in our qualitative analyses, but there were too few respondents in Spanish (n = 94) for meaningful quantitative analyses. Mean age (SD) was 45.7 (10.4), with a range from 20 to 83 (IQR 39, 53).

Fatigue was common in this cohort. Using the HIV Symptoms Index single item, 65% stated they had fatigue (Table 2). Scores from the PROMIS® items mapped closely to these scores from the HIV Symptoms Index. As shown in Fig. 1, median fatigue scores on the PROMIS® metric ranged from just below 40 for those who stated they did not have fatigue to just over 65 for those who stated they had fatigue and that it bothered them a lot.

Dimensionality

A single factor confirmatory factor analysis model did not fit well by RMSEA criteria (CFI 0.98, TLI 0.98, RMSEA 0.103). We assigned items a priori to one of two subdomains, the experience of fatigue vs. the impact of fatigue, based on PROMIS®'s domain framework (see Table 1), but this model did not fit well and had loadings that did not support the theoretical structure, such as negative loadings on a subdomain. A negative loading means that as levels of the item were of increasing severity, the level of fatigue impact was expected to be *lower down*, which is difficult to explain.

We then considered modification indices from a single factor model that suggested candidate pairs of items with residual correlations that would have the greatest impact on model fit. We included 6 such pairs, which resulted in a model with CFI 0.99, TLI 0.99, and RMSEA 0.08. We extracted factor scores for the single factor score and the bifactor score with the six residual correlations. These scores were highly correlated at 0.9999. We compared standardized factor loadings between these models, and the largest difference was 0.020, well lower than the 0.10 threshold that would indicate a salient difference in loadings between the single factor and bifactor models [44]. These findings led us to conclude that the items were sufficiently unidimensional to proceed with IRT analyses.

PROMIS item parameters

The loadings and thresholds for the two anchor items and the five freely estimated items are shown in Additional file 1. The correlation between the score using those parameters and the score based entirely on PROMIS parameters was >0.99. All of the score differences were within the SEM curve thresholds (Additional file 2). These results supported use of PROMIS item parameters for PLWH.

Measurement properties

We show a plot of the SEM for the 24 items administered and for the 7-item PROMIS® Fatigue Short Form subset in Fig. 2. The median SEM was 0.29 (range 0.24–0.57; IQR 0.26–0.34) for the 7-item PROMIS® Fatigue Short Form and 0.15 (range 0.11–0.52; IQR 0.14–0.20) using all 24 items. On the T-score metric, the 7-item PROMIS® Fatigue Short Form has an SEM < 3 over the 45–73 range, while using all 24 items gives an SEM under 3 for all scores 35 and above. We also show a histogram of observed fatigue scores from the 7-item PROMIS® Fatigue Short Form on the same plot. There are very few people with extremely high levels of fatigue (over 73) for whom the 24 items would provide a markedly improved level of precision; most of the people for whom differences in precision between the 7-item short form and the 24-item bank are characterized by low levels of fatigue, with scores 35-45 on the PROMIS® metric. While scores in this range are common, it may not be clinically

Table 2 Participant characteristics (n = 1597)

Characteristic	N	Percent	Recent CD4 <500		Recent CD4 500+	
			N	Percent	N	Percent
Male	1315	82.3	591	84.8	724	80.4
Race						
White	861	53.9	346	49.6	515	57.2
Black	461	28.9	197	28.3	264	29.3
Hispanic	195	12.2	105	15.1	90	10.0
Other	80	5.0	49	7.0	31	3.4
HIV Symptom Index fatigue item						
No fatigue	558	34.9	233	33.4	325	36.1
Doesn't bother me	151	9.5	66	9.5	85	9.4
Bothers me a little	383	24.0	161	23.1	222	24.7
Bothers me	260	16.3	117	16.8	143	15.9
Bothers me a lot	221	13.8	110	15.8	111	12.3
Did not answer	24	1.5	10	1.4	14	1.6
CD4 Nadir						
<200	732	45.8	487	69.9	245	27.2
200 to <350	392	24.6	152	21.8	240	26.7
350 or higher	468	29.3	55	7.9	413	45.9
Missing	5	0.3	3	0.4	2	0.2
Taking anti-HIV meds	1412	88.4	604	86.7	808	89.8

important to measure fatigue levels precisely in these individuals 1.5–2.5 SD below national norms for fatigue.

CAT results

Our first CAT simulation used a minimum of seven items. With this criterion, only people with PROMIS fatigue scores <40 required more than seven items to achieve a SEM < 3 on the T-metric (Table 3). There were two items that were administered in all simulated CATs: *"How run-down did you feel on average"* and *"How fatigued were you on average."* The item *"How often were you physically drained"* was almost always administered. None of the items from the 7-item PROMIS® Fatigue Short Form was routinely selected for CAT administration across all fatigue levels, though *"How often did you feel tired"* and *"How often did you run out of energy"* were always administered to individuals with fatigue scores <40.

As outlined in our previous publication, we developed four new fatigue items based on our qualitative work [25]. In simulated CAT, one of these, *"How often did your body feel exhausted?"* was selected 46% of the time; it was always selected for people with fatigue scores ≤40, 61% of the time for fatigue scores >40–50 and 46% of the time for those with the highest levels of fatigue. In contrast, the other new items we developed were either never or rarely selected for people with fatigue levels >40; these items were *"How often were you too exhausted to carry out your daily responsibilities?", "How often were you too exhausted to chew and swallow food?"* and *"How often were you too exhausted to concentrate?"*

In our secondary analyses, we completed another CAT simulation with no minimum number of items and a stopping rule of either a standard error of measurement <3 points on the T metric or up to 7 items maximum; the median (IQR) number of items administered was 3 (3–4).

Based on the mean time per item for the PROMIS fatigue items (mean 6.73 s, SD 2.74 per item), a person completing the 7-item PROMIS short form or 7-item CAT would be expected to take an average of 47.1 s. Based on the second simulated CAT where people completed a mean of 3 items, the average completion time for the PROMIS fatigue CAT would be 20.2 s. This is in comparison to an estimated time to complete the HIV Symptom Index fatigue screening item of 6 s (mean 6.0 s, SD 10.1).

DIF results

A few items had DIF with respect to age, sex, race, and/or nadir CD4 count with the very sensitive DIF thresholds we used (results not shown). There was negligible DIF impact, and for none of these covariates was there any individual PLWH where accounting for DIF

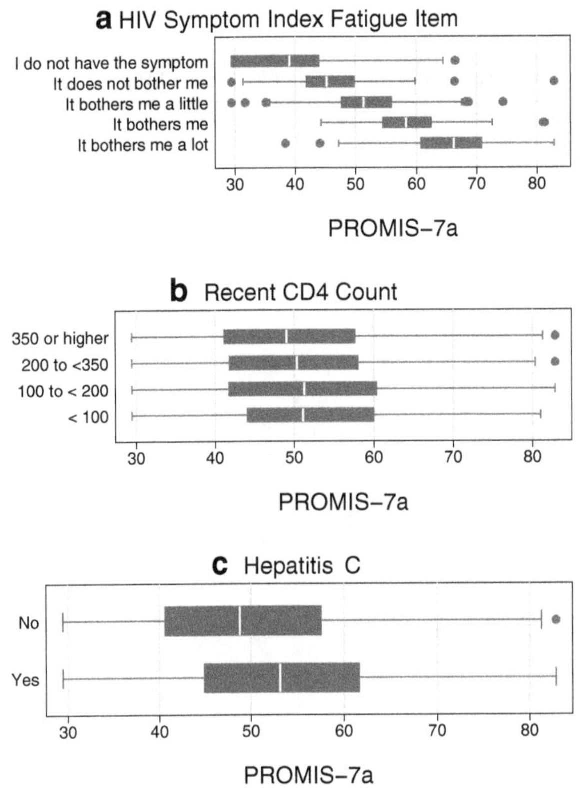

Fig. 1 *Box* and *whisker plots* showing the distribution of PROMIS® 7a fatigue scores on the PROMIS® T score metric for each level of fatigue according to the HIV symptoms inventory fatigue item* (**a**); for people with different recent CD4+ T-cell counts (**b**), and with and without Hepatitis C virus co-infection (**c**). *For these plots, the box shows the 25th and 75th percentile scores, and the median is shown with a *white vertical bar* within the *box*. The *whiskers* show 1.5 times the extent of the *box*. *Dots* show more extreme values. In **a**, the median score for the group who denied having fatigue was around 40; the median for those who had fatigue but stated it did not bother them was around 45; the median score for those who had fatigue that bothered them a little was around 53; the median score for those who had fatigue that bothered them was around 58; and the median score for those who had fatigue that bothered them a lot was around 66

led to a change in score as much as three points on the PROMIS T-score metric. Indeed, when we considered a more stringent 1.7 points PROMIS T-score metric (the median SEM for this sample), only 1–7 people (all <1%) had DIF impact of this magnitude with respect to each of these covariates. We concluded that there was negligible DIF in these items with respect to these covariates.

Associations with clinical characteristics

The HIV Symptom Index single item fatigue score was closely associated with the 7-item PROMIS® Fatigue Short Form ($\rho = 0.82$) and with the score from all of 24

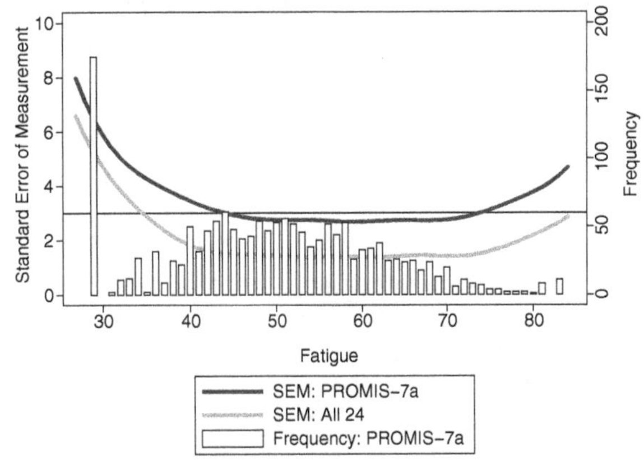

Fig. 2 Histogram of observed fatigue levels (*open bars*) superimposed on standard error of measurement curves for the 24 fatigue items administered to participants (*lower light gray curve*) and for the 7-item PROMIS® Fatigue Short Form (*upper darker gray curve*). A *horizontal line* is at a SEM of 3, which is the common default stopping rule for computerized adaptive testing

items ($\rho = 0.85$) (Table 4). Similarly, the PHQ-9 fatigue item was closely associated with the HIV Symptoms Index fatigue item ($\rho = 0.77$), with the 7-item PROMIS® Fatigue Short Form ($\rho = 0.75$), and with the 24-item score ($\rho = 0.77$). Correlations with clinical characteristics were generally as strong for the HIV Symptom Index fatigue item as they were for either the 7-item PROMIS® Fatigue Short Form or the full 24-item score.

Test–retest reliability

Fifty-one people completed the 7-item PROMIS® Fatigue Short Form again 6–14 days later (median 8, IQR 7–11 days). The ICC was 0.74 (0.55, 0.83). The mean change was −0.17 points, though 4 people had a decrease of at least on point and 2 had an increase of at least one point, either due to true changes in fatigue [43] or measurement error. Among the 31 people who said their level of fatigue was "about the same" as previously, the ICC was similar at 0.66 (0.44, 0.81).

Longitudinal analyses

On average there was little change in level of fatigue over approximately 4 months—the mean change was −0.16. However, this obscures individual variation, in that 9% reported an increase in fatigue of at least one point, and 16% reported a decrease of at least one point. Changes in the PHQ-9 depression score were more highly correlated with changes in the HIV Symptom Index fatigue item (Spearman $\rho = 0.47$) than were changes in the 7-item PROMIS® Fatigue Short Form score ($\rho = 0.39$). Only 13 people changed from using methamphetamines to not, or vice versa, so comparisons of the fatigue measures were not feasible.

Table 3 Frequency of item administration in simulated computerized adaptive testing, by level of fatigue

Item	Overall (n = 1597)	Fatigue score			
		≤40 (n = 246)	>40–50 (n = 561)	>50–60 (n = 556)	>60 (n = 234)
How often did you feel tired?	22.0	100.0	18.4	0.0	1.3
How often did you run out of energy?	57.5	100.0	54.2	45.9	48.7
How often were you too tired to take a bath or shower?	6.6	43.1	0.0	0.0	0.0
How often did you experience extreme exhaustion?	7.3	45.9	0.0	0.0	1.7
How often did your fatigue limit you at work (including work at home)?	8.9	57.7	0.0	0.0	0.0
How often were you too tired to think clearly?	7.8	45.9	0.0	0.0	4.7
How often did you have enough energy to exercise strenuously?	8.7	56.5	0.0	0.0	0.0
How often were you physically drained?	99.7	100.0	100.0	100.0	97.9
To what degree did you have to force yourself to get up and do things?	79.8	46.7	69.5	100.0	91.5
How run-down did you feel on average?	100.0	100.0	100.0	100.0	100.0
How fatigued were you on average?	100.0	100.0	100.0	100.0	100.0
How fatigued were you when your fatigue was at its worst?	11.6	75.2	0.0	0.0	0.0
To what degree did your fatigue interfere with your physical functioning?	70.6	49.6	38.3	100.0	100.0
I felt fatigued	47.3	64.2	82.7	22.1	4.3
I had trouble starting things because I was tired	20.5	48.0	0.0	35.1	6.0
How much were you bothered by your fatigue on average?	85.2	85.4	75.6	89.9	97.0
How often did you wake up feeling exhausted?	7.6	49.2	0.0	0.0	0.0
How often did you feel so exhausted that you stayed in bed all day?	6.9	44.7	0.0	0.0	0.0
How often were you too exhausted to take your medication?	6.2	40.2	0.0	0.0	0.0
How often were you so exhausted that you missed appointments?	6.6	42.7	0.0	0.0	0.0
How often were you too exhausted to carry out your daily responsibilities?	7.0	43.9	0.0	0.0	1.7
How often did your body feel exhausted?	46.1	100.0	61.3	7.0	46.2
How often were you too exhausted to chew and swallow food?	6.1	39.8	0.0	0.0	0.0
How often were you too exhausted to concentrate?	7.0	45.5	0.0	0.0	0.0
Mean number of items	8.3	15.2	7.0	7.0	7.0
Mean standard error of measurement (T-metric)	2.2	3.2	2.1	2.0	2.1

Discussion

In a thorough evaluation of the psychometric properties of the 7-item PROMIS® Fatigue Short Form and additional items selected from the PROMIS® Fatigue Item Bank or items specifically developed for this project, we found that these fatigue items had excellent content validity among PLWH. While the 24 fatigue items did not form a scale that was strictly unidimensional, it was sufficiently unidimensional to use item response theory. Furthermore, our analyses suggested that PROMIS® item parameters were appropriate to use among PLWH. We used very sensitive DIF detection thresholds and identified items with DIF, but did not find salient impact for DIF with respect to age, sex, race, or nadir CD4 count. Scores from the 7-item PROMIS® Fatigue Short Form or from all 24 items from the fatigue item bank had excellent validity in a variety of analyses, but were no better than the HIV Symptom Index single fatigue item measure or the fatigue item from the PHQ-9. The HIV Symptom Index single fatigue item has limited ability to detect change over time, because it has only a few response options. Nevertheless, in the longitudinal sample, we did

Table 4 Spearman correlation coefficients between fatigue measures and clinical characteristics

	HIVSI fatigue		PHQ-9 "tired"		PROMIS-7a		All 24 items	
	Coefficient	P value	Coefficient	P value	Coefficient	P value	Coefficient	P value
Factors related to fatigue itself								
HIV Symptom Index 1-item Fatigue response	–	–	0.77	<0.0001	0.82	<0.0001	0.85	<0.0001
PHQ-9 item "feeling tired or having little energy"	–	–	–	–	0.75	<0.0001	0.77	<0.0001
Hepatitis-C	0.09	0.0004	0.09	0.0002	0.11	<0.0001	0.12	<0.0001
HIV disease severity								
Current CD4 count	−0.04	0.1402	−0.04	0.1562	−0.05	0.0699	−0.04	0.2392
CD4 nadir	0.01	0.8828	0.05	0.0534	0.00	0.8584	0.01	0.3481
Symptom burden								
Number of symptoms in inventory	0.69	<0.0001	0.59	<0.0001	0.64	<0.0001	0.66	<0.0001
Specific symptoms								
Fever, chills or sweats	0.42	<0.0001	0.37	<0.0001	0.64	<0.0001	0.44	<0.0001
Dizzy or lightheaded	0.51	<0.0001	0.46	<0.0001	0.42	<0.0001	0.54	<0.0001
Pain/numbness/tingling in hands/feet	0.44	<0.0001	0.35	<0.0001	0.52	<0.0001	0.49	<0.0001
Having difficulty remembering	0.57	<0.0001	0.48	<0.0001	0.46	<0.0001	0.62	<0.0001
Nausea or vomiting	0.45	<0.0001	0.37	<0.0001	0.63	<0.0001	0.47	<0.0001
Diarrhea or loose bowel movements	0.41	<0.0001	0.34	<0.0001	0.47	<0.0001	0.42	<0.0001
Feeling sad or depressed	0.65	<0.0001	0.55	<0.0001	0.40	<0.0001	0.66	<0.0001
Feeling nervous or anxious	0.57	<0.0001	0.50	<0.0001	0.63	<0.0001	0.61	<0.0001
Difficulty falling or staying asleep	0.57	<0.0001	0.50	<0.0001	0.58	<0.0001	0.59	<0.0001
Coughing or trouble catching breath	0.39	<0.0001	0.36	<0.0001	0.56	<0.0001	0.44	<0.0001
Headaches	0.42	<0.0001	0.35	<0.0001	0.43	<0.0001	0.46	<0.0001
Appetite loss/change taste of food	0.45	<0.0001	0.43	<0.0001	0.44	<0.0001	0.52	<0.0001
Bloating pains or gas in stomach	0.44	<0.0001	0.37	<0.0001	0.51	<0.0001	0.47	<0.0001
Muscle aches or joint pain	0.47	<0.0001	0.42	<0.0001	0.47	<0.0001	0.52	<0.0001
Sex-loss of interest/satisfaction	0.47	<0.0001	0.41	<0.0001	0.50	<0.0001	0.50	<0.0001
Body changes-fat deposits/wt gain	0.46	<0.0001	0.38	<0.0001	0.50	<0.0001	0.49	<0.0001
Weight loss or wasting	0.32	<0.0001	0.30	<0.0001	0.49	<0.0001	0.39	<0.0001
EQ-5D	0.59	<0.0001	0.56	<0.0001	0.38	<0.0001	0.64	<0.0001
PHQ-9	0.75	<0.0001	0.84	<0.0001	0.63	<0.0001	0.77	<0.0001
Self-rated health (EuroQOL)	−0.53	<0.0001	0.50	<0.0001	0.74	<0.0001	−0.57	<0.0001
Among ART users								
Last time missed meds	−0.15	<0.0001	−0.16	<0.0001	−0.18	<0.0001	−0.19	<0.0001
Ability to take meds	−0.19	<0.0001	−0.24	<0.0001	−0.23	<0.0001	−0.23	<0.0001
Take how much of meds	−0.14	0.0001	−0.16	<0.0001	−0.17	<0.0001	−0.17	<0.0001

not find evidence that the PROMIS scores were more responsive to change than was the HIV Symptom Index fatigue item or the PHQ-9 fatigue item.

Fatigue is clearly a relevant consideration for this clinical population. Sizable numbers of PLWH had substantial levels of fatigue. One advantage of the PROMIS® fatigue metric is that we can relate fatigue levels to national averages. As shown in Fig. 1 and in Table 3, substantial numbers of PLWH endorse high levels of fatigue. Those who stated that they have fatigue that bothers them a lot on the HIV Symptom Index have median (IQR) PROMIS® fatigue scores of 66 (IQR 61–71), which is about 1.5 SD (1–2 SD) above the national average.

Our CAT simulations showed a small amount of overlap with the 7-item PROMIS® Fatigue Short Form. We set up the first simulation such that each individual received at least seven items to facilitate comparisons with the short form. Only people with very low fatigue levels received more than 7 items from the simulated CAT; everyone else received exactly 7 items. While the 7-item short form may not include the most informative items from the PROMIS® Fatigue Item Bank, it nevertheless had good measurement precision across a broad range of fatigue levels (see Fig. 2). Furthermore, the 7-item PROMIS® Fatigue Short Form performed well in all of our validity analyses; indeed, scores from the 7-item PROMIS® Fatigue Short Form performed just as well as scores from the entire 24 items we considered. At the same time, briefer instruments, including the fatigue item from the PHQ-9 and the single HIV Symptom Index fatigue item, also did well in all of our validity analyses. We did not find a compelling case to choose the PROMIS® fatigue scores over much shorter instruments. A CAT with different specifications could have arrived at a PROMIS fatigue score in fewer items, but it would be unlikely to have better performance in our validity analyses than the entire scale considered here. Furthermore, the HIV Symptom Index fatigue item required much less time on average for patients to complete than the 7-item PROMIS short form, CAT, or even the shorter CAT with an average of 3 items. While this may be of limited importance in research settings, minimizing patient burden in clinical care settings is important to avoid impacting clinical flow.

Our findings should be considered in the context of strengths and limitations. Our study was performed in CNICS, which is a nationally distributed cohort of PLWH who are in clinical care. Our data were collected from convenience samples of PLWH seen in particular calendar months, and were not purposefully sampled from people particularly likely to have changing fatigue levels. Generalizability is limited as our study was conducted only among PLWH. We did administer the PROMIS fatigue items to Spanish speakers, but had too few of them during the data collection window to facilitate analyses of DIF. We found no evidence of DIF with respect to four covariates, but were not able to evaluate DIF with respect to Spanish vs. English. The CNICS assessment of patient-reported measures now includes Amharic, but unfortunately, an Amharic version of the PROMIS Fatigue Item Bank has not been developed, nor were we able to assess the performance of these items in any other language.

Our ability to evaluate change in fatigue over time was limited, because we had few options for external comparison. One validation option was changes in depression levels as measured by the PHQ-9, where we found that the HIV Symptom Index fatigue item was more closely correlated to changes in depression levels than were PROMIS scores. In theory, IRT scores are more accurate measures of change over time than ordinal scales, because they have linear measurement properties [45], which means that one point of change in a score corresponds to the same amount of change in fatigue regardless of the initial level of fatigue. Indeed, PROMIS® scores may have shown better responsiveness to change than the HIV symptoms index fatigue item scores had we designed our study specifically to collect data on people expected to change [46]. In that setting, a brief CAT may prove to have better responsiveness to change than the single HIV symptoms index fatigue item and may fit in a reasonable time footprint, making this a feasible choice in routine clinical care settings. Firmer conclusions regarding responsiveness of PROMIS® scores among PLWH will require additional data.

This study has several strengths that are also worth noting. It includes a particularly relevant population (PLWH) given the high rates of fatigue experienced by a substantial proportion of this group. We studied the performance of these items in a geographically and racially/ethnically diverse population. We performed a variety of psychometric analyses using state-of-the-art approaches.

Fatigue in PLWH often does not remit [10], suggesting the need for additional research to better understand factors leading to fatigue in PLWH and interventions to successfully address it. Research on fatigue among PLWH will require a sustainable systematic approach to measuring fatigue in clinical care.

Conclusions

The PROMIS® Fatigue Short Form and other fatigue items performed well among PLWH, though we did not find evidence that they performed better than shorter legacy scales in the specific context of routine clinical care. Unless comparison to national norms is needed, the HIV Symptom Index fatigue item may be preferred in HIV clinical care settings due to reduced patient burden.

Abbreviations

CAT: computerized adaptive test; CFI: confirmatory fit index; CNICS: Centers for AIDS Research Network of Integrated Clinical Systems; DIF: differential item functioning; ICC: intraclass correlation coefficient; IQR: interquartile Range; IRT: item response theory; PHQ-9: patient health questionnaire for depression; PLWH: persons living with HIV; PROMIS: Patient Reported Outcomes Measurement and Information System; PROs: patient reported measures, symptoms, and outcomes; RMSEA: root mean squared error of approximation; SEM: standard error of measurement; TLI: Tucker–Lewis Index.

Authors' contributions

LG conducted the statistical analyses and drafted sections of the manuscript. RF conducted all the qualitative analyses and made substantial contributions to the conception and design of the study and acquisition of data. DB, LD, KM, WM, MM, EP, and MK were involved in acquisition of data and critical revision of the manuscript for important intellectual content. TE, LM, and FY, were involved in critical revision of the manuscript for important intellectual content. DP was involved in the conception and design of the study and critical revision of the manuscript for important intellectual content. HC made substantial contributions to the conception and design of the study and acquisition of data and provided important intellectual content. PC made substantial contributions to the conception and design of the study and drafted sections of the manuscript. All authors read and approved the final manuscript.

Author details

[1] Department of Medicine, Harborview Medical Center, University of Washington, 325 9th Ave, Box 359931, Seattle, WA, USA. [2] Department of Social Work, University of Alabama at Birmingham, 900 13th Street S, Suite 203, Birmingham, AL 35294, USA. [3] Fenway Institute, 1340 Boylston Street, Boston, MA 02215, USA. [4] Department of Health Services, University of Washington, 1208 NE 43rd Street, Seattle, WA 98195, USA. [5] Department of Medicine, Harvard Medical School, Boston, MA, USA. [6] Department of Medicine, University of California at San Diego, 4168 Front Street, San Diego, CA 92103, USA. [7] Center for Health Equity, Diversity and Inclusion, School of Medicine, University of Washington, 1959 Pacific Street, Seattle, WA 98195, USA. [8] Department of Medicine, University of Alabama at Birmingham, 908 20th Street S, Suite 250, Birmingham, AL 35205, USA. [9] Department of Biostatistics and Epidemiology, Augusta University, 1120 15th Street, AE-1035, Augusta, GA 30912, USA. [10] Harborview Medical Center, University of Washington, 325 9th Ave, Box MS 35978, Seattle, WA 98104, USA.

Acknowledgements

We would like to thank the patients and clinics across CNICS. This research was funded by a cooperative agreement from the National Institute of Allergy and Infectious Diseases (NIAID) and National Institute of Arthritis and Musculoskeletal and Skin Diseases (NIAMS) (Grant #U01 AR057954). Support was also provided by the National Institute of Allergy and Infectious Diseases (NIAID) University of Washington Center for AIDS Research (Grant #P30 AI027757) and CNICS (R24 AI067039).

Competing interests

The authors declare that they have no competing interests.

Funding

This research was funded by a cooperative agreement from the National Institute of Allergy and Infectious Diseases (NIAID) and National Institute of Arthritis and Musculoskeletal and Skin Diseases (NIAMS) (Grant #U01 AR057954). Support was also provided by the National Institute of Allergy and Infectious Diseases (NIAID) University of Washington Center for AIDS Research (Grant #P30 AI027757) and CNICS (R24 AI067039).

References

1. Jong E, Oudhoff LA, Epskamp C, et al. Predictors and treatment strategies of HIV-related fatigue in the combined antiretroviral therapy era. AIDS. 2010;24(10):1387–405.
2. Barroso J, Voss JG. Fatigue in HIV and AIDS: an analysis of evidence. J Assoc Nurses AIDS Care. 2013;24(1 Suppl):S5–14.
3. daCosta DiBonaventura M, Gupta S, Cho M, Mrus J. The association of HIV/AIDS treatment side effects with health status, work productivity, and resource use. AIDS Care. 2012;24(6):744–55.
4. Sowa NA, Bengtson A, Gaynes BN, Pence BW. Predictors of depression recovery in HIV-infected individuals managed through measurement-based care in infectious disease clinics. J Affect Disord. 2016;192:153–61.
5. O'Brien KK, Solomon P, Bergin C, et al. Reliability and validity of a new HIV-specific questionnaire with adults living with HIV in Canada and Ireland: the HIV disability questionnaire (HDQ). Health Qual Life Outcomes. 2015;13:124.
6. Simmonds MJ, Novy D, Sandoval R. The differential influence of pain and fatigue on physical performance and health status in ambulatory patients with human immunodeficiency virus. Clin J Pain. 2005;21(3):200–6.
7. Al-Dakkak I, Patel S, McCann E, Gadkari A, Prajapati G, Maiese EM. The impact of specific HIV treatment-related adverse events on adherence to antiretroviral therapy: a systematic review and meta-analysis. AIDS Care. 2013;25(4):400–14.
8. Marconi VC, Wu B, Hampton J, et al. Early warning indicators for first-line virologic failure independent of adherence measures in a South African urban clinic. AIDS Patient Care STDS. 2013;27(12):657–68.
9. Fredericksen RJ, Edwards TC, Merlin JS, et al. Patient and provider priorities for self-reported domains of HIV clinical care. AIDS Care. 2015;27(10):1255–64.
10. Barroso J, Leserman J, Harmon JL, Hammill B, Pence BW. Fatigue in HIV-infected people: a three-year observational study. J Pain Symptom Manag. 2015;50(1):69–79.
11. Barroso J, Lynn MR. Psychometric properties of the HIV-related fatigue scale. J Assoc Nurses AIDS Care. 2002;13(1):66–75.
12. Pence BW, Barroso J, Leserman J, Harmon JL, Salahuddin N. Measuring fatigue in people living with HIV/AIDS: psychometric characteristics of the HIV-related fatigue scale. AIDS Care. 2008;20(7):829–37.
13. Justice AC, Holmes W, Gifford AL, et al. Development and validation of a self-completed HIV Symptom Index. J Clin Epidemiol. 2001;54(Suppl 1):S77–90.
14. Lai JS, Cella D, Choi S, et al. How item banks and their application can influence measurement practice in rehabilitation medicine: a PROMIS fatigue item bank example. Arch Phys Med Rehabil. 2011;92(10 Suppl):S20–7.
15. Cella D, Lai JS, Jensen SE, et al. Clinical validity of the PROMIS fatigue item bank across diverse clinical samples. J Clin Epidemiol. 2016;73:128–34.
16. Junghaenel DU, Christodoulou C, Lai JS, Stone AA. Demographic correlates of fatigue in the US general population: results from the patient-reported outcomes measurement information system (PROMIS) initiative. J Psychosom Res. 2011;71(3):117–23.
17. Kitahata MM, Rodriguez B, Haubrich R, et al. Cohort profile: the centers for AIDS research network of integrated clinical systems. Int J Epidemiol. 2008;37(5):948–55.
18. Crane HM, Lober W, Webster E, et al. Routine collection of patient-reported outcomes in an HIV clinic setting: the first 100 patients. Curr HIV Res. 2007;5(1):109–18.
19. Fredericksen RJ, Crane PK, Tufano J, et al. Integrating a web-based patient assessent into primary care for HIV-infected adults. J AIDS HIV Res. 2012;4(2):47–55.
20. Lawrence ST, Willig JH, Crane HM, et al. Routine, self-administered, touch-screen, computer-based suicidal ideation assessment linked to automated response team notification in an HIV primary care setting. Clin Infect Dis. 2010;50(8):1165–73.
21. Spitzer RL, Kroenke K, Williams JB. Validation and utility of a self-report version of PRIME-MD: the PHQ primary care study. Primary care evaluation of mental disorders. Patient health questionnaire. JAMA. 1999;282(18):1737–44.
22. Kroenke K, Spitzer RL, Williams JB. The PHQ-9: validity of a brief depression severity measure. J Gen Intern Med. 2001;16(9):606–13.
23. Newcombe DA, Humeniuk RE, Ali R. Validation of the World Health Organization alcohol, smoking and substance involvement screening test (ASSIST): report of results from the Australian site. Drug Alcohol Rev. 2005;24(3):217–26.
24. WHO Assist Working Group. The alcohol, smoking and substance involvement screening test (ASSIST): development, reliability and feasibility. Addiction. 2002;97(9):1183–94.
25. Edwards TC, Fredericksen RJ, Crane HM, et al. Content validity of Patient-Reported Outcomes Measurement Information System (PROMIS) items in the context of HIV clinical care. Qual Life Res. 2016;25(2):293–302.
26. DeWalt DA, Rothrock N, Yount S, Stone AA. Evaluation of item candidates: the PROMIS qualitative item review. Med Care. 2007;45(5 Suppl 1):S12–21.
27. Garcia SF, Cella D, Clauser SB, et al. Standardizing patient-reported outcomes assessment in cancer clinical trials: a patient-reported outcomes measurement information system initiative. J Clin Oncol. 2007;25(32):5106–12.

28. Stata statistical software: release 14. [computer program]. College Station: StataCorp LP; 2015.
29. Mplus: statistical analysis with latent variables [computer program]. Version 7.11. Los Angeles: Muthén & Muthén; 1998–2013.
30. Reeve BB, Hays RD, Bjorner JB, et al. Psychometric evaluation and calibration of health-related quality of life item banks: plans for the Patient-Reported Outcomes Measurement Information System (PROMIS). Med Care. 2007;45(5 Suppl 1):S22–31.
31. Choi SW. Firestar: computerized adaptive testing simulation program for polytomous item response theory models. Appl Psych Meas. 2009;33(8):644–5.
32. Crane PK, Gibbons LE, Jolley L, van Belle G. Differential item functioning analysis with ordinal logistic regression techniques: DIFdetect and difwithpar. Med Care. 2006;44(11 Suppl 3):S115–23.
33. Wu AW, Jacobson KL, Frick KD, et al. Validity and responsiveness of the euroqol as a measure of health- related quality of life in people enrolled in an AIDS clinical trial. Qual Life Res. 2002;11(3):273–82.
34. Johnson JA, Coons SJ. Comparison of the EQ-5D and SF-12 in an adult US sample. Qual Life Res. 1998;7(2):155–66.
35. Johnson JA, Coons SJ, Ergo A, Szava-Kovats G. Valuation of EuroQOL (EQ-5D) health states in an adult US sample. Pharmacoeconomics. 1998;13(4):421–33.
36. Harding R, Clucas C, Lampe FC, et al. What factors are associated with patient self-reported health status among HIV outpatients? A multi-centre UK study of biomedical and psychosocial factors. AIDS Care. 2012;24(8):963–71.
37. Chesney MA, Ickovics JR, Chambers DB, et al. Self-reported adherence to antiretroviral medications among participants in HIV clinical trials: the AACTG adherence instruments. Patient Care Committee & Adherence Working Group of the Outcomes Committee of the Adult AIDS Clinical Trials Group (AACTG). AIDS Care. 2000;12(3):255–66.
38. Lu M, Safren SA, Skolnik PR, et al. Optimal recall period and response task for self-reported HIV medication adherence. AIDS Behav. 2008;12(1):86–94.
39. Walsh JC, Mandalia S, Gazzard BG. Responses to a 1 month self-report on adherence to antiretroviral therapy are consistent with electronic data and virological treatment outcome. AIDS. 2002;16(2):269–77.
40. Kalichman SC, Cain D, Fuhrel A, Eaton L, Di Fonzo K, Ertl T. Assessing medication adherence self-efficacy among low-literacy patients: development of a pictographic visual analogue scale. Health Educ Res. 2005;20(1):24–35.
41. Giordano TP, Guzman D, Clark R, Charlebois ED, Bangsberg DR. Measuring adherence to antiretroviral therapy in a diverse population using a visual analogue scale. HIV Clin Trials. 2004;5(2):74–9.
42. Feldman BJ, Fredericksen RJ, Crane PK, et al. Evaluation of the single-item self-rating adherence scale for use in routine clinical care of people living with HIV. AIDS Behav. 2012;17(1):307–18.
43. O'Brien KK, Davis AM, Strike C, Young NL, Bayoumi AM. Putting episodic disability into context: a qualitative study exploring factors that influence disability experienced by adults living with HIV/AIDS. J Int AIDS Soc. 2009;12:5.
44. McDonald RP. Test theory: a unified treatment. Mahwah: Lawrence Erlbaum; 1999.
45. Mungas D, Reed BR. Application of item response theory for development of a global functioning measure of dementia with linear measurement properties. Stat Med. 2000;19(11–12):1631–44.
46. Cook KF, Jensen SE, Schalet BD, et al. PROMIS measures of pain, fatigue, negative affect, physical function and social function demonstrate clinical validity across a range of chronic conditions. J Clin Epidemiol. 2016;73:89.

Safety and immunogenicity of the quadrivalent human papillomavirus (qHPV) vaccine in HIV-positive Spanish men who have sex with men (MSM)

Carmen Hidalgo-Tenorio[1*], Jessica Ramírez-Taboada[1], Concepción Gil-Anguita[1], Javier Esquivias[2], Mohamed Omar-Mohamed-Balgahata[3], Antonio SamPedro[4], Miguel Lopez-Ruz[1] and Juan Pasquau[1]

Abstract

Background: Safety and immunogenicity of the quadrivalent human papillomavirus (qHPV) vaccine were evaluated in HIV-positive Spanish MSM. The prevalence of High Squamous Intraepithelial Lesions (HSIL) and genotypes of high-risk human papillomavirus (HR-HPV) were also determined, as well as risk factors associated with the presence of HR-HPV in anal mucosa.

Methods: This is a randomised, double blind, placebo-controlled trial of the quadrivalent HPV (qHPV) vaccine. The study enrolled from May 2012 to May 2014. Vaccine and placebo were administered at 0, 2 and 6 months (V1, V2, V3 clinical visits). Vaccine antibody titres were evaluated at 7 months. Cytology (Thin Prep® Pap Test), HPV PCR genotyping (Linear Array HPV Genotyping Test), and high-resolution anoscopy (Zeiss 150 fc© colposcope) were performed at V1.

Results: Patients (n = 162; mean age 37.9 years) were screened for inclusion; 14.2% had HSIL, 73.1% HR-HPV and 4.5% simultaneous infection with HPV16 and 18. Study participants (n = 129) were randomized to qHPV vaccine or placebo. The most common adverse event was injection-site pain predominating in the placebo group [the first dose (83.6% vs. 56.1%; p = 0.0001]; the second dose (87.8% vs. 98.4%; p = 0.0001); the third dose (67.7% vs. 91.9%; p = 0.0001). The vaccine did not influence either the viral load of HIV or the levels of CD4. Of those vaccinated, 76% had antibodies to HPV vs. 30.2% of those receiving placebo (p = 0.0001). In the multivariate analysis, Older age was associated with lower HR-HPV infection (RR 0.97; 95% CI 0.96–0.99), and risk factor were viral load of HIV >200 copies/μL (RR 1.42 95% CI 1.17–1.73) and early commencement of sexual activity (RR 1.35; 95% CI 1.001–1.811).

Conclusions: This trial showed significantly higher anti-HR-HPV antibody titres in vaccinated individuals than in unvaccinated controls. There were no serious adverse events attributable to the vaccine. In our cohort, 1 of every 7 patients had HSIL and the prevalence of combined infection by genotypes 16 and 18 was low. This suggests that patients could benefit from receiving qHPV vaccine. Older age was the main protective factor against HR-HPV infection, and non-suppressed HIV viremia was a risk factor.

Keywords: Quadrivalent HPV vaccine, High squamous intra-epithelial lesions (HSIL), Low squamous intra-epithelial lesion (LSIL), Human immunodeficiency virus (HIV), Men having sex with men (MSM), Anal cancer

*Correspondence: chidalgo72@gmail.com
[1] Infectious Disease Service, University Hospital Virgen de las Nieves, Granada, Spain
Full list of author information is available at the end of the article

Background

Anal squamous cell carcinoma (ASCC) in HIV patients is, currently, one of the most-frequent non-AIDS-defining cancers [1]. There are several studies that confirm its higher prevalence in HIV-positive individuals compared to the seronegative population; in one of them, the prevalence of anal HPV infection was 60% among HIV-negative men who have sex with men (MSM) and 93% among HIV-positive MSM [2]. However, its special relevance in HIV patients is not only due to its high prevalence, in MSM and women with cervical pathologies [3, 4], but also because of its greater rapidity of progression if not treated early. In a study carried out in Seattle, Washington, in MSM who were free of Anal intraepithelial neoplasia, High Squamous Intraepithelial Lesion (HSIL) developed in 15% of HIV-positive and 8% of HIV-negative men in an average of 21 months [5]. One of the risk factors implicated in the appearance of pre-malignant lesions (HSIL) and ASCC is the chronic infection by high-risk human papillomavirus (HR-HPV) genotypes [6, 7].

The classical risk factors involved in the infection of oncogenic HPV in the anal mucosa include: young age [8], a large number of sexual partners [9], and in HIV-positive MSM patients, low CD4 counts, among others [10].

Several strategies for the prevention of ASCC have been evaluated, including: screening for ASCC/HSIL with anal cytology alone [11, 12], anal cytology and HPV-PCR [13–18], or high-resolution anoscopy (HRA) [19]; and prevention of HPV infection with condom use [20] and vaccination [21].

There have been several trials with the quadrivalent human papillomavirus (qHPV) vaccine carried-out in HIV seronegative MSM. In two of them, MSM were compared to heterosexual males (HM), and they found lower protection rates against external genital lesions (EGL) in MSM (rate of EGL in MSM 0.42/100 person-year at risk, vs. in HM 0.08/100 person-year at risk) [22], and a lower antibody response against the qHPV vaccine (at month 36: Ab of HPV-6 was in HM 89.5% vs. 80% in MSM; Ab HPV-11 94.3% vs. 89.1%; HPV-16 98.3% vs. 93.9%; HPV-18 57.3% vs. 53.6%) [23]. Another trial conducted only in MSM showed effectiveness in preventing the appearance of HSIL in approximately half of patients [24]. Until now, there have only been 2 clinical trials with the qHPV vaccine carried out in adult HIV+ population, one in MSM in which immunogenicity was found to be close to 100% [25]; and another in men and women that was interrupted due to lack of efficacy against the appearance of anal high-grade squamous intraepithelial lesions in anal mucosa [26]. With these data, we decided to conduct a randomised, single-centred, double blind trial of the qHPV vaccine in HIV-positive MSM patients. The main objective of this paper was to assess the safety and immunogenic capacity of the vaccine in adult Spanish HIV-positive MSM patients. The secondary objectives were to evaluate the prevalence of high squamous intraepithelial lesion (HSIL) and HR-HPV, as well as the predictive factors associated with the infection by this virus in anal mucosa.

Patients and methods

Trial design

This is a randomised, double blind, placebo-controlled trial of the quadrivalent HPV (qHPV) vaccine. It was conducted according to the protocols of the Spanish Drugs and Health Products Agency (*Agencia Española del Medicamento y Productos Sanitarios; AEMPS*). The recruitment period was between May 15th 2012 and May 15th 2014. Clinical trial registration: ISRCTNregistry. ISRCTN14732216. DOI 10.1186/ISRCTN14732216. Date assigned 02/08/2016. Retrospectively registered. See clinical trial protocol at http://www.isrctn.com/ISRCTN14732216.

Participants

Inclusion criteria

- HIV-positive MSM patients of ≥18 years of age who, at the time of study inclusion were not infected simultaneously by the four genotypes of HPV that the quadrivalent vaccine addresses.
- Patients who had a normal high-resolution anoscopy (HRA) at screening for inclusion or only had condylomas and/or low squamous intraepithelial lesion (LSIL) in anal biopsy.

Exclusion criteria

- HIV MSM patients who had simultaneous anal infection with the four genotypes addressed by the vaccine, and who at least had HPV genotypes 16 and 18.
- Active opportunist infection at the time of recruitment into the study.
- Patients who, in screening anoscopy had HSIL, or ASCC or had received treatment for these lesions (these patients were excluded because patients with HSIL have a higher probability of progression to ASCC).
- History of allergy to aluminium and/or yeast extract excipient.

Settings and locations

The patients who enrolled were HIV-positive MSM that were attending the Infectious Diseases Service of the "*University Hospital Virgen de las Nieves*", *Granada* (Spain), and *Ciudad de Jaén* (Spain).

The purposes of the study were explained to the potential participants who then underwent screening, and enrolled if they met the inclusion criteria for the trial. They were asked to sign the fully informed consent form. The project received approval from the hospital's Ethics Committee (Institution Review Board) "Comité de Ética de la Investigación Biomédica de la Provincia de Granada (CEI-GRANADA)" University Hospital Virgen de las Nieves. The study was conducted in compliance with ethical and moral principles stated in the Declaration of Helsinki as well as the current Spanish Laws on Biomedical Research. Data were coded to ensure anonymity. The project received funding from the Foundation for Progress and Health (*Fundación Progreso y Salud*) of the Government of Andalucia (2011 convocation). This trial was registered in Clinical trial registration: ISRCTN14732216.

Data collection

All data were collected and coded to ensure anonymity according to the current legal requirements in Spain.

At the initial clinical visit (V1), the conditions and objectives of the study were explained. The details were summarised in a document, which was presented to the patient who then signed the informed consent form.

Clinical-epidemiological variables At the baseline visit (V1), data collected included: age, number of different partners participating in anal intercourse in the previous 12 months, and over the whole sexual life of the participant; use of prophylactics and percentage frequency of their use; work status (actively employed, unemployed, retired), education level, smoking habit (packets/year), alcohol abuse (standard units of alcohol (SUA) consumed per day); intra-venous drug abuse (IVDA); HIV infection route, months since HIV diagnosis, CDC status, CD4 nadir (considered to be the lowest level of CD4 throughout evolution of HIV), months of anti-retroviral therapy (ART), current line of ART, virological failure (considered to be two consecutives viral load of HIV over 50 copies/μL), concomitant treatment. Other diseases included chronic viral hepatitis B infection (VHB), or hepatitis C (VHC), syphilis, other sexually transmitted diseases (STD), history of anal and/or genital condylomas and the therapy employed, current condylomas, latent active or treated tuberculosis infection.

At clinical visits at 2 and 6 months (V2 and V3), the data collected (again) were number of different anal-sex partners, use of condoms, ART therapy (adherence, change, relapse), appearance of STD or condylomas. The adverse events assessment system employed was a questionnaire that included the most frequent local reactions such as fever, nausea, vomiting, dizziness, syncope, headache and others such as allergic reaction, pruritus, difficulty breathing and/or wheezing. Rare occurrences included lymphadenopathies, chest and lower-limb pain, confusion, chills, muscle pain. The adverse events (AE) were graded on a scale of 1–4. In case of AE grade 4, the blind of the vial administered was broken and, if the code identified the vaccine, the reaction was communicated immediately to the relevant drug-vigilance authorities.

Blood analyses At visits V1, V2 and V3 full blood haemogram and blood chemistry analysis were measured, together with CD4, CD8 lymphocytes counts, and HIV viral load (VL).

Antibodies against the 4 genotypes of the qHPV vaccine were determined after the 3rd dose, at 7th month. The analyses were performed in the microbiology department of the hospital by the same microbiologist of the research team (AS). The assays were performed using HPVG ELISA commercial kit (DIA.PRO, Milano, Italy), according to the manufacturer's instructions. The ELISA kit measures antibodies against the major capsidic protein (L1) of HPV types 6, 11, 16, 18. The blood samples collected in the clinic were centrifuged in the laboratory, frozen at −20 °C and thawed for use at the time of the assay. The results were expressed qualitatively as positive or negative.

High-resolution anoscopy (HRA) (at V1) All the recruited patients had an anoscopy performed and a biopsy taken following 3% acetic acid instillation and Lugol. Biopsies were taken of acetic-white change and Lugol-negative zones, and normal mucosa, with a minimum of 1 biopsy in each of the four quadrants (right, left, anterior, posterior). The colposcopy equipment employed was Zeiss 150 fc©.

PCR of the HPV and anal cytology (at V1): 2 mucosa samples were taken from the anal canal with cotton swabs soaked in physiologic saline serum. The samples were stored in liquid medium (Thin Prep® Pap Test) for the detection and genotyping of the HPV using the polymerase chain reaction (PCR) qualitative technique (Linear Array HPV Genotyping Test) performed in a Gene Amp PCR System 9700 thermocycler (Applied Biosystems, Roche, Switzerland). Cytology evaluation was with the Thin Prep® Pap Test (Thin Prep Processor 2000, Hologic Corp, USA). Both samples were sent to the anatomy–pathology laboratory where the same senior pathologist of the research team (JE) carried out the cytology evaluation, validation of PCR methodology, and histology analyses. HPV genotypes 16, 18, 26, 31, 33, 35, 39, 45, 51–53, 56, 58, 59, 66, 68, 73 and 82 were considered high-risk-HPV (HR-HPV). Genotypes 6, 11, 34, 40, 42–44, 54, 55, 57, 61, 70–72, 81, 83, 84 and 89 were considered low-risk-HPV (LR-HPV). The HPV-18 virus species was classified as genotypes 39, 45, 59, 68; and of the HPV-16 species as genotypes 31, 33, 35, 52, 58, 67 [27]. The cytology classification was that of Bethesda [28] which classifies the lesions into 3 types: atypical squamous cells (ASC) (atypical squamous cells undetermined significance [ASC-US], and atypical squamous cells that cannot exclude high grade squamous intraepithelial lesion [ASC-H]), LSIL and HSIL. The histology classification employed was the Squamous Terminology (LAST) Standardization Project for HPV that segregates the lesions as LSIL (AIN1/condyloma), HSIL (AIN2, AIN3), and invasive carcinoma (ASCC) [29].

Quadrivalent (HPVs 6/11/16/18) vaccine and placebo: subjects were randomly assigned in a 1:1 ratio to receive vaccine or placebo at day 1, month 2 and month 6. The HPV vaccine was the quadrivalent HPV vaccine (Gardasil©; Merck Research Laboratories). Vaccine or placebo was administered as a 0.5 ml injection in the deltoid muscle (with all three doses administered in the same arm). Placebo was the same quantity (0.5 mL) of excipient provided to us by the hospital's pharmacy department. The placebo had 0.5 mL of "Solvent for injectable solutions", this is water used in the preparation of injectable with <1 mmol of Na. All vials were numbered according to patient assignment, and kept until the end of the study.

Sample size

Based on our own data, 67.2% of HIV MSM patients have a pathological anal biopsy and, of these, 29.8% have HSIL (≥AIN2) with a rate of colonization by high-risk genotypes of 74.2% [30]. To demonstrate a reduction of at least 50% with the administration of the qHPV vaccine, with a statistical power of 80% and a level of significance of 5%, it would be necessary to include 29 patients per group. Nevertheless, we increased the sample to 60 in each arm with an intention to strengthen the statistical power to 98%.

Randomisation

For allocation of the participants, a computer generated a list of random numbers that was assigned to each patient. Randomization sequence was created using Epidat (Epidat 4.2, 2016. Consellería de Sanidade, Xunta de Galicia, España; Organización Panamericana de la salud (OPS-OMS); Universidad CES, Colombia) statistical software. Participants were randomly assigned following simple randomization procedures to experimental or placebo groups. The person in charge of generating and keeping the list was not part of the research team and did not participate in evaluation or enrollment of patients, therefore guaranteeing patient blinding. This was a double-blind study and randomization was prior to any study interventions.

Statistical methodology

Descriptive analyses

Descriptions of the principal variables collected in the study were, for the quantitative variables, measures of central tendencies and dispersion: mean, standard deviation, median, percentiles, and for the qualitative variables, absolute and relative frequencies. The prevalence with 95% confidence interval (CI) was calculated for HPV and the dysplastic lesions of anal mucosa.

Bivariate analysis was employed to assess the different factors associated with infection by HR-HPV genotypes. For quantitative variables, the Student t test for independent variables with a normal distribution, or the Mann–Whitney test in case of non-normal distribution were used to compare means. The χ^2 test of Pearson or Fisher test was used to compare qualitative variables, depending on the criteria for use. The Kolmogorov–Smirnov test was applied to compare different variables fulfilling the hypothesis of normality of distribution. The FDR correction for multiple comparisons was applied [31].

Multivariate analyses were applied using Poisson regression analysis. Variables that were statistically significant in the bivariate analysis and those that were considered clinically relevant were introduced into the model. The variables were entered into the model using a forward stepwise selection with a probability of between 0.05 and 0.10 for each entry.

All the tests had a probability level of 0.05 for statistical significance. The SPSS package (version 19) and Stata Statistical Software: Release 12 was used throughout.

Results

Study population: screening

Between May 15th, 2012 and May 15th, 2014, 162 subjects were screened. Mean age was 37.9 years; CD4 nadir was 337.8 cells/μL; 91.4% of the patients were receiving ART and had a mean CD4 of 688.5 cells/μL; only 3.3% of patients were in virological failure. The epidemiological, clinical and analytical variables are summarised in Table 1.

In anal mucosa, 26.3% of patients had genotype HPV16, 12.8% HPV18, 17.3% HPV6, 13.5% HPV11, 4.5% had simultaneous infection with oncogenic genotypes 16 and 18. 36.9% had HPV18 species and 50% HPV16 species. Finally, anal mucosa biopsy analysis showed that 40.1% were normal, 45.7% LSIL and 14.2% HSIL (Table 2). The cytology, PCR of HPV and anal biopsy results are summarised in Table 2.

Of the 162 patients, 129 (79.6%) were finally included in the trial; 30 (18.5%) were excluded for not fulfilling the selection criteria and 3 (1.8%) for withdrawal of consent; 66 (51.2%) were vaccinated while 63 (48.8%) received placebo; 128 (99.2%) received 3 doses of the vaccine (or placebo) and completed the first 6 months of follow-up. One participant left the country following the 1st vaccination, and was lost to follow-up (Fig. 1).

Table 1 Baseline demographic of HIV-positive MSM screened

Variables	HIV-MSM patients n = 162
Mean age; years ±SD	37.9 ± 10.2
Spanish, n (%)	153 (94.2)
Primary school, n (%)	21 (13)
Secondary school; technical school, n (%)	53 (32.7)
University, n (%)	88 (54.3)
Median months of sexual activity (P_{25}–P_{75})	216 (120–300)
Median of anal-receptive sexual partners in previous 12 months (P_{25}–P_{75})	1 (1–5)
Overall median number of sexual partners, (P_{25}–P_{75})	70 (20–250)
Condom users, n (%)	127 (78.4)
Median percentage of condom use, (P_{25}–P_{75})	100% (50–100%)
History of condylomatosis, n (%)	47 (29)
Current condylomatosis, n (%)	48 (29.6)
Syphilis treated, n (%)	35 (21.6)
Latent treated tuberculosis, n (%)	10 (11.8)
Chronic HCV infection, n (%)	4 (4.7)
Chronic HBV infection, n (%)	1 (1.2)
Smoking habit, n (%)	33 (38.8)
Ex-smoker, n (%)	12 (14.1)
Ex-IVDA, n (%)	1 (1.2)
Alcohol, median SUA, (P_{25}–P_{75})	1 (0–1)
Prior AIDS diagnosis, n (%), 95% CI	27.8 (45)
Median time of HIV duration, months (P_{25}–P_{75})	57 (24.5–120)
CD4 nadir, cells/μL, (±SD)	337.8 (±205)
Treatment naïve, n (%)	14 (8.6)
Median ART, months (P_{25}–P_{75})	37 (13–88)
Median lines of ART, n (P_{25}–P_{75})	1 (1–2)
Virological failure, n (%), 95% CI	5 (3.3)
Baseline CD4, cells/μL (±SD)	688 (±256.4)
Baseline CD8, cells/μL (±SD)	976.5 (±399.4)
Baseline viral load, log10 (±SD)	3.74 (±4.5)

HCV hepatitis C virus, *HBV* hepatitis B virus, *LSIL* low-squamous intra-epithelial lesion, *HSIL* high-squamous intra-epithelial lesion, *ASC* indeterminate lesion, *HPV* human papilloma virus, *SUA* standard unit of alcohol, *Ex-IVDA* ex-intravenous drug abuser, *HR-HPV* high risk HPV, *LR-HPV* low risk HPV, *SD* standard deviation, *IQR* interquartile range

Patients enrolled in clinical trial

The patients who received placebo were similar to those who received the vaccine with respect to age, variables related to HIV, ART, others STD, number of lifetime sexual partners, years of sexual relationships and tobacco consumption. The variables are summarised in Table 3.

The group of patients receiving the vaccine and the placebo were similar in relation to the PCR of HPV, cytology and anal histology (Table 4).

Table 2 HPV PCR, cytology and anoscopy variables of the screening population

Variables	n = 162
HPV PCR positive, n (%)	n = 156
LR-HPV	90 (57.7)
HR-HPV	71 (73.7)
HR and LR-HPV	76 (48.7)
Vaccine genotypes, n (%)	
HPV6	27 (17.3)
HPV11	21 (13.5)
HPV16	41 (26.3)
HPV18	20 (12.8)
HPV16 and HPV18	7 (4.5)
HPV of the HPV16 species (31, 33, 35, 52, 58, 67)	80 (50%)
HPV of the HPV18 species (39, 45, 59, 68)	59 (36.9%)
Anal cytology, n (%)	n = 160
Normal	62 (38.8)
LSIL	76 (47.5)
HSIL	9 (5.6)
ASCUS	13 (8.1)
Anoscopy histology, n (%)	n = 162
Normal	65 (40.1)
LSIL	74 (45.7)
HSIL	23 (14.2)
ASCC	0

LSIL low squamous intra-epithelial lesion, *HSIL* high squamous intra-epithelial lesion, *ASC-US* atypical squamous cells undetermined significance, *HPV* human papillomavirus, *HR-HPV* high-risk HPV, *LR-HPV* low-risk HPV

Safety of qHPV vaccine

Adverse events (AEs) were higher in the placebo group compared to vaccine group at the time of the first dose (87% vs. 54%; p = 0.0001); the most common being injection-site pain (83.6% vs. 56.1%; p = 0.0001). As for the second dose, there were no significant differences in the frequencies of AEs in general between the Vaccine vs. placebo arms (89.4% vs. 98.4%; p = 0.06), but there were differences once more in regards to pain (87.8% vs. 98.4%; p = 0.0001). Finally, at the third dose, the AEs were higher in the placebo arm again (66.7% vs. 91.9%; p = 0.0001), with pain being significantly greater in this arm (67.7% vs. 91.9%; p = 0.0001). No other AEs were observed. Based on our laboratory values, we observed no patients in either arm with grade 3–4 analytical abnormalities (Table 5).

Similarly, there were no statistically significant differences with respect to the levels of CD4 (at V1: vaccine 668 cells/μL vs. placebo 772 cells/μL, p = 0.5; at V2: vaccine 733 cells/μL vs. placebo 692 cells/μL, p = 0.89; at V3: vaccine 705 cells/μL vs. placebo 702 cells/μL, p = 0.94) and HIV viral load [(at V1: median vaccine 0 copies/mL (IQR 0–0) vs. median placebo 0 (IQR 0–20.5), p = 0.38;

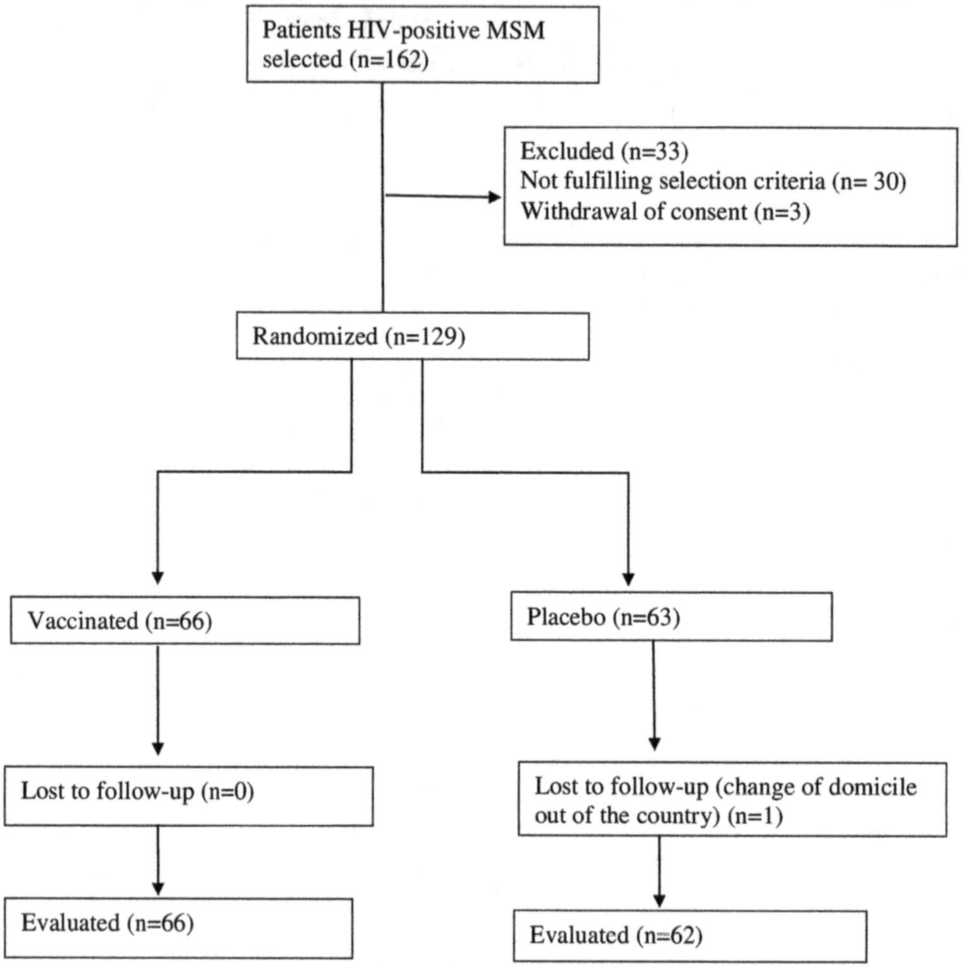

Fig. 1 Flow of subjects through the study

at V2: median vaccine 0 (IQR 0–0) vs. median placebo 0 (IQR 0–20.5), p = 0.9; and at V3: median vaccine 0 (IQR 0–0) vs. median placebo 0 (IQR 0–10.5), p = 0.98)].

Immunogenicity of qHPV vaccine

Of those vaccinated, 76% had antibodies (Ab) against HPV at 7 month vs. 30.2% of those receiving placebo (p = 0.0001). There was no record of the baseline (V0/screening) HPV antibody status of the patients.

Risk factors associated with the presence of HR-HPV genotypes

Bivariate analysis

The following variables were observed to be protective factors against the infection of genotypes of HR-HPV in the anal mucosa: age, i.e. being older (without HR-HPV: 42.1 years vs. with HR-HPV 36.3, p = 0.02); duration of ART (without HR-HPV: 60.5 months vs. 28 months; p = 0.008); and months since HIV diagnosis (without HR-HPV: 74 vs. 54; p = 0.02). Conversely, we found the following predictive factors: early age of sexual activity commencement (without HR-HPV: 21 years vs. 17 years; p = 0.017); and HIV viral load ≥200 copies/mL (without HR-HPV: 2.3% vs. 17.9%, p = 0.01) (Table 6).

Multivariable analysis

In the multivariate analyses were applied using Poisson regression analysis., we only observed older age to be a protective factor against infection by oncogenic virus (RR: 0.97; 95% CI 0.96–0.99) and, as a risk factors the early commencement of sexual activity (RR: 1.35; 95% CI 1.001–1.811) and viral load >200 copies/mL (RR: 1.42; 95% CI 1.172–1.732) (Table 6).

Discussion

In this clinical trial conducted in Spanish HIV-positive MSM population, no patients had grade 3–4 adverse events (AE) related to the vaccine administration. The

Table 3 Baseline demographics of HIV-positive MSM enrolled in clinical trial

	HIV-MSM vaccine (n = 66)	HIV-MSM placebo (n = 63)	p*
Age, years; mean (±SD)	37.3 (±10.6)	40.5 (±10.02)	0.082
Spanish nationality, n (%)	63 (95.5)	60 (95.2)	0.2
University education, n (%)	34 (51.5)	35 (55.5)	0.56
Partners in the previous 12 months; median (IQR)	1 (1–3)	1 (1–5)	0.8
Life-time partners; n, median (IQR)	50 (20–300)	100 (45–350)	0.041*
Years of sexual activity; median (IQR)	17 (9–24)	21 (13–27)	0.025*
Condom use, n (%)	53 (80.3)	47 (74.6)	0.4
Perianal/genital condylomas at screening, n (%)	20 (30.3)	20 (31.7)	0.86
History of condylomas, n (%)	19 (28.8)	15 (23.8)	0.52
Duration of HIV; mean months (IQR)	58 (26–120)	77 (37–138)	0.2
History of AIDS; n (%)	19 (28.8)	21 (33.3)	0.58
CD4 mean nadir; cells/μL, (±SD)	336 (±227.3)	334.2 (±193.7)	0.96
CD4 mean; cells/μL (±SD)	733 (±252.7)	710.4 (±266.6)	0.62
CD8 mean; cells/μL (±SD)	999.9 (±463.6)	992.2 (±374.9)	0.98
VL of HIV log10; copies/mL (±SD)	3.76 (±4.5)	3.67 (±4.46)	0.8
VL <50 copies/mL, n (%)	53 (80.3)	53 (84.1)	0.57
Virological failure, n (%)	1 (1.5)	3 (4.8)	0.29
Median duration of ART; months (IQR)	42 (17–86)	43 (17–129)	0.42
Number of lines of ART, median (IQR)	1 (1–2)	1 (1–2)	0.56
Syphilis treated, n (%)	16 (24.2)	12 (19.1)	0.47
Other STD, n (%)	11 (16.6)	12 (19.1)	0.72
Latent tuberculosis treated, n (%)	5 (7.6)	10 (15.9)	0.14
HCV, n (%)	2 (3)	2 (3.2)	1
HBV, n (%)	2 (3)	0 (0)	0.49
Smoking, packets/year, median (IQR)	0.2 (0–1)	6.5 (0–18)	0.008*
Ex-smoking, n (%)	10 (15)	13 (20.6)	0.0.42
Ex-IVDA, n (%)	1 (1.5)	0 (0)	0.42
Alcohol (standard units of alcohol; SUA)	0 (0–1)	0.4 (0–1.4)	0.15

p*: $p < 0.05$

* After applying the FDR correction for multiple comparisons, none of the 3 variables we statistically significant

commonest AE was local injection-site pain which was more frequent in the placebo group. In a contrasting result [22] a different (vaccine adjuvant) placebo was used, but this result is negligible. There were no changes in the HIV viral load or levels of CD4 with any of the doses used, consistent with another study [25]. Finally, in another randomized, double-blind clinical trial that compared the bivalent vs. quadrivalent vaccine (Cervarix© vs. Gardasil©, is the one we employed) in HIV-infected adults; mild injection site reactions were more common in the Cervarix© group than in the Gardasil© group (91.1% vs. 69.6%; $p = 0.02$) and no serious EA occurred [32], despite the fact that both had a similar adjuvant.

With respect to immunogenicity, in our study 76% of patients receiving the vaccine had measurable antibody levels at the 1th month following administration of the 3rd dose of the vaccine. Although this was significantly higher in the vaccine arm, the lack of baseline antibody levels precludes a definite conclusion that the vaccine is immunogenic. The prevalence of patients with detectable antibody against HPV is lower than in a previous clinical trial carried-out in HIV MSM patients in whom 98% of the patients developed antibodies against the four HPV genotypes in the quadrivalent vaccine [25]. These differences could result from different assay sensitivities, and there is a lack of a standardized diagnostic test to measure Ab of HPV in blood; the different study design in that trial limits direct comparison with this study; the clinical significance of antibodies following qHPV vaccination is not known. On the other hand, there is no established relationship between antibody titres and vaccine efficacy in EGL, anal intra-epithelial neoplasia, and cervix, vulva or vaginal cancer [25, 26]. The response rates in this study were lower than previously reported [33], though they

Table 4 Baseline HPV PCR and HRA results of patients enrolled

Variable	HIV-MSM vaccine (n = 66)	HIV-MSM placebo (n = 63)	p*
PCR of HPV			
LR-HPV, n (%)	39 (59)	34 (53.9)	0.63
HR-HPV, n (%)	46 (69.7)	44 (69.8)	0.87
HR and LR HPV, n (%)	28 (42.4)	31 (49.2)	0.39
Number of HR-HPV (IQR)	1 (0–2)	2 (0–3)	0.22
Number of LR-HPV (IQR)	1 (0–2)	1 (0–2)	0.94
Genotypes, n (%)			
HPV6	11 (16.6)	8 (12.6)	0.55
HPV11	8 (12.1)	7 (11.1)	0.88
HPV16	15 (22.7)	15 (23.8)	0.85
HPV16 species	22 (33.3)	24 (38.1)	0.49
HPV18	4 (6.1)	5 (7.9)	0.74
HPV18 species	18 (27.3)	22 (34.9)	0.35
Cytology, n (%)			
Normal	26 (39.4)	27 (42.9)	0.69
LSIL	34 (51.5)	26 (41.3)	0.24
HSIL	1 (1.5)	4 (6.3)	0.21
ASC	5 (7.6)	6 (9.5)	0.69
HRA, n (%)			
Normal	33 (0.5)	29 (46)	0.65
LSIL	33 (0.5)	34 (53.9)	0.65

HRA high resolution anoscopy

* $p < 0.05$

Table 5 On-treatment safety and tolerability

Adverse events	V1: vaccine vs. placebo N (%) p*	V2: vaccine vs. placebo N (%) p*	V3: vaccine vs. placebo N (%) p*
Total AE	36 (54.4) vs. 55 (87.3) 0.0001	59 (89.4) vs. 62 (98.4) 0.06	44 (66.7) vs. 57 (91.9) 0.0001
Injection-site pain	37 (56.1) vs. 53 (83.6) 0.0001	58 (87.8) vs. 62 (98.4) 0.0001	45 (67.7) vs. 57 (91.9) 0.0001
Local itching	10 (15.1) vs. 5 (8) 0.13	1 (1.5) vs. 1 (1.6) 0.37	1 (1.5) vs. 0 0.33
Syncope	2 (3) vs. 0 0.5	1 (1.5) vs. 0 0.33	1 (1.5) vs. 0 0.33
AE leading to treatment discontinuation	0 vs. 0	0 vs. 0	0 vs. 0
Deaths	0 vs. 0	0 vs. 0	0 vs. 0
Serious AE	0 vs. 0	0 vs. 0	0 vs. 0
Grade 3 or 4 abnormalities	0 vs. 0	0 vs. 0	0 vs. 0

Treatment-emergent grade 3 or 4 abnormalities defined by laboratory values: ALT >5.0 × upper limit of normal (ULN); AST >5.0 × ULN; total bilirubin >2.5 × ULN

* $p < 0.05$

were obtained in an older population and using a different assay technique. Possible causes for a lower antibody titre include prior infection not detectable by anal HPV DNA testing or serology [26], and being MSM [34].These patients may have a worse immunogenic response to the vaccine compared to heterosexuals as implied in a previous clinical trial with the nine-valent HPV vaccine [34] in which, for all HPV genotypes, the geometric mean titers at month 7 were numerically lower in MSM than in heterosexual men [34].

The prevalence of HR-HPV in the anal mucosa in our group of HIV-positive MSM patients was 73.7%. Similar percentages have been communicated in previous research in seropositive MSM [31]. However, in a

Table 6 Bivariate and multivariable analysis of factors associated with HR-HPV infection

Factors	HIV-MSM with HR-HPV (n = 117)	HIV-MSM without HR-HPV (n = 43)	p*	RR; (95% CI)
Age; mean years (±SD)	36.3 (9.7)	42.1 (10.4)	0.001	0.98; (0.96–0.99)
Age ≥ 50 years, n (%)	12 (10.3)	11 (25.6)	0.014	
University education, n (%)	68 (58.1)	19 (44.1)	0.2	
Partners in the previous 12 months; median (IQR)	1 (1–5)	1 (0.75–4.25)	0.24	
Life-time partners; median (IQR)	80 (25–300)	50 (19–212.5)	0.38	
Time since commencement of sexual activity (years); median (IQR)	17 (9–24)	21 (13–27)	0.036	1.35; (1.001–1.811)
Condom use, n (%)	96 (82.1)	29 (67.4)	0.048	1.14; (0.857–1.509)
% condom use; median (IQR)	100 (70–100)	98 (0–100)	0.066	
Perianal/genital warts, n (%)	31 (26.5)	16 (37.2)	0.19	1.57; (0.466–1.716)
History of warts, n (%)	34 (29.1)	13 (30.2)	0.8	
Smoking, packets/year; median (IQR)	1.8 (0–12)	0.7 (0–16)	0.8	
	21 (17.9)	7 (16.3)	0.8	
Ex-smoker, n (%)	1 (0.85)	0 (0)	1	
Ex-IVDA, n (%)	0.14 (0–1)	0 (0–1.3)	0.66	
Duration of HIV; mean (IQR)	54 (19–118)	74 (49.2–139.7)	0.002	0.998; (0.995–1.002)
CD4 mean nadir; cells/μL (± SD)	345.9 (±217.9)	323.1 (±164.5)	0.54	
Treatment naïve	12 (10.3)	2 (4.6)	0.35	1.33; (0,99–1.77)
VL of HIV, log10 (±SD)	3.8 (±4.5)	3.4 (±4.2)	0.8	
VL <50 copies/mL, n (%)	90 (76.9)	39 (90.7)	0.051	
VL ≥200 copies/mL, n (%)	21 (17.9)	1 (2.3)	0.01	1.42; (1.172–1.732)
CD4 mean; cells/μL, (±SD)	683.7 (±263.6)	717.3 (±228.3)	0.46	
CD8 mean; cells/μL (±SD)	984.1 (±407.2)	996.9 (±402.7)	0.86	
Prior AIDS diagnosis; n (%)	33 (28.2)	11 (25.6)	0.74	
Median duration of ART; months (IQR)	28 (10–95)	60.5 (31.5–124.5)	0.08	1.002; (0.998–1.005)
	1 (1–2)	1 (1–2)	0.59	
Syphilis, n (%)	28 (23.9)	7 (16.2)	0.29	
Others STD, n (%)	22 (18.8)	7 (16.3)	0.8	
HCV, n (%)	4 (3.4)	1 (2.3)	1	
HBV, n (%)	1 (0.85)	2 (4.6)	0.49	

* $p < 0.05$

population of HIV-negative MSM patients, the prevalence of HPV in anal mucosa was much lower, around 40% [35]. Our patients, similar to others who are immunocompromised, present a higher number of viruses, possibly due to the lower capacity of clearance of the virus from the anal mucosa [36].

With respect to the genotypes against which the qHPV generates immunity, in our cohort we found, in the pre-vaccination analyses, that the most frequent of all was genotype 16, which was present in 1 of every 4 patients, and only 4.5% of our patients had a simultaneous infection by two oncogenic genotypes (16 and 18). On analysing the combinations of viruses pertaining to the species 16 and 18, we observed that up to 50% of the study participants were infected by the viral species HPV16 and 37% by the species HPV18. HPV16 is the genotype that has been shown most frequently, in the majority of published studies, to be associated with anogenital pathology in both genders [37, 38]. HIV infection is among the associated risk factors in MSM patients [39]. This low level of simultaneous infection by HPV16 and 18 of only 4.5%, and for both viruses separately >30%, implies that an important proportion of MSM seropositive patients of this cohort could benefit from the HPV vaccine. This hypothesis will be tested at the conclusion of the current, ongoing, trial. However, we must take into account that the ACTG A5298 study carried out in both seropositive men and women did not support routine vaccination of older HIV-positive adults for prevention of anal HPV infection or improving anal HSIL [26]. The main disadvantage of this clinical trial was that data concerning effectiveness of the vaccine in both women and men were analyzed together. Considering some clinical trials detected differences in the formation of antibodies between genders, being lower in older males, this could translate into lower global efficacy rates [27]. Patients in this study also had a higher median age compared to previous studies [26].

We observed that only 14.2% had HSIL lesions at V1; results similar to those communicated by other authors [31, 40], and much lower than the earlier findings of other studies in which the level was 54% [41]. These differences are possibly due to the historical period in which the researches were conducted. Not only our study but also those cited above [30, 37] were conducted in the period of late ART (after 2005) and another in the era of early ART (before 2005) [42].

In relation to the risk-factors associated with the infection of HR-HPV in the anal mucosa, multivariate analyses identified viral load ≥200 copies/mL as risk predictor for HR-HPV infection, whilst older age was protective. A study, that analysed the incidence and clearance of anal high-risk human papillomavirus in HIV-positive MSM, found that those with low HIV-RNA-viral load had the highest clearance [43]. Classically, youth has been associated with the infection of HPV in anal mucosa [8]. Data have been presented showing that, in patients >50 years of age, the virus prevalence is only 5.9% [44]. In our study patients over 50 years had a prevalence of HR-HPV infection of only 10%, being statistically significant ($p = 0.014$). In other hand, there are evidences that naturally acquired antibodies to HPV-16, and to a lesser extent HPV-18, are associated with some reduced risk of subsequent infection with the same HPV type [45, 46].

The principal limitations of our study that need to be highlighted derive from the exclusion criteria which do not permit generalisation of data; 18.7% of patients who underwent screening were excluded because of HSIL (14.2%) or because of simultaneous infection by genotypes 16 and 18 (4.5%). Baseline Ab were also not determined and this event is a potential weakness. The results of our study suggest immunogenicity, but without baseline differences to compare we can't be certain.

Consequently, a further study would be necessary to demonstrate the usefulness of the vaccine in these subsets of patients who had been excluded.

Conclusions

This trial of qHPV vaccine conducted in Spanish HIV-positive MSM patients showed significantly higher anti-HR-HPV antibody titres in vaccinated individuals than in unvaccinated controls. There were no serious adverse events attributable to the vaccine. Although current prevalence of HPV 16/18 is low, a large proportion of men likely have had incident HPV 16/18 infections and cleared them; therefore, they may have natural immunity that protect against subsequent infection. Older age was the protective factor against HR-HPV infection and HIV no suppressed was the risk factor.

Abbreviations

qHPV vaccine: quadrivalent human papillomavirus vaccine; MSM: men having sex with men; HR-HPV: high-risk human papillomavirus; HSIL: High Squamous Intraepithelial Lesions; HIV: human immunodeficiency virus; LSIL: low squamous intra-epithelial lesion; ASCC: anal squamous cell carcinoma; HRA: high-resolution anoscopy; HM: heterosexual males; STD: Sexually Transmitted Diseases; AE: adverse events; VL: viral load; PCR: polymerase chain reaction; ART: anti-retroviral therapy; HBV: hepatitis B viral; HCV: hepatitis C viral.

Authors' contributions

CH-T: conceptualization, methodology; investigation, writing (original draft preparation), and funding adquisition. JE: writing (review), resources, and investigation. AS: resources and investigation. MOM-G, JP, ML-R: supervision, visualization. JR-T and CG-A: software. All authors read and approved the final manuscript.

Author details

[1] Infectious Disease Service, University Hospital Virgen de las Nieves, Granada, Spain. [2] Pathology Service, University Hospital Virgen de las Nieves, Granada, Spain. [3] Infectious Disease Unit of the Hospital Ciudad de Jaén, Jaén, Spain. [4] Microbiology Service, University Hospital Virgen de las Nieves, Granada, Spain.

Acknowledgements

We thank Manuela Expósito for her expert statistical help; Mercedes Álvarez-Romero for specialist nursing care and data collection; Marina Gutierrez-Ariza for expertise with the HPV PCR technology; Rosario Javier-Martínez and Antonio Tapia-Gomez for patient management.

Editorial assistance by D. Samantha Elizabeth de Jesus.

Competing interests

The authors affirm that there were no conflicts of interest in the conduct of the study.

Funding

The study was supported by a grant (#PI-0615-2011) from the Public Health and Social Progress Foundation of the Government of Andalucia [*La Fundación Pública Andaluza Progreso y Salud de la Consejería de Igualdad Salud y Política Social*] in its 2011 convocation.

References

1. Shiels MS, Cole SR, Kirk GD, Poole C. A meta-analysis of the incidence of non-AIDS cancers in HIV-infected individuals. J Acquir Immune Defic Syndr. 2009;52:611–22.
2. Palefsky JM, Holly E, Ralston MR, et al. Prevalence and risk factors for human papillomavirus infection of the anal canal in human immunodeficiency virus (HIV)-positive and HIV-negative homosexual men. J Infect Dis. 1998;177:361–7.
3. Pinzone MR, Fiorica F, Di Rosa M, et al. Non-AIDS-defining cancers among HIV-infected people. Eur Rev Med Pharmacol Sci. 2012;16:1377–88.
4. Fraunhoiz IB, Harberl A, Klauke S, Gute P, Rodel CM. Long-term effects of chemotherapy for anal cancer in patients with HIV infection: oncological outcomes, immunological status, and the clinical course of HIV disease. Dis Colon Rectum. 2014;57:423–31.
5. Critchlow CW, Surawicz CM, Holmes KK, Kuypers J, Daling JR, Hawes SE, et al. Prospective study of high grade anal squamous intraepithelial neoplasia in a cohort of homosexual men: influence of HIV infection, immunosuppression and human papillomavirus infection. AIDS. 1995;9:1255–62.

6. Hidalgo-Tenorio C, Rivero-Rodriguez M, Gil-Anguita C, et al. Antiretroviral therapy as a factor protective against anal dysplasia in HIV-infected males who have sex with males. PLoS ONE. 2014;27:e92376. doi:10.1371/journal.pone.0092376.
7. Salati SA, Al Kadi A. Anal cancer—a review. Int J Heal Sci. 2012;6:206–30.
8. Nyitray AG, Carvalho da Silva RJ, Baggio ML, et al. Six-month incidence, persistence, and factors associated with persistence of anal human papillomavirus in men: the HPV in Men Study. J Infect Dis. 2011;204:1711–22.
9. Piketty C, Darragh TM, Da Costa M, et al. High prevalence of anal human papillomavirus infection and anal cancer precursors among HIV-infected persons in the absence of anal intercourse. Ann Intern Med. 2003;183:453–9.
10. Hidalgo-Tenorio C, Rivero Rodríguez M, Concha A, et al. CD4 lymphocytes as a protective factor against infection by oncogenic genotypes of human papillomavirus in the anal mucosa of men who have sex with human immunodeficiency virus positive men. Med Clin (Barc). 2013;140:193–9.
11. Chin-Hong PV, Berry JM, Cheng SC, et al. Comparison of patient- and clinician-collected anal cytology samples to screen for human papillomavirus-associated anal intraepithelial neoplasia in men who have sex with men. Ann Intern Med. 2008;149:300–6.
12. Nathan M, Singh N. Performance of anal cytology in a clinical setting when measured against histology and high-resolution anoscopy findings. AIDS. 2010;24:373–9.
13. Salit IE, Lytwyn A, Raboud J, et al. The role of cytology (Pap test) and human papillomavirus testing in anal cancer screening. AIDS. 2011;24:1307–13.
14. Walts AE, Thomas P, Bose S. Anal cytology: is there a role for reflex HPV DNA testing? Diagn Cytopathol. 2005;33:152–6.
15. Goldstone SE, Enyinna ChS, Davis TW. Detection of oncogenic human papillomavirus and other predictors of anal high-grade dysplasia in men who have sex with men with abnormal cytology. Dis Colon Rectum. 2009;52:31–9.
16. Berry JM, Palefsky JM, Jay N, Cheng SC, Darragh TM, Chin-Hong PV. Performance characteristics of anal cytology and human paillomavirus testing in patients with high resolution anoscopy-guided biopsy of high grade anal intraepithelial neoplasia. Dis Colon Rectum. 2009;52:239–47.
17. Padilla-España L, Repiso-Jiménez B, Fernández-Sánchez F, et al. Usefulness of human papillomavirus testing in anal intraepithelial neoplasia screening in a risk behaviour population. Enferm Infecc Microbiol Clin. 2014. doi:10.1016/j.eimc.2014.03.008.
18. Hidalgo-Tenorio C, Rivero-Rodriguez M, Gil-Anguita C, et al. The role of polymerase chain reaction of high-risk human papilloma virus in the screening of high-grade squamous intraepithelial lesions in the anal mucosa of human immunodeficiency virus-positive males having sex with males. PLoS ONE. 2015;10:e0123590. doi:10.1371/journal.pone.0123590.
19. Lam JM, Hoch JS, Tinmouth J, Sano M, Raboud J, Salit IE. Cost-effectiveness of screening for anal precancers in HIV-positive men. AIDS. 2011;25:635–42.
20. Lam JU, Rebolj M, Dugué PA, Bonde J, von Euler-Chelpin M, Lynge E. Condom use in prevention of human papillomavirus infections and cervical neoplasia: systematic review of longitudinal studies. J Med Screen. 2014;21:38–50. doi:10.1177/0969141314522454.
21. de Sanjosé S, Bruni L, Alemany L. HPV in genital cancers (at the exception of cervical cancer) and anal cancers. La Presse Med. 2014;43(12P2):e423–8. doi:10.1016/j.lpm.2014.10.001.
22. Giuliano AR, Palefsky JM, Goldstone S, Moreira ED, Penny ME, Aranda C, et al. Efficacy of quadrivalent HPV vaccine against HPV Infection and disease in males. N Engl J Med. 2011;364:401–11.
23. Hillman RJ, Giuliano AR, Palefsky JM, Goldstone S, Moreira ED Jr, Vardas E, et al. Immunogenicity of the quadrivalent human papillomavirus (type 6/11/16/18) vaccine in males 16 to 26 years old. Clin Vaccine Immunol. 2012;19:261–7.
24. Palefsky JM, Giuliano AR, Goldstone S, et al. HPV vaccine against anal HPV infection and anal intraepithelial neoplasia. N Engl J Med. 2011;365:1576–85.
25. Wilkin T, Lee JY, Lensing SY, Stier EA, Goldstone SE, Berry JM. Safety and immunogenicity of the quadrivalent human papillomavirus vaccine in HIV-1-infected men. J Infect Dis. 2010;202:1246–53.
26. Wilkin T, Chen H, Cespedes M, Paczuski P, Godefrey C, Luque A, et al. ACTG A5298: a phase 3 trial of the quadrivalent HPV vaccine in older HIV + Adults. CROI, febrero 22–25. Boston. USA; 2016.
27. Muñoz N, Bosch FX, de Sanjose S, et al. Epidemiologic classification of human papillomavirus types associated with cervical cancer. N Engl J Med. 2003;348:518–27.
28. Solomon D, Davey D, Kurman R, et al. The 2001 Bethesda system: terminology for reporting results of cervical cytology. JAMA. 2002;287:2114–9.
29. Darragh TM, Colgan TJ, Cox JT, et al. The Lower Anogenital Squamous Terminology Standardization Project for HPV-Associated Lesions: background and consensus recommendations from the College of American Pathologists and the American Society for Colposcopy and Cervical Pathology. J Low Genit Tract Dis. 2012;16:205–42.
30. Hidalgo-Tenorio C, Rivero-Rodriguez M, Gil-Anguita C, et al. Antiretroviral therapy as a factor protective against anal dysplasia in HIV-infected males who have sex with males. PLoS ONE. 2014;27:e92376.
31. Benjamini Y, Hochberg Y. Series B (methodological). J R Stat Soc. 1995;57:289–300.
32. Toft L, Storgaard M, Müller M, Sehr P, Bonde J, Tolstrup M, et al. Comparison of the immunogenicity and reactogenicity of Cervarix and Gardasil human papillomavirus vaccines in HIV-infected adults: a randomized, double-blind clinical trial. J Infect Dis. 2014;209:1165–73.
33. Giuliano AR, Isaacs-Soriano K, Torres BN, Abrahamsen M, Ingles DJ, Sirak BA, et al. Immunogenicity and safety of Gardasil among mid-adult aged men (27–45 years)—the MAM Study. Vaccine. 2015;33:5640–6.
34. Castellsagué X, Giuliano AR, Goldstone S, Guevara A, Mogensen O, Palefsky JM, et al. Immunogenicity and safety of the 9-valent HPV vaccine in men. Vaccine. 2015;33:6892–901.
35. Sendagorta E, Herranz P, Guadalajara H, et al. Prevalence of abnormal anal cytology and high grade squamous intraepithelial lesions among a cohort of HIV-infected men who have sex with men. Dis Colon Rectum. 2014;57:475–81.
36. Goldstone S, Palefsky JM, Giuliano AR, et al. Prevalence of and risk factors for human papillomavirus (HPV) infection among HIV-seronegative men who have sex with men. J Infect Dis. 2011;203:66–74.
37. Kreuter A, Wieland U. Human papillomavirus-associated diseases in HIV-infected men who have sex with men. Curr Opin Infect Dis. 2009;22:109–14.
38. Slama J, Sehnal B, Dusek L, Zima T, Cibula D. Impact of risk factors on prevalence of anal HPV infection in women with simultaneous cervical lesion. Neoplasma. 2015;62:308–14.
39. Li Z, Zhang H, Li X, et al. Anal human papillomavirus genotyping among HIV-positive men who have sex with men in Xi'an, China. PloS ONE. 2015;10:e0125120. doi:10.1371/journal.pone.0125120.
40. Alberts CJ, van Rooijen MS, Prins M, Pawlita M, van der Loeff MFS, Waterboer T. HIV is an important risk factor for human papillomavirus types 16 and 18 seropositivity among sexually active men who have sex with men. Sex Transm Dis. 2015;42:129–34.
41. van der Snoek EM, van der Ende ME, den Hollander JC, Schutten M, Neumann HA, van Doornum GJ. Use of highly active antiretroviral therapy is associated with lower prevalence of anal intraepithelial neoplastic lesions and lower prevalence of human papillomavirus in HIV-infected men who have sex with men. Sex Transm Dis. 2012;39:495–500. doi:10.1097/OLQ.0b013e31825aa764.
42. Palefsky JM, Holly EA, Efirdc JT, et al. Anal intraepithelial neoplasia in the highly active antiretroviral therapy era among HIV-positive men who have sex with men. AIDS. 2005;19:1407–14.
43. Geskus RB, González C, Torres M, Del Romero J, Viciana P, Masiá M, et al. Incidence and clearance of anal high-risk human papillomavirus in HIV-positive men who have sex with men: estimates and risk factors. AIDS. 2016;30:37–44.
44. Parisi SG, Cruciani M, Scaggiante R, et al. Anal and oral human papillomavirus (HPV) infection in HIV infected subjects in Northern Italy: a longitudinal cohort study among men who have sex with men. BMC Infect Dis. 2011;11:150.
45. Castellsagué X, Naud P, Chow SN, Wheeler CM, Germar MJ, Lehtinen M, et al. Risk of newly detected infections and cervical abnormalities in women seropositive for naturally acquired human papillomavirus type 16/18 antibodies: analysis of the control arm of PATRICIA. J Infect Dis. 2014;210:517–34.

10

Comparison of six methods to estimate adherence in an ART-naïve cohort in a resource-poor setting: which best predicts virological and resistance outcomes?

Catherine Orrell[1,6*], Karen Cohen[2], Rory Leisegang[2], David R. Bangsberg[3,4,5], Robin Wood[1†] and Gary Maartens[2†]

Abstract

Background: Incomplete adherence to antiretroviral therapy (ART) results in virologic failure and resistance. It remains unclear which adherence measure best predicts these outcomes. We compared six patient-reported and objective adherence measures in one ART-naïve cohort in South Africa.

Methods: We recruited 230 participants from a community ART clinic and prospectively collected demographic data, CD4 count and HIV-RNA at weeks 0, 16 and 48. We quantified adherence using 3-day self-report (SR), clinic-based pill count (CPC), average adherence by pharmacy refill (PR-average), calculation of medication-free days (PR-gaps), efavirenz therapeutic drug monitoring (TDM) and an electronic adherence monitoring device (EAMD). Associations between adherence measures and virologic and genotypic outcomes were modelled using logistic regression, with the area under the curve (AUC) from the receiver operator characteristic (ROC) analyses derived to assess performance of adherence measures in predicting outcomes.

Results: At week 48 median (IQR) adherence was: SR 100% (100–100), CPC 100% (95–107), PR-average 103% (95–105), PR-gaps 100% (95–100) and EAMD 86% (59–94), and efavirenz concentrations were therapeutic (>1 mg/L) in 92%. EAMD, PR-average, PR-gaps and CPC best predicted virological outcome at week 48 with AUC ROC of 0.73 (95% CI 0.61–0.83), 0.73 (95% CI 0.61–0.85), 0.72 (95% CI 0.59–0.84) and 0.64 (95% CI 0.52–0.76) respectively. EAMD, PR-gaps and PR-average were highly predictive of detection of resistance mutations at week 48, with AUC ROC of 0.92 (95% CI 0.87–0.97), 0.86 (0.67–1.0) and 0.83 (95% CI 0.65–1.0) respectively. SR and TDM were poorly predictive of outcomes at week 48.

Conclusion: EAMD and both PR measures predicted resistance and virological failure similarly. Pharmacy refill data is a pragmatic adherence measure in resource-limited settings where electronic monitoring is unavailable.

Keywords: HIV, Antiretroviral therapy, Adherence, Electronic monitoring, Virological outcome, HIV-1 resistance, Genotyping

*Correspondence: catherine.orrell@hiv-research.org.za
†Robin Wood and Gary Maartens contributed equally to this work
[6] Desmond Tutu HIV Centre, Werner Beit Building North, UCT Faculty of Health Science, Anzio Road, Observatory, Cape Town 7925, South Africa
Full list of author information is available at the end of the article

Background

Adherence is critical to realising the clinical and prevention benefits of ART [1–3]. Despite this, there is no gold standard identifying adherence levels and patterns that place individuals at risk for virologic failure and/or drug resistance [4–6].

A variety of ART adherence measures have been used in both observational and intervention studies. Self-report is the most frequently used method, but is often imprecise and overestimates adherence, similar to clinic-based pill count [4–7]. Pharmacy refill data also overestimate adherence, but have been consistently associated with virological failure and mortality [8–10]. Electronic drug monitoring methods have been closely associated with virologic failure, despite underestimating adherence due to storage and ingestion of medications outside of the device (pocket-doses) [6, 11, 12]. Therapeutic drug concentration monitoring has been associated with virologic outcomes, though its precision relative to other adherence monitoring approaches is poorly understood [3, 13, 14].

Few studies have directly compared the ability of multiple adherence monitoring methods to predict virological failure in one cohort [15–17] or explored their relationship with drug resistance [18].

Our study compared a variety of adherence measures, three widely accessible to clinicians in a resource-poor setting: self-report (SR), clinic-based pill count (CPC) and pharmacy refill data (PR-average); and three requiring additional technology or calculation: therapeutic drug monitoring (TDM), calculation of medication free days or gaps (PR-gaps) and real-time electronic drug monitoring. All adherence measures were collected in a prospective ART-naïve cohort starting first-line ART, in order to explore which measure best predicted virological or resistance outcome at 16 and 48 weeks into treatment.

Methods

Participants and setting

This study is a sub-study of a randomised controlled trial recruited at the Hannan Crusaid Treatment Centre, an outpatient antiretroviral treatment centre in Cape Town, South Africa. This site and the study have been described elsewhere [19, 20]. The cohort included ART-naïve adults and adolescents (≥12 years) starting first-line ART. Participants were eligible for the parent study if they had their own mobile phone, signed an informed consent, and had either a baseline CD4 count below 350 cells/μl or a stage 3 or 4 AIDs-defining illness in keeping with the national HIV guidelines for starting ART [20]. All patients on the parent study with viral load data available at week 16 or week 48 were included in this sub-study.

Standard of care (SoC)

All participants received three group counsellor-driven treatment preparedness sessions prior to commencing ART [21, 22]. They were visited at home by a community care worker to confirm address and ascertain home circumstances. All participants commenced a non-nucleoside reverse transcriptase inhibitor (NNRTI)-based first-line ART regimen. SoC visit frequency and procedures are detailed in Additional file 1: Table S1. *Counts of pill returns* were done at each scheduled clinic visit. Those with a raised HIV-RNA (>1000 copies/ml) or non-optimal clinic-based pill count adherence (<90%) received additional adherence support, which included tailored counselling, monthly drug dispensing and follow-up home-visits. Participants were traced by phone and home visit if they were more than 4 weeks late in attending a scheduled clinic visit.

Study design and procedures

The parent study was a randomised controlled trial, with primary outcome at 48 weeks, investigating the impact of mobile phone message reminders when missed doses were detected by a real-time electronic adherence monitoring device (EAMD) on adherence to ART [20]. This device has been used in other resource-limited settings [23, 24]. This sub-study includes data from participants without reference to study arm.

There were five study visits: screening (week-4), baseline (week 0), weeks 16, 32 and 48, detailed in Table 1. Participants were reimbursed for local travel (~US$2) at each visit and for the three on-study visits (weeks 16, 32 and 48) were given a gift of a T-shirt, bag or mug valued at R80 (~US$8) or less. If participants came to a SoC clinic visit but did not attend the corresponding study visit, tablet return and virological data were extracted from their clinic folder.

Demographic and psychosocial details, including age, gender, weight, height as well as assessments for depression, anxiety and alcohol use, were collected at screening. The 14-question Hospital Anxiety and Depression Score (HADS) was used to assess anxiety and depression and the CAGE score used to assess alcoholism [25, 26]. Blood was drawn for CD4 cell count (FACS Count™, Beckton Dickinson, NJ, USA) and HIV-RNA (HIV-1 RNA 3.0 assay®, Bayer Healthcare, Leverkusen, Germany) at baseline, 16 week and 48 week visits. Mid-dose efavirenz concentrations were determined at weeks 16 and 48. The time of blood draw, and the self-reported time of most recent ART dosing were recorded.

Table 1 Baseline demographic, clinical treatment and psychosocial characteristics of participants

Variable	Full cohort	With VL at week 16	With VL at week 48
Number: *n*	230	160	180
Female sex: *n* (%)	150 (65.2)	108 (67.5)	121 (67.2)
Age in years: mean (SD)	34.5 (9.1)	34.8 (8.9)	35.0 (9.4)
Height (cm): mean (SD)	164.0 (8.6)	164.1 (8.2)	164.0 (8.1)
Weight (kg): median (IQR)	67.3 (57.8–79.6)	67.2 (58.0–80.0)	68.1 (58.7–80.4)
BMI: median (IQR)	24.3 (21.3–29.8)	24.2 (21.5–29.9)	24.6 (21.5–30.7)
WHO stage: *n* (%)			
1	84 (36.5)	58 (36.3)	73 (40.6)
2	47 (20.4)	34 (21.3)	39 (21.7)
3	75 (32.6)	54 (33.8)	51 (28.3)
4	24 (10.4)	14 (8.8)	17 (9.4)
CD4 count (cells/mm^3): median (IQR)	225 (133–287)	229 (132–288)	233 (144–287)
Log HIV-RNA (copies/ml): median (IQR)	4.9 (4.4–5.4)	4.9 (4.4–5.4)	4.8 (4.4–5.4)
NNRTI at start: *n* (%)			
Efavirenz	228 (99.1)	(98)	
Nevirapine	2 (0.9)	2 (1.2)	2 (1.1)
NRTI at start[a]: *n* (%)			
Tenofovir	225 (97.8)	159 (99.4)	177 (98.3)
Zidovudine	4 (1.7)	1 (0.6)	3 (1.7)
Stavudine	1 (0.4)	–	–
HADS depression score of 8 or above (borderline or case)[b]: *n* (%)	74 (32.1)	55 (34.3)	58 (32.2)
HADS anxiety score of 8 or above (borderline or case)[b]: *n* (%)	89 (38.7)	64 (40.0)	70 (38.9)
Non-disclosure: *n* (%)	11 (4.7)	8 (5.0)	7 (3.9)
CAGE score ≥ 2: *n* (%)	35 (15.2)	22 (13.8)	25 (13.9)

[a] All were taking 3TC or FTC as a second NRTI

[b] 14-question Hospital Anxiety and Depression Score

Adherence data

For pill counts, average pharmacy refill data and self-recall, the data used was that typically available to clinic staff during a consultation with a patient.

Three-day self-recall (SR)

At weeks 16 and 48, study staff asked each participant: "Did you swallow your pills yesterday/2 days ago/3 days ago?" Percent doses taken over 3 days was calculated from the participants' responses. Study staff were not part of the clinical team. Data were only available if a participant attended the study visit.

Clinic-based pill count (CPC)

Participants were instructed to bring any remaining tablets to each study visit. CPC adherence was calculated using the difference between the number of tablets dispensed and the number returned and dividing by the number of days between the date of dispensing and the current visit date (adjusted for the number of doses per day). At week 16 this would give adherence over the previous 1 month period (last dispensing visit was the SoC visit a week 12) and at week 48 adherence over the previous 2 month period (last dispensing visit was the SoC visit at week 40). For the analyses, only the tablet count related to dosing efavirenz, nevirapine or, for those who switched to second-line, lopinavir/r dosing was used.

Pharmacy refill: average method (PR-average)

An electronic dispensing system (iDART) was used at the site to record the date of ART dispensed and the quantity given to each participant [27, 28]. Obvious errors, such as date and dispensing duplications were removed. A cumulative PR-average measure was obtained at week 16 and week 48 visits by dividing the number of days of efavirenz, nevirapine or lopinavir/r tablets each patient received between study randomisation date and the visit date, by the number of days they were in care over the same period. This method averages adherence across the whole period in question.

Pharmacy refill: gaps method (PR-gaps)

This measure used pharmacy dispensing quantities and refill visit dates to determine the number of medication-free days (days when the participant could not have had medication in hand) in each dispensing period. The number of medication-free days are subtracted from the number of days in the period, and the result divided by the number of days in the period (up to week 16 or up to week 48) to give an adherence percentage [10]. This method identifies days when it was not possible for a patient to have taken medication; and might be expected to yield lower but potentially more accurate median adherence values than the average method.

Therapeutic drug measuring (TDM)

At weeks 16 and 48 visits a sample was taken to quantify mid-dosing interval efavirenz concentrations. Mid-dosing interval samples were drawn in the morning, after dosing the previous evening. Self-reported time of the evening dose was recorded. Samples were kept cold (4 °C) until transfer to the laboratory within 2–3 h of blood draw. Samples were centrifuged at 3500 revolutions/min for 10 min and plasma pipetted into cryovials which were labelled and frozen at −80 °C. Efavirenz concentrations were analysed using a validated LC–MS/MS method. The therapeutic range for mid-dose EFV concentrations is 1–4 mg/L.

EAMD data

All participants received the EAMD on study entry to record daily ART dosing times. The device (Wisepill®) held a week of medication in an internal and removable seven compartment pill box container. Participants were trained to fill these pill boxes themselves and replace them once a week at the same time as they dosed. On opening, a signal was sent via the mobile-phone network to a secure central computer, thus recording tablet taking or treatment interruptions in real time. An adherent day was defined as any recorded EAMD opening from 06h00am on that day to 05h59am the following day. Days with battery voltage <3660 V or no heartbeat were censored (dead battery days). The daily EAMD data for each participant were downloaded from the Wisepill® server. Cumulative adherence data for EAMD was calculated as the number of adherent days divided by the number of days in care, from date of randomisation to either weeks 16 or 48.

Study outcomes

Virological failure

Failure was defined as a single HIV RNA of >400 copies/ml at week 16 or >40 copies/ml at week 48 [29, 30].

HIV-1 drug resistance

Genotype resistance tests were done on those with HIV RNA >500 copies/ml (the minimum HIV-RNA for amplification) at weeks 16 or 48. Nucleic acid was extracted with the NucliSens EasyMag automated extraction system (bioMérieux, Boxtel, The Netherlands). Genotyping was performed by RT-PCR followed by a nested PCR and sequencing of the complete PR gene and RT codons 1–262 (HXB2 numbering: HIV-1 nucleotide positions 2250–4229) and using gene-specific sequencing primers [31]. Participants with one or more major resistance mutation as defined by the 2014 IAS update of drug resistance in HIV-1, causing resistance to ≥1 of the three drugs in their regimen were classified as resistant [32].

Statistical analysis

Data were analysed using Stata 13.0 (Stata Corporation, College Station, USA). Descriptive statistics (number, percentage, median and interquartile ranges) were used to summarise the baseline characteristics of the participant group and to tabulate the adherence data.

All available adherence data were used from each individual who had a HIV-RNA drawn within a 4 week window around week 16 (weeks 12–20) or a 16 week window around week 48 (weeks 32–64) in a per-protocol analysis from the time they entered care until the date of the respective viral load.

Univariate and multivariable logistic regression models were used to explore each adherence measure's relationship to virological failure and genotypic resistance at weeks 16 and 48. Both outcomes were binary, categorised as described above. The data for each adherence variable was continuous, although models were repeated using categorical variables (binary or quartiles) to assess linearity. For the TDM models, the $\log_{10}$ values of EFV mid-dose drug concentrations were used, as $\log_{10}$ values shift the distribution curve of the EFV concentration values toward normal for regression modelling.

Other variables included in the models (age, baseline CD4 cell count and baseline HIV-RNA) were specified prior to the analysis. Receiver Operator Characteristics (ROC) were generated to view the overall predictive power of the univariate and multivariable models. The area under the curve derived from the ROC (AUC ROC), with 95% confidence intervals, was used to compare the prediction of virological failure or resistance by each adherence measure. AUC ROCs were compared using non-parametric methods.

Results

Two-hundred-thirty antiretroviral naïve HIV-positive participants were recruited onto the study between 09 July 2012 and 09 April 2013. Figure 1 is a flow diagram of study participants. Baseline characteristics are described

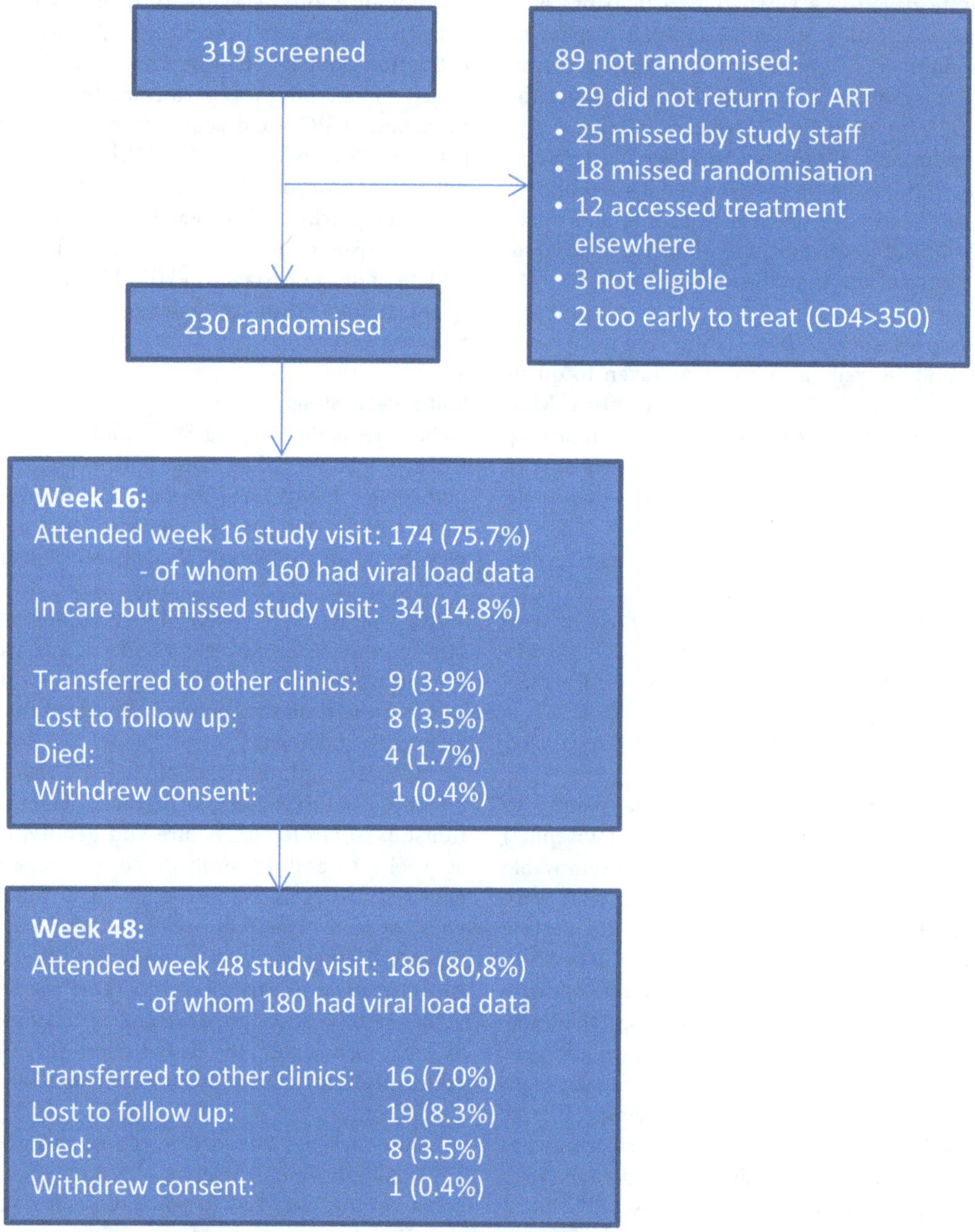

Fig. 1 Flow diagram describing the outcome of the 319 individuals screened and the 230 individuals randomised to the study

in Table 1. The cohort is typical of other African ART cohorts, with a predominance of women. The majority were clinically well. More than a third of the cohort had anxiety or depression scores (>8) that required further assessment and 15% were alcoholic on CAGE (score of ≥2). These data did not significantly impact on adherence in the parent study [20]. A minority had not disclosed their HIV-status to any other person.

Antiretroviral therapy

Efavirenz-based ART was initiated in 228 participants and the remaining two started twice-daily nevirapine-based ART. Both regimens were given with two background nucleoside reverse transcriptase inhibitors. Tenofovir/3TC were used in 97.8% (Table 1). The majority of participants were taking three tablets once a day during the study period.

Retention in care (Fig. 1)

At the end of the study 186 participants remained in care (80.8%) at the study site and a further 16 (7.0%) had transferred to care elsewhere. Eight participants (3.5%) had died and 19 (8.3%) were lost to follow up i.e. had not attended the clinic for more than 12 weeks and were not known to have transferred out or to have died. One participant withdrew consent.

Adherence measures

Table 2 describes the median adherence by each measure at weeks 16 and 48, for all participants with a HIV-RNA drawn at that visit. Three-day self-recall (SR) and efavirenz therapeutic drug monitoring (TDM) data were only available if study visits were completed. Clinic-based pill count (CPC) and pharmacy refill data (PR-gaps and PR-average) were available for all those who attended the clinic. EAMD data were available for all study participants. There were 82,311 participant dosing days recorded, and of these, 8362 (10.1%) were dead battery days.

The subjective measure, SR, gave the highest adherence with the most individuals reporting 100% adherence (median 100%, IQR 100–100%). CPC, PR-gaps and PR-average also gave perfect or close to perfect adherence at week 16 and 48, but widened inter-quartile ranges highlighted some variations within the participants. Cumulative adherence by EAMD showed the lowest median adherence at both visits: 93% (IQR 74–98%) at week 16 and 86% (IQR 59–94%) at week 48. Median efavirenz concentrations were 2.3 (IQR 1.6–4.4) mg/L at week 16, and 2.1 (IQR 1.5–3.4) mg/L at week 48, within the currently recognised therapeutic range of 1.0–4.0 mg/L at both time points.

Table 2 Median adherence percentage with inter-quartile range at each study visit, by adherence measure

	n	Week 16	*n*	Week 48
Self-report (%): median (IQR)	140	100 (100–100)	169	100 (100–100)
Pill count (%): median (IQR)	160	100 (92–100)	178	100 (95–107)
Average pharmacy refill (%): median (IQR)[a]	158	104 (101–105)	178	103 (95–105)
Gaps pharmacy refill (%): median(IQR)[a]	158	100 (100–100)	178	100 (95–100)
EAMD adherence (%): median (IQR)[a]	160	93 (74–98)	180	86 (59–94)
EFV concentration (mg/L): median(IQR)	136	2.3 (1.6–4.4)	156	2.1 (1.5–3.4)
Viral suppression: *n* (%)	160	146 (91.2)	180	153 (85.0)

Self-report and EFV concentrations are measured on the date of the visit. Tablet counts cover the 30 days (week 16) or 60 days (week 48) before the visit. Pharmacy refill and EAMD adherence are cumulative data from baseline to latest time in care

[a] Cumulative per protocol measures

Virological outcome

At week 16, 160 participants had HIV-RNA available within the 12–20 week window and 146 (91.2%) were suppressed to ≤400 copies/ml (Table 1). At week 48, 180 had a HIV-RNA available, of whom 153 (85.0%) were suppressed to ≤40 copies/ml (Table 1). Three participants switched to second-line therapy between weeks 32 and 48 of the study.

Virological failure prediction models

At week 48, adherence measured by EAMD, PR-average, PR-gaps and CPC significantly predicted virological failure both in univariate and multivariable analyses. The odds ratio for these models gives the reduction in the risk of failure for each 10% increase in adherence as quantified by the specified method (Table 3). Neither TDM nor SR adherence predicted failure. For all multivariable models, an increased CD4 cell count at baseline was associated with reduced odds of failure (continuous model examples are presented in Additional file 1: Table S2; and categorical model examples in Additional file 1: Table S3).

ROC curves were generated from the univariate models at 48 weeks, and AUC ROCs were derived to allow for comparison of predictive value across adherence methods (Fig. 2a). Cumulative measures EAMD (ROC AUC 0.73, 95% CI 0.61–0.83), PR-average (ROC AUC 0.73, 95% CI 0.61–0.85), PR-gaps (ROC AUC 0.72, 95% CI 0.59–0.84) and CPC (ROC AUC 0.64, 95% CI 0.52–0.76) best predicted failure at week 48.

At week 16, analyses showed that both PR-average and PR-gaps were predictive of failure, in both univariate and multivariable models. Log_{10} EFV concentration also reached significance in the univariate model (for every 10 times or 1 log increase in EFV concentration, the odds of failure reduced by 83%), but the other adherence measures, including EAMD, did not significantly predict failure at week 16 (Table 3).

Resistance outcome

Twelve of the fourteen participants whose HIV-RNA was >400 copies/ml at week 16 were successfully amplified when sent for HIV-1 resistance genotyping. Two participants had no major resistance mutations. Eight (66.7%) participants expressed the K65R mutation-conferring resistance to tenofovir, and three the M184 V mutation-conferring resistance to lamivudine/emtricitabine. All 10 who expressed resistance had NNRTI mutations, including L100I, K101E, K103N, V106M, Y181C, Y188C/Y/L, G190A/G/S and H221HY. Despite only efavirenz and nevirapine being used, mutations conferring resistance to etravirine and rilpivirine were noted in three participants: one each of V90I, E138A and V179D.

Table 3 The table below presents odds ratios (OR) or adjusted odds ratios (aOR) with 95% confidence intervals (CI) for failure or resistance given a 10% increase in the adherence variable (or a 1 log increase in EFV concentration) in each logistic regression model

Adherence measure	Univariate model		Multivariable model	
	OR (95% CI)	p value	aOR (95% CI)	p value
Virological failure (>40 copies/ml) at week 48				
EAMD[a]	0.87 (0.82–0.94)	*<0.001*	0.89 (0.82–0.95)	*0.001*
PR-average	0.78 (0.70–0.88)	*<0.001*	0.78 (0.69–0.87)	*<0.001*
PR-gaps	0.69 (0.56–0.82)	*<0.001*	0.68 (0.56–0.82)	*<0.001*
CPC	0.89 (0.82–0.96)	*0.004*	0.88 (0.80–0.96)	*0.004*
$Log_{10}EFV$	0.40 (0.16–1.03)	0.059	0.52 (0.19–1.37)	0.184
SR	0.98 (0.89–1.08)	0.698	0.98 (0.88–1.09)	0.720
Resistance (presence of ≥1 major mutation) at week 48				
EAMD	0.74 (0.64–0.87)	*<0.001*	0.68 (0.53–0.88)	*0.003*
PR-average	0.77 (0.69–0.87)	*<0.001*	0.77 (0.66–0.89)	*<0.001*
PR-gaps	0.74 (0.65–0.85)	*<0.001*	0.77 (0.66–0.89)	*0.001*
CPC	0.85 (0.77–0.94)	*0.002*	0.82 (0.69–0.98)	*0.031*
$Log_{10}EFV$	0.14 (0.04–0.45)	*0.001*	0.14 (0.02–0.78)	*0.025*
SR	0.92 (0.83–1.02)	0.102	0.92 (0.78–1.08)	0.316
Virological failure (>400 copies/ml) at week 16				
EAMD	0.93 (0.86–1.01)	0.085	0.96 (0.87–1.06)	0.459
PR-average	0.68 (0.55–0.83)	*<0.001*	0.66 (0.50–0.73)	*0.004*
PR-gaps	0.64 (0.51–0.82)	*<0.001*	0.64 (0.47–0.88)	*0.006*
CPC	0.89 (0.78–1.03)	0.133	0.94 (0.78–1.13)	0.491
$Log_{10}EFV$	0.17 (0.04–0.75)	*0.020*	0.20 (0.03–1.47)	0.115
SR	0.92 (0.83–1.03)	0.163	0.98 (0.83–1.01)	0.765
Resistance (presence of ≥1 major mutation) at week 16				
EAMD	0.93 (0.85–1.01)	0.085	0.96 (0.86–1.07)	0.435
PR-average	0.85 (0.72–0.99)	*0.036*	0.87 (0.72–1.06)	0.171
PR-gaps	0.85 (0.71–1.01)	0.066	0.88 (0.69–1.11)	0.287
CPC	0.90 (0.80–1.01)	0.069	0.93 (0.82–1.06)	0.316
$Log_{10}EFV$	0.34 (0.08–1.81)	0.228	0.43 (0.07–2.66)	0.362
SR	0.93 (0.83–1.03)	0.147	0.97 (0.85–1.11)	0.647

Univariate models use only the adherence variable in the model with the outcome variable, multivariable models include the adherence variable and three baseline variables (CD4 cell count, log HIV-RNA and age) with the outcome variable. There are four outcome variables: the risk of virological failure to >40 copies/ml at week 48, the risk of virological failure to >400 copies/ml at week 16, the risk of resistance (presence of ≥1 IAS major mutation at genotyping) at weeks 16 and 48

[a] EAMD = electronic adherence monitoring device data; PR-average = average pharmacy refill data; PR-gaps = pharmacy refill gaps data; CPC = clinic-based pill count data; EFV = efavirenz mid-dosing interval data; SR = 3-day self-recall data

Those results that are significant ($p < 0.05$) are in italics

Twenty-seven participants had a HIV RNA of >40 copies/ml at week 48. Eleven of the fourteen (51.9%) who had HIV RNA >500 copies/ml had resistance genotyping successfully completed. One had no major resistance mutations. Two (18%) participants expressed the K65R mutation and four (36%) the M184 V mutation. As at week 16, the majority of the remaining mutations, in all 11 who expressed resistance, were NNRTI mutations, including L100I, K101E, K103N, V106M, Y181C, G190A, H221HY and F227L. Again, mutations to etravirine and rilpivirine were noted in 3 participants: one with E138A and two with V179D.

Resistance prediction models

As for virological failure, each adherence variable was modelled against the risk of resistance using both univariate and multivariate logistic regression models for prediction. Adherence as quantified by EAMD, PR-average, PR-gaps, TR and $\log_{10}$ EFV concentration were all significantly predictive of resistance in both univariate and multivariable analyses at week 48 (Table 3). SR was non-significant in either model. Reduced age and decreased CD4 cell count at baseline significantly increased the odds of resistance in all multivariable models (data not shown). AUC ROC values were obtained to allow for inter-measure comparison of resistance prediction at weeks 48 and 16. While cumulative EAMD best predicted resistance with the narrowest confidence intervals (AUC ROC 0.92, 95% CI 0.87–0.97), it was not significantly better than either PR measure (PR-average AUC ROC 0.86, 95% CI 0.67–1.0; PR-gaps AUC ROC 0.83, 95% CI 0.65–1.00) at week 48.

In contrast, only PR-average predicted resistance at week 16 (AUC ROC 0.72, 95% CI 0.57–0.90) (Table 3). Reduced age and decreased CD4 cell count at baseline significantly increased the odds of resistance in all multivariable models at week 16. All data on which theses analyses are based are available in Additional file 2.

Discussion

We found high levels of adherence using both short-term and cumulative measures. Three-day SR yielded the highest adherence estimate, but was not a significant predictor of either viral suppression or resistance. This is consistent with findings which show that while short-term SR measures are widely utilised and useful for clinical intervention [33], they overestimate adherence, likely due to recall and social desirability bias [34–37], and are unreliable measures for research purposes.

In contrast, four of the five objective adherence measures effectively predicted virological failure: CPC, PR-average, PR-gaps and EAMD data. Cumulative PR measures (PR-average and PR-gap) were among the best predictors of virological failure and resistance at 48 and, of note, PR-average was the only predictor of resistance at week 16. PR-average has previously been reported to be a reliable predictor of virological outcomes and mortality [3, 8, 9], while our group demonstrated that short term PR-gap can predict failure on second-line ART [10]. Software to calculate PR-average or PR-gaps could

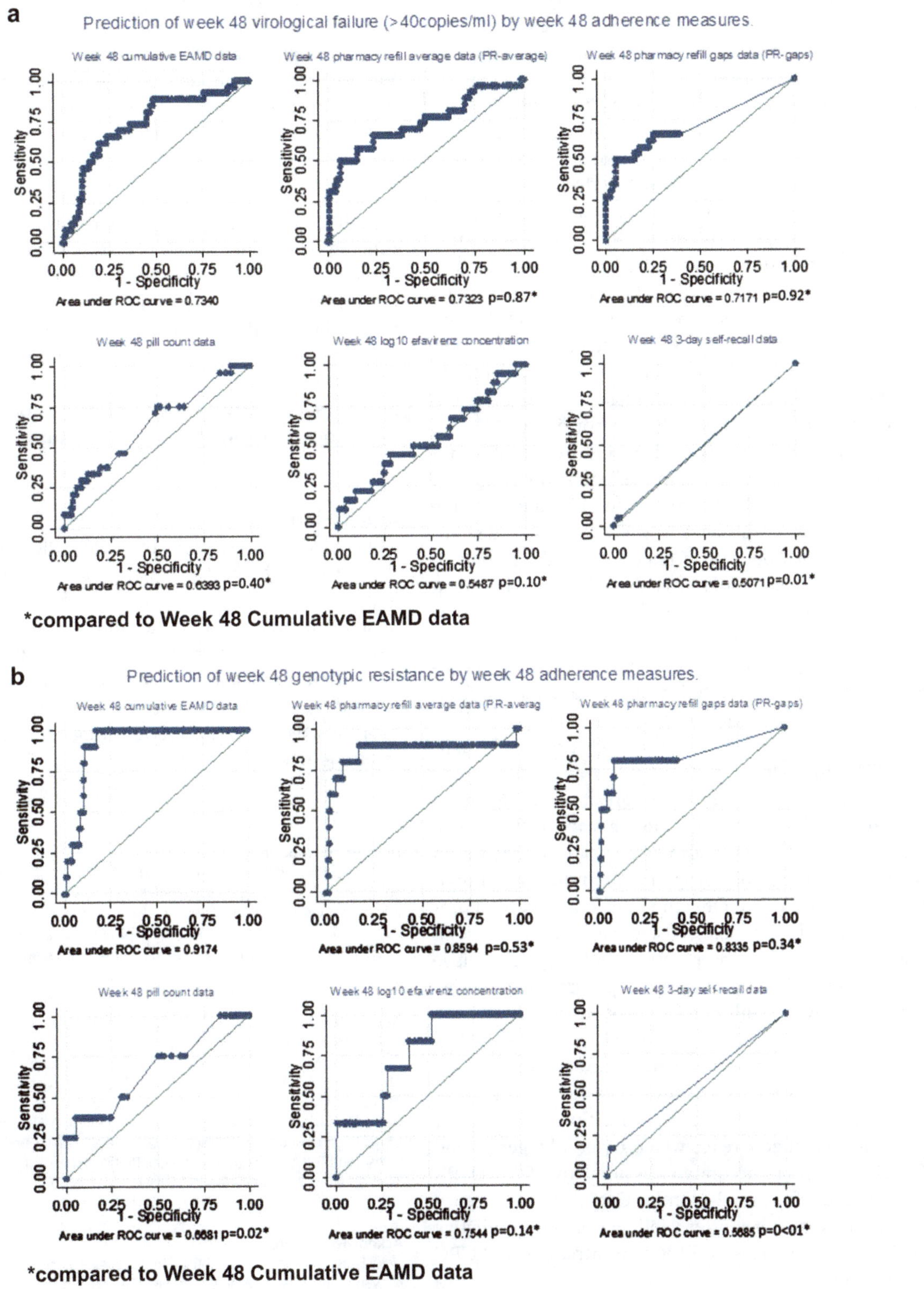

Fig. 2 Prediction of virological failure or resistance by each adherence measure at week 48. Receiver operating characteristic (ROC) curves showing prediction of virological failure (>40 copies/ml) and resistance at week 48 by six adherence measures. Univariate model data are shown. **a** Prediction of virological failure to <40 copies/ml at week 48 using adherence measures at week 48. **b** Prediction of resistance at week 48 using adherence measures at week 48. *Compared to week 48 cumulative EAMD data

easily be added to electronic dispensing systems, which are widely used in resource-limited settings. Programmatic review of adherence using PR methods could be implemented immediately.

CPC is not widely recommended as it is subject to "pill dumping" and can be complex to perform in a large clinic [3]. Nonetheless, CPC, which is a standard of care procedure in our clinic, performed well in this study and was predictive of virological failure and resistance at week 48.

While EAMD data were among the best at predicting outcome in this study at week 48, EAMDs are not routinely used in clinical care. However, recent data shows EAMD can reduce costs associated with HIV-RNA monitoring and real-time devices can detect early virologic rebound before established failure [3, 38, 39]. With the availability of newer, more affordable real-time technologies, electronic strategies should be reconsidered [40].

By altering the distribution of efavirenz concentrations through the use of log values in the regression model, we found that the log values of mid-dose EFV concentration were predictive of resistance at week 48, with wide confidence intervals, but not of failure. Most drug concentrations were therapeutic, possibly reflecting white coat pre-visit dosing, leaving few with concentrations below therapeutic where virological failure would be more likely. The few participants with sub-therapeutic concentrations limit the interpretation of this data. Larger studies including more participants with sub-therapeutic EFV concentrations are needed to adequately explore the ability of TDM to predict virological failure and resistance.

Most participants remaining in care at weeks 16 and 48 had virological suppression. The majority of those who had detectable HIV RNA also had resistance that would compromise at least one drug in their antiretroviral regimen, even at 16 weeks. Only the PR-average method predicted this early resistance. Using early pharmacy refill data to predict failure is practical and easy to achieve both for an individual and on a programmatic level. EAMD data was highly predictive of resistance at week 48, as were both PR measures and, to a lesser extent CPC.

It is interesting that while many of the adherence measures are predictive of viral or resistance outcomes at week 48, far fewer are predictive at week 16. This might suggest that measures of adherence which cover a longer period of dosing are more accurate e.g. cumulative EAMD, PR methods and CPC over 2-months. Conversely, adherence data collected over a shorter window were not predictive e.g. 3-day self-report, spot EFV concentrations and CPC over 1 month.

The prospective collection of multiple adherence measures in a single cohort is the strength of our study as it has allowed direct comparison of these measures—a comparison rarely achieved [13, 16]. Our study was based on maximum use of existing adherence data and used a per protocol approach to analysis, with those who did not have virological data at weeks 16 or 48 treated as missing for the predictive models. Losses to care in this cohort were similar to those previously reported at this site. All participants had data included in the cumulative adherence measures [41, 42].

Both genotyping and viral load testing are costly and funding to conduct baseline resistance testing and confirmatory viral loads at week 48 was not available. This is a study limitation. In addition, SR data was only collected as a 3-day recall at each visit and CPC data were only available for the 1 or 2 months preceding the week 16 or 48 visit and not over the complete study period. These measures may have performed better being collected over a longer or cumulative period of time.

Conclusion

Adherence as measured by CPC, PR measures and EAMD were the best predictors of resistance and virological failure in this prospective study. Pill counting can be implemented at any clinic, and pharmacy refill data is already widely available and an immediately implementable option, particularly in resource-poor settings. Consideration should also be given to the use of electronic measures as adherence monitoring strategies as costs reduce [40].

Authors' contributions

CO, KC, DB, RW and GM conceptualised the study. CO ran the study and collected/collated the data. CO, RL and KC analysed the data. CO wrote the original manuscript and all authors read and contributed to each version. All authors had full access to the study data. All authors have approved this final version. All authors read and approved the final manuscript.

Author details

[1] Department of Medicine, Desmond Tutu HIV Centre, Institute of Infectious Disease and Molecular Medicine, University of Cape Town, Cape Town, South Africa. [2] Division of Clinical Pharmacology, Department of Medicine, University of Cape Town, Cape Town, South Africa. [3] Harvard Medical School, Boston, MA, USA. [4] Massachusetts General Hospital Center for Global Health, Boston, MA, USA. [5] Ragon Institute of Massachusetts General Hospital, Boston, MA, USA. [6] Desmond Tutu HIV Centre, Werner Beit Building North, UCT Faculty of Health Science, Anzio Road, Observatory, Cape Town 7925, South Africa.

Acknowledgements

Heidi Freislich, Monica Vogt, Christie Heiberg, Alienah Mpahleni, Nomsa Ngwenya and Speech Mzamo for their time and dedication throughout the study. Cathy Kalombo, Liz Seabe and their teams at the HCTC. Anna Arnaudo for her proficient editing skills. Jennifer Norman and the team at the Clinical Pharmacology Laboratory, Division of Clinical Pharmacology, Dept. of Medicine, UCT for the drug assays. Lloyd Marshall and the team at Wisepill. Gert van Zyl and Mathilda Claassen, National Health Laboratory Service, Tygerberg, for HIV drug resistance genotyping. Funding for this work was provided by the European and Developing Countries Clinical Trials Partnership (EDCTP; TA.2011.40200.015) and the Discovery Foundation.

Competing interests

The authors declare that they have no competing interests.

Funding

The Discovery Foundation supported CO through an Academic Fellowship Award in 2013 and EDCTP awarded CO a senior fellowship from 2012 to 2014: TA.2011.40200.015. The sponsors of the study had no role in the design and implementation of this study, nor in manuscript preparation.

References

1. Paterson DL, Swindells S, Mohr J, Brester M, Vergis EN, Squier C, et al. Adherence to protease inhibitor therapy and outcomes in patients with HIV infection. Ann Intern Med. 2000;133(1):21–30.
2. Bangsberg DR, Perry S, Charlebois ED, Clark RA, Roberston M, Zolopa AR, et al. Non-adherence to highly active antiretroviral therapy predicts progression to AIDS. AIDS. 2001;15(9):1181–3.
3. Thompson MA, Mugavero MJ, Amico KR, Cargill VA, Chang LW, Gross R, et al. Guidelines for improving entry into and retention in care and antiretroviral adherence for persons with HIV: evidence-based recommendations from an International Association of Physicians in AIDS Care panel. Ann Intern Med. 2012;156(11):817–33.
4. Glass T, Cavassini M. Asking about adherence—from flipping the coin to strong evidence. Swiss Med Wkly. 2014;144:w14016.
5. Marcellin F, Spire B, Carrieri MP, Roux P. Assessing adherence to antiretroviral therapy in randomized HIV clinical trials: a review of currently used methods. Expert Rev Anti Infect Ther. 2013;11(3):239–50.
6. Gill CJ, Hamer DH, Simon JL, Thea DM, Sabin LL. No room for complacency about adherence to antiretroviral therapy in sub-Saharan Africa. AIDS. 2005;19(12):1243–9.
7. Williams AB, Amico KR, Bova C, Womack JA. A proposal for quality standards for measuring medication adherence in research. AIDS Behav. 2013;17(1):284–97.
8. Bisson GP, Gross R, Bellamy S, Chittams J, Hislop M, Regensberg L, et al. Pharmacy refill adherence compared with CD4 count changes for monitoring HIV-infected adults on antiretroviral therapy. PLoS Med. 2008;5(5):e109.
9. Nachega JB, Hislop M, Dowdy DW, Lo M, Omer SB, Regensberg L, et al. Adherence to highly active antiretroviral therapy assessed by pharmacy claims predicts survival in HIV-infected South African adults. J Acquir Immune Defic Syndr. 2006;43(1):78–84.
10. Court R, Leisegang R, Stewart A, Sunpath H, Murphy R, Winternheimer P, et al. Short term adherence tool predicts failure on second line protease inhibitor-based antiretroviral therapy: an observational cohort study. BMC Infect Dis. 2014;14(1):664.
11. Marcellin F, Spire B, Carrieri MP, Roux P. Assessing adherence to antiretroviral therapy in randomized HIV clinical trials: a review of currently used methods. Expert Rev Anti-Infect Ther. 2013;11(3):239–50.
12. Haberer JE, Kiwanuka J, Nansera D, Muzoora C, Hunt PW, So J, et al. Real-time adherence monitoring of antiretroviral therapy among HIV-infected adults and children in rural Uganda. AIDS. 2013;27(13):2166–8.
13. Liu X, Ma Q, Zhang F. Therapeutic drug monitoring in highly active antiretroviral therapy. Expert Opin Drug Saf. 2010;9(5):743–58.
14. Kredo T, Van der Walt JS, Siegfried N, Cohen K. Therapeutic drug monitoring of antiretrovirals for people with HIV. Cochrane Database Syst Rev. 2009. (3):CD007268. doi:10.1002/14651858.CD007268.pub2.
15. Liu H, Golin CE, Miller LG, Hays RD, Beck CK, Sanandaji S, et al. A comparison study of multiple measures of adherence to HIV protease inhibitors. Ann Intern Med. 2001;134(10):968–77.
16. Oyugi JH, Byakika-Tusiime J, Charlebois ED, Kityo C, Mugerwa R, Mugyenyi P, et al. Multiple validated measures of adherence indicate high levels of adherence to generic HIV antiretroviral therapy in a resource-limited setting. J Acquir Immune Defic Syndr. 2004;36(5):1100–2.
17. Muller AD, Jaspan HB, Myer L, Hunter AL, Harling G, Bekker LG, et al. Standard measures are inadequate to monitor pediatric adherence in a resource-limited setting. AIDS Behav. 2011;15(2):422–31.
18. Bangsberg DR, Hecht FM, Charlebois ED, Zolopa AR, Holodniy M, Sheiner L, et al. Adherence to protease inhibitors, HIV-1 viral load, and development of drug resistance in an indigent population. AIDS. 2000;14(4):357–66.
19. Ncaca LN, Kranzer K, Orrell C. Treatment interruption and variation in tablet taking behaviour result in viral failure: a case-control study from Cape Town, South Africa. PLoS ONE. 2011;6(8):e23088.
20. Orrell C, Mauff K, Bangsberg D, Maartens G, Wood R. A randomised controlled trial of real-time electronic adherence monitoring with text message dosing reminders in people starting first-line antiretroviral therapy. J Acquir Immune Defic Syndr. 2015;70(5):495–502.
21. Orrell C, Kaplan R, Wood R, Bekker LG. Virological breakthrough: a risk factor for loss to followup in a large community-based cohort on antiretroviral therapy. AIDS Res Treat. 2011;2011:469127.
22. Orrell C, Harling G, Lawn SD, Kaplan R, McNally M, Bekker LG, et al. Conservation of first-line antiretroviral treatment regimen where therapeutic options are limited. Antivir Ther. 2007;12(1):83–8.
23. Haberer JE, Kahane J, Kigozi I, Emenyonu N, Hunt P, Martin J, et al. Real-time adherence monitoring for HIV antiretroviral therapy. AIDS Behav. 2010;14(6):1340–6.
24. Sabin LL, Bachman DeSilva M, Gill CJ, Zhong L, Vian T, Wubin X, et al. Improving adherence to antiretroviral therapy with triggered real time text message reminders: the China through technology study (CATS). J Acquir Immune Defic Syndr. 2015;69(5):551–9.
25. National Insititute on Alcohol Abuse and Alcoholism. CAGE questionnaire. http://pubs.niaaa.nih.gov/publications/inscage.htm. 2002.
26. Herrmann C. International experiences with the Hospital Anxiety and Depression Scale—a review of validation data and clinical results. J Psychosom Res. 1997;42(1):17–41.
27. Nglazi MD, Kaplan R, Wood R, Bekker LG, Lawn SD. Identification of losses to follow-up in a community-based antiretroviral therapy clinic in South Africa using a computerized pharmacy tracking system. BMC Infect Dis. 2010;10:329.
28. Orrell C, Dipenaar R, Killa N, Tassie JM, Harries AD, Wood R. Simplifying HIV cohort monitoring–pharmacy stock records minimize resources necessary to determine retention in care. J Acquir Immune Defic Syndr. 2013;62(3):e106–8.
29. van Leth F, Phanuphak P, Ruxrungtham K, Baraldi E, Miller S, Gazzard B, et al. Comparison of first-line antiretroviral therapy with regimens including nevirapine, efavirenz, or both drugs, plus stavudine and lamivudine: a randomised open-label trial, the 2NN Study. Lancet. 2004;363(9417):1253–63.
30. Puls R, Amin J, Losso M, Phanuphak P, Nwizu C, Orrell C, et al. Efficacy of 400 mg efavirenz versus standard 600 mg dose in HIV-infected, antiretroviral-naive adults (ENCORE1): a randomised, double-blind, placebo-controlled, non-inferiority trial. Lancet. 2014;383(9927):1474–82.
31. van Zyl GU, Claassen M, Engelbrecht S, Laten JD, Cotton MF, Theron GB, et al. Zidovudine with nevirapine for the prevention of HIV mother-to-child transmission reduces nevirapine resistance in mothers from the Western Cape, South Africa. J Med Virol. 2008;80(6):942–6.
32. Wensing AM, Calvez V, Gunthard HF, Johnson VA, Paredes R, Pillay D, et al. 2014 Update of the drug resistance mutations in HIV-1. Top Antivir Med. 2014;22(3):642–50.
33. Wu P, Johnson BA, Nachega JB, Wu B, Ordonez CE, Hare AQ, et al. The combination of pill count and self-reported adherence is a strong predictor of first-line ART failure for adults in South Africa. Curr HIV Res. 2014;12(5):366–75.
34. Lester RT, Ritvo P, Mills EJ, Kariri A, Karanja S, Chung MH, et al. Effects of a mobile phone short message service on antiretroviral treatment adherence in Kenya (WelTel Kenya1): a randomised trial. Lancet. 2010;376(9755):1838–45.
35. Hardy H, Kumar V, Doros G, Farmer E, Drainoni ML, Rybin D, Myung D, Jackson J, Backman E, Stanic A, Skolnik PR. Randomized controlled trial of a personalized cellular phone reminder system to enhance adherence to antiretroviral therapy. AIDS Patient Care STDS. 2011;25(3):153–61. doi:10.1089/apc.2010.0006.
36. Da Costa TM, Barbosa BJP, E Costa DAG, Sigulem D, De Fátima Marin H, Filho AC, et al. Results of a randomized controlled trial to assess the

effects of a mobile SMS-based intervention on treatment adherence in HIV/AIDS-infected Brazilian women and impressions and satisfaction with respect to incoming messages. Int J Med Inform. 2012;81(4):257–69.

37. Maduka O, Tobin-West CI. Adherence counseling and reminder text messages improve uptake of antiretroviral therapy in a tertiary hospital in Nigeria. Niger J Clin Pract. 2013;16(3):302–8. doi:10.4103/1119-3077.113451.
38. Petersen ML, LeDell E, Schwab J, Sarovar V, Gross R, Reynolds N, et al. Super learner analysis of electronic adherence data improves viral prediction and may provide strategies for selective HIV RNA monitoring. J Acquir Immune Defic Syndr. 2015;69(1):109–18.
39. Haberer JE, Musinguzi N, Boum Y 2nd, Siedner MJ, Mocello AR, Hunt PW, et al. Duration of antiretroviral therapy adherence interruption is associated with risk of virologic rebound as determined by real-time adherence monitoring in rural Uganda. J Acquir Immune Defic Syndr. 2015;70(4):386–92.
40. Phillips AN, Cambiano V, Nakagawa F, Bansi-Matharu L, Sow PS, Ehrenkranz P, et al. Cost effectiveness of potential ART adherence monitoring interventions in Sub-Saharan Africa. PLoS ONE. 2016;11(12):e0167654.
41. Nglazi MD, Kaplan R, Orrell C, Myer L, Wood R, Bekker LG, et al. Increasing transfers-out from an antiretroviral treatment service in South Africa: patient characteristics and rates of virological non-suppression. PLoS ONE. 2013;8(3):e57907.
42. Nglazi MD, Lawn SD, Kaplan R, Kranzer K, Orrell C, Wood R, et al. Changes in programmatic outcomes during 7 years of scale-up at a community-based antiretroviral treatment service in South Africa. J Acquir Immune Defic Syndr. 2011;56(1):e1–8.

11

Distribution and fate of HIV-1 unintegrated DNA species

Faysal Bin Hamid, Jinsun Kim and Cha-Gyun Shin*

Abstract

Reverse transcription of viral RNA and the subsequent integration of reverse transcripts are the classical early events of the HIV-1 life-cycle. Simultaneously, abundant unintegrated DNAs (uDNAs), are formed in cells ubiquitously. The uDNAs either undergo recombination or degradation or persist inactively for long periods in the nucleus as future resources. Among them, 2-LTR circles are considered a dead-end for viral spread. Their contribution to the HIV-1 infection is still poorly understood. Nevertheless, the preintegration transcription of the aberrant DNAs and the consequent alterations of cellular factors have already been reported. Since the major fate of the viral genome is to persist as episomal DNA, precise characterization is required for studying the biology of HIV-1. This review compiles the biochemical and genetic updates on uDNA in the HIV-1 life cycle and could provide direction to further study of their roles in HIV-1 replication and application in HIV-1 pathogenesis.

Keywords: Retrovirus, HIV-1, Nuclear import, 2-LTR, Unintegrated DNA

Background

Conversion of single-stranded RNAs to linear double-stranded reverse transcripts and their subsequent integration into host chromosomes are signature features of the early stage of the human immunodeficiency virus (HIV) lifecycle [1, 2]. Reverse transcription occurs in the cytoplasm, and the translocation of cDNA to the nucleus gives rise to at least two types of cDNA: linear and circular. Linear cDNA is integrated into host DNA and is transcribed into viral mRNA used in making viral progeny. However, circular forms of viral DNA, containing either one or two copies of the long terminal repeat (LTR) region, accumulate in the infected cells because of abortive integration processes. Although different studies report that they can express a limited range of early genes [3–8], the role of these unintegrated DNAs is still unclear.

Retroviruses enter host cells by endocytosis or by binding to glycoproteins on their surface. Specifically, HIV-1 binds to the receptor CD4 and co-receptors CCR5 and CXCR4 on T lymphocytes and macrophages [9, 10]. After the reverse transcription of viral RNA, which occurs in the endocytosed viral core and uses free cytoplasmic nucleotides and ions, the viral envelope is gradually released in a process known as uncoating [11]. The viral reverse transcripts then bind to at least four viral proteins: matrix (MA), integrase (IN), reverse transcriptase (RT), viral protein (Vpr), and/or capsid (CA), as well as several host proteins. These form a ribonucleoprotein complex, called the pre-integration complex (PIC), which enters the nucleus [10, 12]. After nuclear import, the cDNA either becomes integerated, or fails to integrate and may become circularized to form episomal DNA [3, 13, 14]; circular episomal DNA has in some cases been found in the cytoplasm as well [15, 16]. Delelis et al. [15] hypothesized that in prototype foamy virus-infected cells, it may be either that the 2-LTR circles formed in the nucleus are unable to be exported into the cytoplasm or that they might be yielded in the cytoplasm and be imported into the nucleus and accumulated. Either of these two events can explain the higher amount of 2-LTR circles detected in the nucleus and their higher stability.

*Correspondence: chagshin@gmail.com
Department of Systems Biotechnology, Chung-Ang University, Anseong, Kyunggido 456-756, South Korea

Although linear DNA is considered as a substrate for provirus production, its ends can also be ligated to form 2-LTR circles by host non-homologous DNA end joining (NHEJ), one of the cellular repair systems. Another form, 1-LTR circles, can result from defective reverse transcription [17], auto-integration from the rearrangement of circular forms [1, 18], or homologous recombination between 2-LTR circles [1]. Several proteins of NHEJ have been reported to be involved in this process, such as the Ku70/80 heterodimer, ligase 4, XRCC4, and RAD52 [18–20]. Another type of unintegrated DNA, also known as autointegrants, is formed through the ligation of the internal region of viral DNA to the IN-processed 3′-end [3, 21–24]. The presence of autointegrants has been confirmed in HIV-1, as well as in other retroviruses, e.g. Moloney murine leukemia virus (MoMLV) and Rous sarcoma virus (RSV) [1, 18, 21].

Distribution

After entry into cells, the reverse transcription of HIV-1 RNA occurs in the cytoplasm. Once inside the cytoplasm, viral reverse transcripts form PICs with host proteins. These complexes containing viral double stranded DNA (dsDNA), which has the triple stranded DNA structure called DNA flap, are able to be integrated into the host dsDNA in vitro. This is mediated by IN, which can cleave the 3′-ends of both LTRs of the blunt (or unprocessed) DNA, named linear unintegrated DNA ($uDNA_L$), and results in 3′-processed linear DNA ($pDNA_L$) [25]. The cleavage is occurred by tetrameric IN in case of both palindromic LTR-LTR junction and 2-LTR circle internally [26]. The DNA in PICs may either undergo circularization or remain in the form of linear dsDNA. Munir et al. [27] updated the order of the persistence of viral DNA forms as follows: provirus > circular DNA (1-LTRc and 2-LTRc) > $uDNA_L$ > $pDNA_L$. The $pDNA_L$ is less stable than $uDNA_L$ and can therefore persist a shorter period than $uDNA_L$. The HIV-1 infection causes the accumulation of unintegrated DNAs in any cell type or cellular status in vivo [8, 27–29] or in vitro [1, 30–32] (Table 1). Gene expression from uDNA is higher than integrated proviruses in non-dividing cells compared to dividing cells [14]. The reason is likely due to lack of dilution of uDNA templates, the transcripts and proteins [3, 14, 33]. Interestingly, several groups have shown that the unintegrated circular forms of HIV-1 are present prominently in the nucleus and can be considered as markers of the active transport of the PIC into the nucleus [3, 29, 34]. Avian sarcoma virus was first reported to form circular DNA in infected cells, particularly in the nucleus [35, 36] (Table 1). However, unintegrated DNA was first reported in brain and blood tissue of HIV-1 infected dementia patients [37]. Later, high levels of unintegrated DNA were found in HIV-1 infected cells, both in in vivo on human patients and animals [38, 39] and in in vitro experiments on lymphocytic and monocytic cell lines [1, 35]. This was expected, as the ratio of linear to 1-LTR circular to 2-LTR circular HIV DNA was previously approximated

Table 1 Examples of unintegrated DNAs in virus-infected cells and their fates

Virus	Cell line	Cell number	hpi (hours per infection)	Methods	Consequence		Ref.
Avian sarcoma virus	QT-6		5 hpi		Closed circular DNA		[34]
MLV	NIH 3T3, TE671, ARPE-19	1×10^6 cells	2 hpi	qPCR	2-LTR		[16]
HIV-1	MT-2	5×10^5 cells	2 hpi	PCR and Southern hybridization	1-LTR		[31]
			12 hpi		2-LTR		
	Monocyte	1×10^6 cells	2 hpi	PCR and Southern hybridization	1-LTR		
			12 hpi		2-LTR		
	Macrophage	3×10^5 cells	4 dpi	qPCR	2-LTR	30–35 copies/100cells	[45]
			21 dpi			6 copies/100cells	
	CD4+ T lymphocytes	3×10^5 cells	4 dpi		2-LTR	11 copies/100cells	
			14 dpi			X	
	Jurkat	1×10^7	3 dpt		2-LTR	8.97%	[36]
					1-LTR	46.21%	
	293T				2-LTR	5.42%	
					1-LTR	40.16%	
	SupT1 (lymphoid cells)	5×10^6 cells	15 hpi		2-LTR	0.01 copy/cell	[46]
			12 hpi			40 copies/cells	

dpt days post-transduction, *dpi* days post infection

as 20:9:1 [40, 41]. Interestingly, 1-LTR circles appeared earlier; at approximately at 2 h post infection (hpi) in HIV-1 infected MT-2 cell lines, while 2-LTR circles were found at about 12 hpi [35]. However, the 2-LTR circles were detected at 1–2 h hpi in the cytoplasm of murine leukemia virus (MLV)-infected cells [16] and after 72 hpi in prototype foamy virus-infected cells, although they started to accumulate already at 3 hpi in the infected cells [15]. Initially, it was thought that this was due to the lack of cell division in aphidicolin-treated NIH 3T3 cells, but 2-LTR circles also formed in arrested and non-arrested TE671 human medulloblastoma cells and ARPE-19 human retinal epithelial cells [17] (Table 1). It is considered that 1-LTR circles are more abundant than 2-LTR in infected cells both in vitro and in vivo [42, 43]. The relative abundance is cytoplasmic linear DNA > proviruses > 1-LTR circles > 2-LTR circles [42]. However, the autointegration of the HIV-1 genome produces cDNA products either containing nicked, inverted, or modified dsDNA circles [43]. This cytoplasmic DNA is detected by DNA sensors and secreted interferons [23, 44].

In the infected cells, non-integrating HIV-1 and HIV-1-based vectors are organized into chromatin structures and enriched with histone modifications typical of silenced chromatins that can be reactivated upon exposure to histone deacetylase (HDAC) inhibitors. [47]. Surprisingly, 1-LTR circles are formed earlier than 2-LTR ones [27]. However, a significant amount, i.e. around 10%, of 1-LTR circles is formed during reverse transcription in the cytoplasm [14, 27]. Kilzer and his colleagues demonstrated that a high level of 1-LTR circles (90%) is generated after nuclear import by homologous recombination between two flanked LTR regions of linear DNA and that most of the 1-LTR circles are found in the nucleus [13]. The mechanism of 1-LTR circle formation and the subcellular localization points at its plausible significance in viral replication, mainly in the step of viral integration [27]. The strand-transfer inhibitor raltegravir (RAL) and the catalytic mutation of IN affected 3′-LTR processing differently: the comparison of 2-LTR circle accumulation mediated by either indicated that 3′-end processing has no role in 2-LTR circle accumulation, while the type of the LTR–LTR junction formation is considerably affected. The formation of 2-LTR circles containing original palindromic sequence junctions (40%) in RAL-treated cells were similar to that in wild type cells, but was nearly doubled in D116N mutants [27]. The pattern of 3′-end processing in circular DNA could be useful in designing the IN-targeting therapeutic agents.

Role of cellular proteins in unintegrated DNA formation

Integration is required for successful retroviral replication. Cellular proteins RAD50, MRE11, and NBS1 are nuclease components that reportedly participate in 1-LTR circle formation [3, 13]. DNA-dependent protein kinase (DNA-PK), a nuclear serine-threonine protein kinase that can phosphorylate downstream proteins after sensing DNA breaks, is essential in the repair of dsDNA breaks by NHEJ. It is composed of a DNA-binding Ku70/Ku86 heterodimer and a 469 kDa catalytic subunit, DNA-PK_{cs} [48]. It has a significant role in V(D)J recombination as well. The RAG1/RAG2 proteins generate breaks in the strands of dsDNA. At the break-sites, the Ku70/Ku80 heterodimer binds to the free DNA termini, keeping them localized. DNA-PK_{cs} binds the DNA-bound Ku to form the DNA-PK complex, which stimulates DNA-PK_{cs} activity through phosphorylation [49]. It is known that 2-LTR circles are products of DNA repair mechanisms in the nucleus as a host reaction to foreign dsDNA [50]. Viral cDNA replication intermediates have been found to interact with host Ku components of the NHEJ pathway [51, 52]. Silencing of the NHEJ components Ku, ligase 4, or XRCC4 decreases the number of 2-LTR circles. Interestingly, the absence of DNA-PKcs, a component of the NHEJ machinery, showed the opposite effect [13, 52].

Fate

Degradation

Circular DNAs are considered as replicative dead end. Linear DNA, the substrate of integration, is degraded in dividing T cells within hours [53], but persists for several days in resting T cells; it may even persist up to one month in macrophages [8, 54, 55] (Fig. 1). In the pre-integration state, viruses express their genes and produce half of the rescuable virions in resting CD4+ T cells [55]. The shortage of the virus production may be due to the virus-induced programmed cell death (apoptosis) or blockage of reverse transcription. In addition to these fates, in the high-titer infections of cultured cells, the majority of viral DNA undergoes intracellular degradation after synthesis [41, 46, 56, 57]. Several further proposals have also been made for DNA repair factors acting on retroviral DNA [58, 59].

Highly active antiretroviral therapy (HAART) causes a dramatic reduction in HIV-1 replication during the first 3 years and lowers the level of 2-LTR circles as well [60]. Furthermore, after 7–8 years of uninterrupted therapy, 2-LTR circles were almost undetectable in peripheral blood mononuclear cells (PBMCs) of most of the patients. These observations indicate the labile nature of 2-LTR circles, which may be subject to continuous HAART therapy. However, HIV-1 DNA was still detectable in the infected patients [60], probably due to the ongoing viral replication in newly infected dividing cells. Previously, it was demonstrated that the gradual decrease of the amount of circular DNA in proliferating cells occurs due to the absence of an origin of replication and is a function of dilution resulting from cell division [53]. IN mutant-infected macrophages produce DNA that persists at low levels even after 2 weeks, most of which is presumably unintegrated DNA. It was confirmed that the stability of 2-LTR was not due to viral replication [61].

Reservoirs

Latent unintegrated genomes present in viremic HIV-1 patients after HAART treatment act as reservoirs and are an obstacle to effective treatment. 2-LTR circles persist in HIV-1 infected, growth-arrested T cell lines beyond their estimated half-life as previously determined in dividing cell populations [45, 56]. The drop of 2-LTR circle levels in dividing cells might be due to cell division, not due to degradation [54, 62]. In non-dividing macrophages, the 2-LTR circle levels remained the same for up to 21 days post infection (dpi) (Fig. 1). The unvarying 2-LTR circle level indicates their high stability in macrophages [45]. Moreover, macrophages are resistant to cytopathic effects caused by HIV-1, which makes macrophages a suitable reservoir for further infection [8, 33, 45, 62]. This stability in non-replicating cells may be due to their association with host proteins, e.g. histones, which protects them from decay [62]. E-DNA would be diluted out with successive rounds of cell division. In contrast to highly-active antiretroviral therapy (HAART)-treated HIV-1 patients, elite controllers, a group of HIV-1 infected persons who can control HIV-1 replication naturally in the absence of antiretroviral therapy and maintain untraceable viral loads, had higher 2-LTR circles than integrated proviruses in Ex Vivo experiments [63, 64].

Gene expression

The integrated HIV-1 provirus is transcribed into new genomic RNA, also serving as mRNA, which is in turn translated into viral proteins [2–6, 65] (Fig. 1). Although it is speculated that the integrated copies of viral DNA are the sole template for viral gene expression, there is also evidence of preintegration transcription from unintegrated DNA [5, 65] (Fig. 1). Most recently, it has been shown that the transcriptional interplay is regulated oppositely between integrated and unintegrated DNA following NF-κB pathway modulation [66]. Upon various pharmacological treatments of NF-κB pathway activation, transcription factors such as NF-κB p65 and AP-1

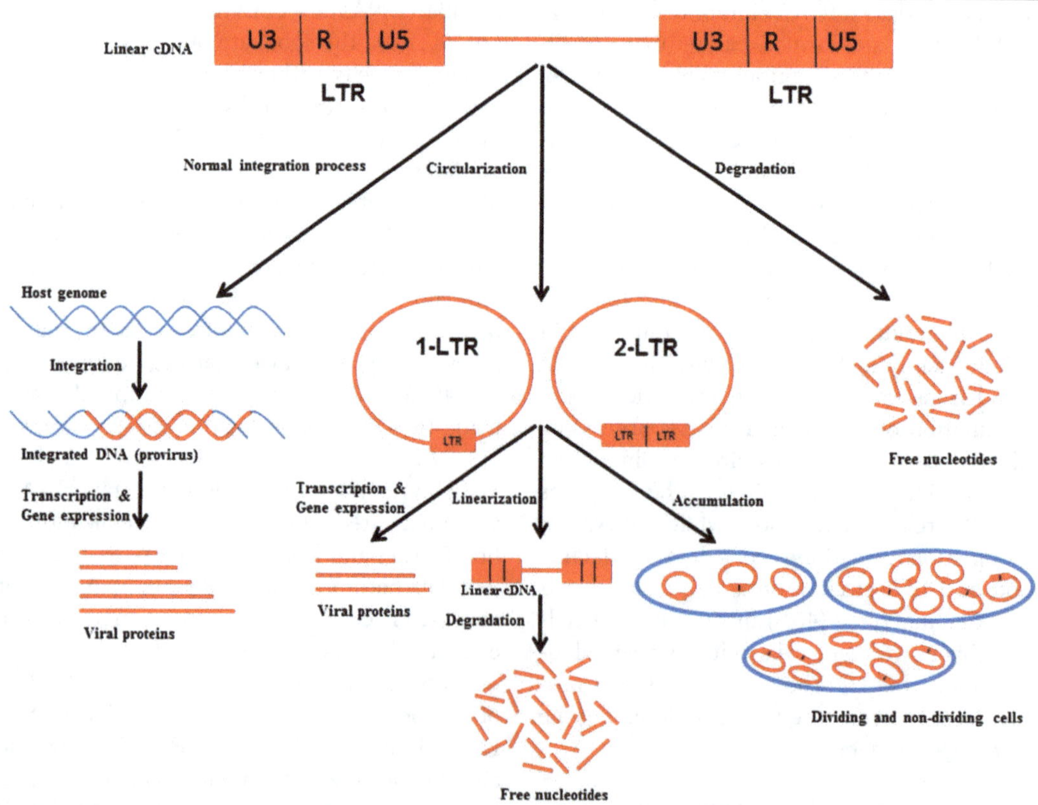

Fig. 1 Fates of viral cDNAs (reverse transcripts) after reverse transcription. After reverse transcription, HIV-1 produces cDNAs that may either be integrated into host genome or circulate themselves. Otherwise, they are degraded into free nucleotides. Circular DNAs have been reported to actively participate in current gene expression similar to the integrated DNAs followed by linearization, degradation, or accumulation as a reservoir

(cFos/cJun) binds to integrated DNA and increases its expression, though the uDNA expression is declined. On the other hand, inhibition of the NF-κB pathway supports the expression of circular uDNA, and Bcl-3 and AP-1 is associated with its LTR region [66]. However, the persistent expression of HIV-1 proteins has already been reported not only in vitro in non-dividing cells, such as primary rat neurons and growth arrested fibroblasts, and dividing cells, such as SV40 T-antigen expressing cells [67–70], but also in vivo in rodent ocular and brain tissues [69]. Even IN-mutant HIV-1 or integration-arrested viruses produce transcriptionally active circular DNA [4, 5, 67, 71]. It is already established that HIV-1 circular unintegrated DNA can promote viral replication itself, but several groups disapproved the notion [40, 47]. Most recently, Shimura et al. [72] reported that the expression of circular DNA genes is possible even after IN strand-transfer inhibitor treatment, probably due to cell-to-cell infection. Particularly, 2-LTR circles can express not only early viral genes, such as *Nef* [5, 65, 72], *Tat* [40, 73], and *Rev* [5, 40, 72], but also late, non-spliced, singly- or multiply-spliced transcripts prior to integration. Among them, the *Nef* and *Tat* proteins are translated only from the fully spliced mRNA [4]. It has been reported that the expression of circular DNA genes, especially *Nef*, is augmented by *Vpr* in HIV-1 infected cells [74]. Interestingly, *Nef* can stimulate T cell activation and decrease the expression of co-receptors CD4, CXCR4, and CCR5, thus increasing HIV-1 infectivity [75]. In addition, *Tat*, a transactivator protein of HIV-1, can activate the transcription from LTRs of both unintegrated and integrated viral DNA [76]. Particularly, viral transcripts are expressed from the upstream promoter, probably from the beginning of the R region located within the tandem LTR repeats of a 2-LTR circle [72]. In non-dividing cells, such as macrophages, gene expression is induced by *Vpr* only when it is driven by the HIV-1 LTR promoter, but not by the cytomegalovirus promoter [45]. However, after integration, Rev activity increases in order to support the production of late genes, such as *Vpu*, both from spliced and unspliced genes [5, 75]. Recently, Emeagwali and his colleagues (2012) showed that *Vpu* and the antagonistic host protein TWIK-related acid sensitive K+ channel 1 (TASK1) can preferentially downregulate the transcription of episomal DNA [75]. However, a greater part of nonintegrated viral DNA might be inactive templates for the transcription machinery. When it was observed experimentally, the *Rev* transcripts were synthesized from nonintegrated DNA, although the expression level was not high (approximately 0.03–5% of total viral DNA) and was transient. Inadequate *Rev* expression was likely the result of the activity of the late structural gene *gag* in nonintegrated HIV-1 DNA, which was similar to IN defective virus-infected, inhibitor-treated, or quiescent cells [5]. Upon latency reversing agents including PKC activators, histone deacetylase inhibitors and P-TEFb agonists) treatment, latent uDNA was reported to initiate lately virus production as well as the latent integrated proviruses [14].

Surprisingly, 2-LTR circles can be used as a substrate for integration by IN and contribute to the spumaviral lifecycle, even after integration [77]. Previously, spleen necrosis virus (SNV), Rous sarcoma virus (RSV), avian sarcoma virus (ASV), and avian leukosis virus (ALV) were assumed to generate the LTR–LTR circles that are used as templates for integration [19, 77]. Generally, IN can cleave the viral double stranded cDNA ends in a staggered manner, which then undergoes covalent transesterification to the 5′ phosphates of the host dsDNA [2, 21]. However, IN also shows the novel pleiotropic action in the mechanism underlying the requirement in the circular DNA integration: it can directly cleave the conserved palindromic sequence found at LTR–LTR junctions and produce linear DNA from 2-LTR circles [77]. Most recently, it has been reported that HIV-1 PIC, specifically IN, can also cleave 2-LTR circles in a similar way [78]. HIV-1 IN required for linearization of 2-LTR circles was found at the palindromic junction, recognized as integration site, and subsequently executed a de novo integration process. It can explain the decrease in the amount of 2-LTR circles and surge of linear DNA, as well as proviral DNA, after the withdrawal of raltegravir in vitro [78] or HAART administration in vivo [39].

Despite the expression level of circular DNA that was reported previously, improved efficiency was observed in the long U3 deletion mutants, both in vivo and in vitro [32]. The U3-region truncation does not alter the diversity of the four types of episomal DNA. Interestingly, the U3 deletion causes high transgene expression from episomes in different levels in non-dividing brain cells and slowly dividing liver cells of rats. The effect of the large U3 deletion on episomal expression indicates that the *cis*-acting elements of the retroviral genome can regulate the extrachromosomal transcriptional activity and that the cell-specific *trans*-acting factors are presumably implicated in negatively regulated transgene expression from lentiviral episomes [32]. Moreover, the addition of HDAC inhibitors in the form of short-chain fatty acids can also induce gene expression, as well as replication, from episomal DNA. To crosstalk genetically and functionally between integrated and unintegrated DNA, it has been found that HIV-1 gene expression, such as of *Vpr*, from unintegrated DNA can be complemented by co-infection with the integrated viral genome [47, 79].

Table 2 Different assays used to measure different analytes

Analytes	Assays	Advantages	Problems	References
Resting CD4+ T cells	PCR	Considered as 'gold-standard' for measuring latently infected cells	Low accuracy, slow, costly	[28, 80]
Total DNA	qPCR	Integrated and unintegrated HIV-DNA per million in peripheral blood mononuclear cells (PBMC) or CD4+ T cells	Unknown	[80]
Total HIV-DNA and 2-LTR circles	Droplet digital PCR	More sensitive and precise comparing to real time *pol* PCR	Short life span of 2-LTR; low accuracy	[80]
Provirus	*Alu–gag* PCR and qPCR	Conventional method to detect integrated proviruses.	Nonspecific, low accuracy	[80]
Intracellular HIV-RNA	PCR	Detection of 1 copy per million resting CD4+ T cells	Unknown	[80]
Viral RNA	HIV-RNA single copy assay (SCA)	Ultrasensitive method to quantify HIV-RNA in plasma	Unknown	[80]

Cytocidal effect on host cells

The cytocidal effect of retroviruses is thought to exist due to the rapid accumulation of unintegrated viral DNA in the cells. The reinfection property might be the reason of cytopathogenesis. Most acutely and chronically infected cells show the cytocidal effect [35]. A lower level of unintegrated DNA indicates that the cells are resistant to superinfection and maintain a persistent infection [35].

Measurement of the HIV-1 reservior and its eradication

The durable nature of HIV-1 reservoir in all CD4+ T-cell subsets, including naïve and memory cells is a key problem to eradication. The establishment of the pool starts from the very initial time of primary infection associated with cytopathic effect and rounds of new infection. CD4+ T cells are reported to maintain high levels of HIV DNA even after HAART and it can resume high levels of new replication following ART withdrawal [64, 80]. However, the samples, the analytes, and the assays must be taken into consideration during the measurement of the reservoir. To date, several assays have been used to measure the different analytes which are considered as the HIV reservoirs (Table 2), but shortage of standardization and validation have made the assessment difficult. The problem of all PCR-based assays is that they can not discriminate between the infectious virion producing cells and latent viral reservoir containg cells (Table 2) [80]. So different real time PCRs have been used to measure the analytes such as viral RNA, 2-LTR and proviruses more accurately. But they are still lack of fidelity of quality and accuracy. Some of the current techniques used to measure the analytes that reflect the HIV-1 reservior have been discussed in Table 2.

Conclusions

The 2-LTR circles are formed at the initial period of infection in vivo. Most of the cells undergo cell death, while some survive [53] and remain viral reservoirs. The longevity of these cells is due to the "intrinsic stability", which is not identical in all cell types. The viral infection may induce cell survival factors, but the complete molecular mechanisms are still unknown. 2-LTR circles are a clear indication of foregoing viral replication, and the question of using them as valid markers of nuclear import for real time measurement arises [53, 81]. Many groups have reported on the significance of 2-LTR circle gene expression [3, 4, 7, 8], while the mechanisms of formation and gene expression and the fate of 1-LTR is in most cases omitted. The nuclear import of HIV-1 is not dependent on any particular viral or cellular karyophilic proteins [10, 82]. Since the study of the nuclear import and 2-LTR circles are closely related, the roles of these proteins should be observed more carefully. The complete characterization of the uDNAs might be convenient to understanding the HIV-1 viremia better. Moreover, the pleotropic fate of uDNA renders it a more eligible candidate for gene therapy and drug delivery.

Abbreviations

uDNAs: unintegrated DNAs; HIV: human immunodeficiency virus; LTR: long terminal repeat; MA: matrix; IN: integrase; RT: reverse transcriptase; Vpr: viral protein; CA: capsid; PIC: pre-integration complex; MoMLV: Moloney murine leukemia virus; RSV: Rous sarcoma virus; uDNAL: linear unintegrated DNA; pDNAL: 3′-processed linear DNA; hpi: post infection; MLV: Murine leukemia virus; RAL: raltegravir; DNA-PK: DNA-dependent protein kinase; HAART: highly active antiretroviral therapy; PBMCs: peripheral blood mononuclear cells; dpi: days post infection; TASK1: TWIK-related acid sensitive K+ channel 1.

Authors' contributions

FBH wrote the manuscript and designed the artwork. Both JSK and CGS revised the text and made valuable suggestions. All authors read and approved the final manuscript.

Acknowledgements
None.

Competing interests
The authors declare that they have no competing interests.

Funding
This study was supported by a grant from the National Research Foundation of Korea (NRF), funded by the Korean government (NRF-2015R1D1A1A01059592).

References

1. Farnet CM, Haseltine WA. Circularization of human immunodeficiency virus type 1 DNA in vitro. J Virol. 1991;65:6942–52.
2. Varmus HE, Brown PO. Retroviruses. In: Berg DE, Howe MM, editors. Mobile DNA. Washington, D.C.: American Society for Microbiology; 1989. p. 53–108.
3. Sloan RD, Wainberg MA. The role of unintegrated DNA in HIV infection. Retrovirology. 2011;8:52.
4. Wu Y, Marsh JW. Selective transcription and modulation of resting T cell activity by preintegration HIV DNA. Science. 2001;293:1503–6.
5. Wu Y, Marsh JW. Early transcription from nonintegrated DNA in human immunodeficiency virus infection. J Virol. 2003;77:10376–82.
6. Wu Y. HIV-1 gene expression: lessons from provirus and non-integrated DNA. Retrovirology. 2004;1:13.
7. Wu Y. The second chance story of HIV-1 DNA: unintegrated? Not a problem! Retrovirology. 2008;5:61.
8. Kelly J, Beddall M, Yu D, et al. Human macrophages support persistent transcription from unintegrated HIV-1 DNA. Virology. 2008;372:300–12.
9. Overbaugh J, Miller AD, Eiden MV. Receptors and entry cofactors for retroviruses include single and multiple transmembrane-spanning proteins as well as newly described glycophosphatidyl inositol-anchored and secreted proteins. Microbiol Mol Biol Rev. 2001;65:371–89.
10. Hamid FB, Kim J, Shin CG. Cellular and viral determinants of retroviral nuclear entry. Can J Microbiol. 2016;62:1–15.
11. Lukic Z, Dharan A, Fricke T, et al. HIV-1 uncoating is facilitated by dynein and kinesin 1. J Virol. 2014;88:13613–25.
12. Arhel N. Revisiting HIV-1 uncoating. Retrovirology. 2010;7:96.
13. Kilzer JM, Stracker T, Beitzel B, et al. Roles of host cell factors in circularization of retroviral dna. Virology. 2003;314:460–7.
14. Chan CN, Trinité B, Lee CS, et al. HIV-1 latency and virus production from unintegrated genomes following direct infection of resting CD4 T cells. Retrovirology. 2016;13:1.
15. Delelis O, Saïb A, Sonigo P. Biphasic DNA synthesis in spumaviruses. J Virol. 2003;77:8141–6.
16. Serhan F, Penaud M, Petit C, et al. Early detection of a two-long-terminal-repeat junction molecule in the cytoplasm of recombinant murine leukemia virus-infected cells. J Virol. 2004;78:6190–9.
17. Miller MD, Wang B, Bushman FD. Human immunodeficiency virus type 1 preintegration complexes containing discontinuous plus strands are competent to integrate in vitro. J Virol. 1995;69:3938–44.
18. Cara A, Klotman ME. Retroviral E-DNA: persistence and gene expression in nondividing immune cells. J Leukoc Biol. 2006;80:1013–7.
19. Li L, Olvera JM, Yoder KE, et al. Role of the non-homologous DNA end joining pathway in the early steps of retroviral infection. EMBO J. 2001;20:3272–81.
20. Lau A, Kanaar R, Jackson SP, et al. Suppression of retroviral infection by the RAD52 DNA repair protein. EMBO J. 2004;23:3421–9.
21. Coffin JM, Hughes SH, Varmus HE. Retroviruses. New York: Cold Spring Harbor Laboratory Press; 1997.
22. Shoemaker C, Hoffman J, Goff SP, et al. Intramolecular integration within Moloney murine leukemia virus DNA. J Virol. 1981;40:164–72.
23. Yan YM, Coffin JM. Efficient autointegration of avian retrovirus DNA in vitro. J Virol. 1990;64:5958–65.
24. Yan N, Cherepanov P, Daigle JE, et al. The SET complex acts as a barrier to autointegration of HIV-1. PLoS Pathog. 2009;5:e1000327.
25. Lesbats P, Engelman AN, Cherepanov P. Retroviral DNA integration. Chem Rev. 2016;116:12730–57.
26. Delelis O, Parissi V, Leh H, et al. Efficient and specific internal cleavage of a retroviral palindromic DNA sequence by tetrameric HIV-1 integrase. PLoS ONE. 2007;2(7):e608.
27. Munir S, Thierry S, Subra F, et al. Quantitative analysis of the time-course of viral DNA forms during the HIV-1 life cycle. Retrovirology. 2013;10:87.
28. Vatakis DN, Bristol G, Wilkinson TA, et al. Immediate activation fails to rescue efficient human immunodeficiency virus replication in quiescent CD4+ T cells. J Virol. 2007;81:3574–82.
29. Badralmaa Y, Natarajan V. Impact of the DNA extraction method on 2-LTR DNA circle recovery from HIV-1 infected cells. J Virol Methods. 2013;193:184–9.
30. Olivares I, Sánchez-Jiménez C, Vieira CR, et al. Evidence of ongoing replication in a human immunodeficiency virus type 1 persistently infected cell line. J Gen Virol. 2013;94:944–54.
31. Sonza S, Kiernan RE, Maerz AL, et al. Accumulation of unintegrated circular viral DNA in monocytes and growth-arrested T cells following infection with HIV-1. J Leukoc Biol. 1994;56:289–93.
32. Bayer M, Kantor B, Cockrell A, et al. A large U3 deletion causes increased in vivo expression from a nonintegrating lentiviral vector. Mol Ther. 2008;16:1968–76.
33. Kumar A, Herbein G. The macrophage: a therapeutic target in HIV-1 infection. Mol Cell Ther. 2014;2:10.
34. Cara A, Reitz MS Jr. New insight on the role of extrachromosomal retroviral DNA. Leukemia. 1997;11:1395–9.
35. Guntaka RV, Richards OC, Shank PR, et al. Covalently closed circular DNA of avian sarcoma virus: purification from nuclei of infected quail tumor cells and measurement by electron microscopy and gel electrophoresis. J Mol Biol. 1976;106:337–57.
36. Shank P, Hughes S, Kung H, et al. Mapping unintegrated avian sarcoma virus DNA: termini of linear DNA bear 300 nucleotides present once or twice in two species of circular DNA. Cell. 1978;15:1383–95.
37. Pang S, Koyanagi Y, Miles S, et al. High levels of unintegrated HIV-1 DNA in brain tissue of AIDS dementia patients. Nature. 1990;343:85–9.
38. Casabianca A, Orlandi C, Canovari B, et al. A real time PCR platform for the simultaneous quantification of total and extrachromosomal HIV DNA forms in blood of HIV-1 infected patients. PLoS ONE. 2014;9:e111919.
39. Meyerhans A, Breinig T, Vartanian J, et al. Forms and function of intracellular HIV DNA. In: Leitner T, Foley B, Hahn B, Marx P, McCutchan F, Mellors JW, Wolinsky S, Korber B, editors. HIV sequence compendium 2003. Los Alamos: Theoretical Biology and Biophysics Group; 2004. p. 14–21.
40. Gelderblom HC, Vatakis DN, Burke SA, et al. Viral complementation allows HIV-1 replication without integration. Retrovirology. 2008;5:60.
41. Butler SL, Hansen MS, Bushman FD. A quantitative assay for HIV DNA integration in vivo. Nat Med. 2001;7:631–4.
42. Vandegraaff N, Kumar R, Burrell CJ, et al. Kinetics of human immunodeficiency virus type 1 (HIV) DNA integration in acutely infected cells as determined using a novel assay for detection of integrated HIV DNA. J Virol. 2001;75:11253–60.
43. Lee MS, Craigie R. Protection of retroviral DNA from autointegration: involvement of a cellular factor. Proc Natl Acad Sci USA. 1994;91:9823–7.
44. Stetson DB, Medzhitov R. Recognition of cytosolic DNA activates an IRF3-dependent innate immune response. Immunity. 2006;24:93–103.
45. Gillim-Ross L, Cara A, Klotman ME. HIV-1 extrachromosomal 2-LTR circular DNA is long-lived in human macrophages. Viral Immunol. 2005;18:190–6.
46. Butler SL, Johnson EP, Bushman FD. Human immunodeficiency virus cDNA metabolism: notable stability of two-long terminal repeat circles. J Virol. 2002;76:3739–47.
47. Kantor B, Ma H, Webster-Cyriaque J, et al. Epigenetic activation of unintegrated HIV-1 genomes by gut-associated short chain fatty acids and its implications for HIV infection. Proc Natl Acad Sci USA. 2009;106:18786–91.
48. Ruis BL, Fattah KR, Hendrickson EA. The catalytic subunit of DNA-dependent protein kinase regulates proliferation, telomere length, and genomic stability in human somatic cells. Mol Cell Biol. 2008;28:6182–95.
49. Collis SJ, DeWeese TL, Jeggo PA, et al. The life and death of DNA-PK. Oncogene. 2005;24:949–61.

50. Shoemaker C, Goff S, Gilboa E, et al. Structure of a cloned circular Moloney murine leukemia virus DNA molecule containing an inverted segment: implications for retrovirus integration. Proc Natl Acad Sci USA. 1980;77:3932–6.
51. Jeanson L, Subra F, Vaganay S, et al. Effect of Ku80 depletion on the preintegrative steps of HIV-1 replication in human cells. Virology. 2002;300:100–8.
52. Zheng Y, Ao Z, Wang B, et al. Host protein Ku70 binds and protects HIV-1 integrase from proteasomal degradation and is required for HIV replication. J Biol Chem. 2011;286:17722–35.
53. Pierson TC, Kieffer TL, Ruff CT, et al. Intrinsic stability of episomal circles formed during human immunodeficiency virus type 1 replication. J Virol. 2002;76:4138–44.
54. Swiggard WJ, O'Doherty U, McGain D, et al. Long HIV type 1 reverse transcripts can accumulate stably within resting CD4+ T cells while short ones are degraded. AIDS Res Hum Retroviruses. 2004;20:285–95.
55. Zhou Y, Zhang H, Siliciano JD, et al. Kinetics of human immunodeficiency virus type 1 decay following entry into resting CD4+ T cells. J Virol. 2005;79:2199–210.
56. Bell P, Montaner LJ, Maul GG. Accumulation and intranuclear distribution of unintegrated human immunodeficiency virus type 1 DNA. J Virol. 2001;75:7683–91.
57. Zennou V, Petit C, Guetard D, et al. HIV-1 genome nuclear import is mediated by a central DNA flap. Cell. 2000;101:173–85.
58. Brin E, Yi J, Skalka AM, et al. Modeling the late steps in HIV-1 integrase-catalyzed DNA integration. J Biol Chem. 2000;275:39287–95.
59. Mulder LC, Chakrabarti LA, Muesing MA. Interaction of HIV-1 integrase with DNA repair protein hRad18. J Biol Chem. 2002;277:27489–93.
60. McDermott JL, Martini I, Ferrari D, et al. Decay of human immunodeficiency virus type 1 unintegrated DNA containing two long terminal repeats in infected individuals after 3 to 8 years of sustained control of viremia. J Clin Microbiol. 2005;43:5272–4.
61. Nakajima N, Lu R, Engelman A. Human immunodeficiency virus type 1 replication in the absence of integrase-mediated DNA recombination: definition of permissive and nonpermissive T-cell lines. J Virol. 2001;75:7944–55.
62. Stein J, Storcksdieck Genannt Bonsmann M, Streeck H. Barriers to HIV cure. HLA. 2016;88:155–63.
63. Graf EH, Mexas AM, Yu JJ, et al. Elite suppressors harbor low levels of integrated HIV DNA and high levels of 2-LTR circular HIV DNA compared to HIV+ patients on and off HAART. PLoS Pathog. 2011;7:e1001300.
64. Buzon MJ, Seiss K, Weiss R, et al. Inhibition of HIV-1 integration in ex vivo-infected CD4 T cells from elite controllers. J Virol. 2011;85:9646–50.
65. Sloan RD, Donahue DA, Kuhl BD, et al. Expression of Nef from unintegrated HIV-1 DNA downregulates cell surface CXCR4 and CCR5 on T-lymphocytes. Retrovirology. 2010;7:44.
66. Thierry S, Thierry E, Subra F, et al. Opposite transcriptional regulation of integrated vs unintegrated HIV genomes by the NF-κB pathway. Sci Rep. 2016;6:25678.
67. Saenz DT, Loewen N, Peretz M, et al. Unintegrated lentivirus DNA persistence and accessibility to expression in nondividing cells: analysis with class I integrase mutants. J Virol. 2004;78:2906–20.
68. Vargas J Jr, Gusella GL, Najfeld V, et al. Novel integrase-defective lentiviral episomal vectors for gene transfer. Hum Gene Ther. 2004;15:361–72.
69. Yáñez-Muñoz RJ, Balaggan KS, MacNeil A, et al. Effective gene therapy with nonintegrating lentiviral vectors. Nat Med. 2006;12:348–53.
70. Lu R, Nakajima N, Hofmann W, et al. Simian virus 40-based replication of catalytically inactive human immunodeficiency virus type 1 integrase mutants in nonpermissive T cells and monocyte-derived macrophages. J Virol. 2004;78:658–68.
71. Brussel A, Sonigo P. Evidence for gene expression by unintegrated human immunodeficiency virus type 1 DNA species. J Virol. 2004;78:11263–71.
72. Shimura K, Miyazato P, Oishi S, et al. Impact of HIV-1 infection pathways on susceptibility to antiviral drugs and on virus spread. Virology. 2015;484:364–76.
73. Engelman A, Englund G, Orenstein JM, et al. Multiple effects of mutations in human immunodeficiency virus type 1 integrase on viral replication. J Virol. 1995;69:2729–36.
74. Poon B, Chang M, Chen I. Vpr is required for efficient Nef expression from unintegrated human immunodeficiency virus type 1 DNA. J Virol. 2007;81:10515–23.
75. Emeagwali N, Hildreth JE. Human immunodeficiency virus type 1 Vpu and cellular TASK proteins suppress transcription of unintegrated HIV-1 DNA. Virol J. 2012;9:277.
76. Iyer SR, Yu D, Biancotto A, et al. Measurement of human immunodeficiency virus type 1 preintegration transcription by using Rev-dependent Rev-CEM cells reveals a sizable transcribing DNA population comparable to that from proviral templates. J Virol. 2009;83:8662–73.
77. Delelis O, Petit C, Leh H, et al. A novel function for spumaretrovirus integrase: an early requirement for integrase-mediated cleavage of 2 LTR circles. Retrovirology. 2005;2:31.
78. Thierry S, Munir S, Thierry E, et al. Integrase inhibitor reversal dynamics indicate unintegrated HIV-1 dna initiate de novo integration. Retrovirology. 2015;12:24.
79. Poon B, Chen I. Human immunodeficiency virus type 1 (HIV-1) Vpr enhances expression from unintegrated HIV-1 DNA. J Virol. 2003;77:3962–72.
80. Rouzioux C, Richman D. How to best measure HIV reservoirs? Current opinion in HIV and AIDS. 2013;8(3):170–5.
81. Bushman F. Measuring covert HIV replication during HAART: the abundance of 2-LTR circles is not a reliable marker. AIDS. 2003;17:749–50.
82. Rivière L, Darlix J-L, Cimarelli A. Analysis of the Viral Elements Required in the Nuclear Import of HIV-1 DNA. J Virol. 2010;84:729–39.

12

Bone mineral density in people living with HIV

M. J. Kruger* and T. A. Nell

Abstract

Bone health status is largely absent in South Africa, the main reasons being the absence and cost-effectiveness of specific screening equipment for assessing bone mineral density (BMD). Various risk factors seem to play a role, some of which can be modified to change bone health status. Urbanisation is also a public health concern. Changing nutritional, as well as social behaviour, play integral roles in the prevalence and incidence of decreased BMD. Furthermore, human immunodeficiency virus (HIV) specifically, has a negative impact on BMD and although highly active antiretroviral therapy increases the prognosis for HIV-infected individuals, BMD still seem to decrease further. Dual energy X-ray absorptiometry is considered the gold standard for BMD assessment; however, recent developments have provided more cost-effective screening methods, among which heel quantitative ultrasound appears to be the most widely used in resource limited countries such as South Africa.

Keywords: HIV, Body composition, Bone mineral density, QUS, DEXA

Background

Osteoporosis, the most common metabolic bone disease, affects almost a quarter of all postmenopausal Caucasian women, the lifetime risk of fracture in these women being 30–40% compared to 20% in men (Fig. 1a) [1]. Worldwide, this risk can vary up to tenfold, depending on the country of origin—the greatest risk reported for the United States of America (USA) [2]. Global statistics regarding the prevalence of osteoporosis, bone mineral density (BMD) and fracture risk are readily available for international countries due to the continuous access to expensive equipment that can screen for bone mass.

The World Health Organization (WHO) developed the Fracture Risk Assessment Tool (FRAX) in order to determine a 10-year probability of the potential risk for future hip fractures or major osteoporotic fractures in women and men between the ages of 40 and 90 years, by using different risk factors related to BMD [3]. In 2000, the incidence of osteoporotic fractures was estimated to be nine million worldwide, with hip fractures contributing 1.6 million (Fig. 1b) [4]. In 2010, projections for the USA (according to FRAX) indicated that approximately 52.4 million individuals older than the age of 50 years would develop low bone mass and osteoporosis [5]. Furthermore, it was predicted that approximately 14 million individuals would be diagnosed with osteoporosis, whereas 47 million will be more likely to have low bone mass in 2020 (Fig. 1c). Since osteoporosis is the most common cause for fractures, it accounts for approximately 1.5 million fractures each year—hip fractures is projected to increase to 6.3 million by 2050, while osteoporosis is projected to increase exponentially due to the aging of the population (Fig. 1b) [6]. Fragility fractures, fractures that occur as a result of a fall from a standing height, lower, or from no trauma at all, can also impact FRAX scoring, although this is poorly understood.

According to the clinical guideline published by the National Osteoporosis Foundation of South Africa (NOFSA) in 2010, the incidence of osteoporosis in white, Asian and mixed race populations in South Africa (SA) seems to be similar to that observed in developed countries, although no accurate fracture data exists for SA [1]. Osteoporosis appears to be less prevalent in SA black populations, similar to data for the USA, although some studies show contradictory results [7–9]. The reasoning

*Correspondence: maritza@sun.ac.za
Department of Physiological Sciences, Stellenbosch University Main Campus, Stellenbosch 7602, Western Cape Province, Republic of South Africa

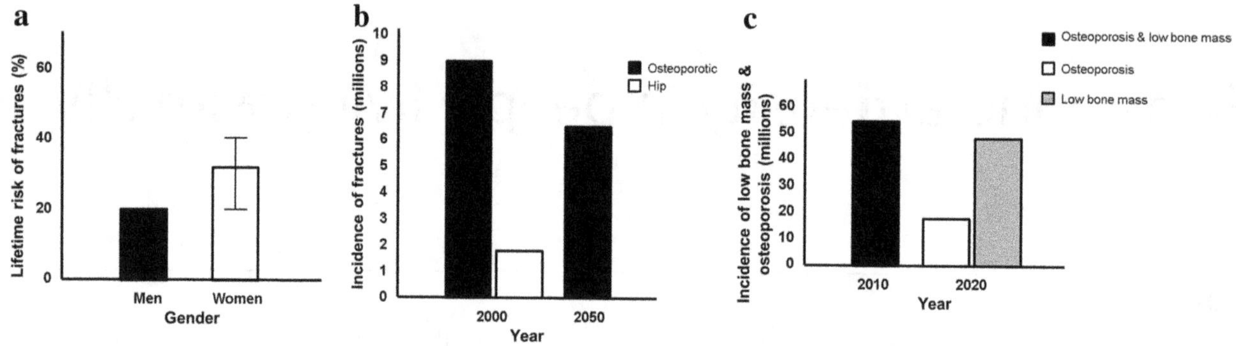

Fig. 1 Representative data indicating (**a**) the lifetime risk of fractures, (**b**) the incidence of fractures and (**c**) the incidence of low bone mass and osteoporosis

behind this being the contribution of fat mass, more specifically visceral adipose tissue (VAT), compared to skeletal muscle mass. What is somewhat concerning is that according to a recent extended report by Sanchez-Riera et al. on the global burden attributable to low BMD as measured by dual energy X-ray absorptiometry (DEXA), no data on BMD at the femoral neck is available for sub Saharan Africa (East and Central), whereas only two studies have reported on BMD in West sub Saharan Africa, and one in South sub Saharan Africa [10].

Bone mineral density (BMD)

Definition, classification and guidelines

Bone mineral density (or bone density), a quantitative measurement of bone mass referring to the amount of mineral matter (calcium) in grams per square centimetre (cm^2) of bones [11, 12], is used in clinical medicine as a surrogate indicator of osteoporosis and fracture risk. According to the National Institutes of Health Consensus Development Panel on Osteoporosis Prevention, Diagnosis, and Therapy, osteoporosis can be defined as a skeletal disorder characterized by increased fracture risk and low bone strength [13].

Several guidelines for the diagnosis and management of osteoporosis have been proposed in 1994 by the WHO. Hough et al. summarized these guidelines into one document for NOFSA [14]. According to the WHO, a subject's BMD is expressed in relation to a young adult reference mean for female Caucasians (T-score) and grouped accordingly into either normal, low bone mass or osteopenia, osteoporotic, and severe osteoporotic categories [14].

The WHO's diagnostic criteria for osteoporosis is a BMD measurement equal to or more than 2.5 standard deviations (SD) below the young female (aged 20–29 years) reference mean (T-score ≤ -2.5 SD), whereas a patient is diagnosed with osteopenia if they have a T-score between -1.0 and -2.5, and as normal if they have a T-score between 1.0 and -0.9 [14].

According to the WHO, T-scores should be reserved for diagnostic use in postmenopausal women and men aged 50 years or more only [14]. For all other populations, Z-scores should be used instead, although categorising individuals as either osteopenia or osteoporotic should still be acceptable for the femoral neck. The Z-score, calculated in the same manner as the T-score, compares a person's bone density to that of an age-, sex-, and race-matched population. This scoring system is usually reserved for youngsters and adolescents; however, considering that these individuals are still growing, the Z-score should also account for pubertal stage and body size. Specialists should also be cautious when diagnosing osteoporosis (a Z-score of ≤ -2.0) in children with this scoring system, as one also needs to consider the presence of at least one fragility fracture [15]. Seeing that the Z-score is age-matched, it can also point to a secondary cause of osteoporosis, other than age in older individuals [16].

Physiology and pathophysiology

In order to fully comprehend the debilitating effects of osteoporosis, a short summary of the natural life history of BMD acquisition and loss is included. Normally, during childhood and the teenage years, bone density accumulates and bone grows in both size and strength (*growth phase*), as new bone is added to the skeleton faster than old bone is removed or resorbed (Fig. 2) [17]. After the growth spurt stops, bone formation continues faster than resorption until *peak bone mass* is reached at about age 25–30 [18, 19]. Bone density is then maintained for about 10 years, at which point bone mass may remain relatively stable (*remodelling phase*), whereafter the age of 35, both men and women will gradually lose 0.3–0.5% of their bone density per year as part of the aging process [20,

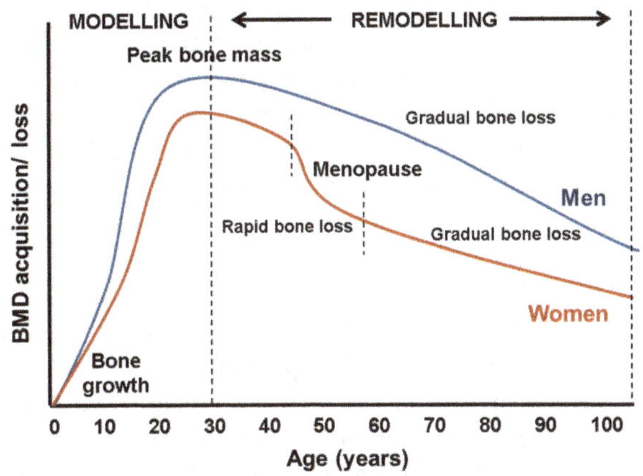

Fig. 2 The general pattern of bone development and loss over time. During years 0–20, bone starts to grow, during the ages of 20–30 years, modelling takes place and peak bone growth is reached. This is followed by the remodelling phase where bone loss is evident

21]. Between the ages of 45 and 55, the menstrual cycle in women ceases, at which point women start to loose bone rapidly in the first 4–8 years thereafter, as a result of decreased oestrogen production [22]. By age 65, men and women tend to lose bone tissue at the same rate, which is much more gradual and continues throughout life.

Considering normal bone growth, osteoporosis is thought of as a silent disease, since bone loss usually occurs without any signs or symptoms. It is also characterized by low BMD, increased bone turnover and deterioration of bone microarchitecture [23]. Although BMD is used in the diagnosis of osteoporosis, low BMD is not the only risk factor for fractures and is not often used on its own to identify fracture risk [24].

Various risk factors are associated with the development of osteoporosis. These include unmodifiable risk factors such as age (the older, the more at risk), sex (females are more at risk), ethnicity (variable results, but pointing towards non-caucasians being more at risk), family history of osteoporosis (immediate family) and prior vertebral fracture or fragility fracture [24–26]. Modifiable risk factors include low body mass index (BMI), particularly in postmenopausal women, exposure to oestrogen, physical activity, long-term glucocorticoid treatment and long-term anticonvulsant therapy (phenytoin, phenobarbital and carbamazephine) [24–26]. Additionally, nutritional status also plays a significant role—impaired absorption or low dietary intake of vitamin D and calcium and excessive use of alcohol (>3 units per day) and tobacco are also risk factors for low BMD [27]. Secondary causes for osteoporosis also exist and include type 1 diabetes, rheumatoid arthritis *osteogenesis imperfect* (brittle bone disease) in adults, *anorexia nervosa*, hyperparathyroidism, untreated long-standing hyperthyroidism, hypogonadism or premature menopause (<45 years), chronic malnutrition or malabsorption (e.g. coeliac disease, inflammatory bowel disease) and chronic liver disease.

Currently, the WHO uses the FRAX index assessment tool to predict fracture risk for a 10 year period in people with low BMD by incorporating various clinical risk factors in its calculation [28]. These include age, sex, race, height, weight, body mass index, fracture history of the patient and parent, current smoking, glucocorticoid usage, the presence of rheumatoid arthritis, secondary causes of osteoporosis, alcohol intake and the BMD measure of the femoral neck. It has been suggested that FRAX only be used to calculate fracture risk for patients who have T-scores between −1.0 and −2.5 in the spine, femoral neck, or total hip region, but not when patients are already on pharmacologic treatment for osteoporosis. According to NOFSA, treatment should also only be considered when the 10-year risk of major-osteoporotic-related fractures as calculated by FRAX are ≥20% [29, 30]. Although FRAX includes a vast number of risk factors, it neglects other important factors, such as 25-hydroxyvitamin D [25(OH)D], physical activity, risk of falls, and biochemical bone markers. Furthermore, multiple risk factors could account for the presence of secondary osteoporosis; however, the risk score does not distinguish between any of these risk factors, which could impact the predicted risk differently.

Different methods exist to assess BMD. These methods will be discussed in the next section, with specific focus on the advantages and disadvantages of each.

Bone mineral density assessment methods

Dual energy X-ray absorptiometry (DEXA)

The use of DEXA in the diagnosis and management of osteoporosis is considered the gold standard to determine loss of BMD [31]. Despite being considered the best clinical tool for diagnosing osteoporosis, DEXA does have some limitations. The biggest critique is that it is influenced by bone size, which suggests that the larger the bone, the greater the BMD, irrespective of its volume. This poses a potential problem since men display higher BMD, even though they might have similar or lower volumetric bone mineral density (vBMD) [32]. Furthermore, two-dimensional (2D) DEXA can also be influenced by artefacts such as aortic calcification and degenerative changes in the spine [23]. Nonetheless, and even though a skilled operator is necessary for its interpretation, DEXA is known for its speed, low radiation dose, moderate cost and ease of operation [33]. In the SA setting specifically, DEXA is not readily available in all clinics; therefore, various other diagnostic assessment tools are implemented to determine BMD. Although BMD can be assessed with other imaging tools, the DEXA T-score must be used as reference standard to compare and validate other BMD modalities.

Quantitative computed tomography (QCT)

In contrast to DEXA which provides 2D scans of bone, quantitative computed tomography (QCT) provides three-dimensional (3D) measures of vBMD with the potential to examine specific compartments within the body separately, such as trabecular and cortical bone, as well as provides a better estimate of the bones' cross-sectional geometry (bone shape and size) [34, 35]. This technique is usually used in conjunction with DEXA for better prediction of fracture risk and osteoporosis, as QCT is predominantly perceived as a research tool [34].

Volumetric QCT is regarded as a quicker and technically less demanding acquisition tool, even though skill is required for its interpretation, and is more widely available since a whole body scanner can be used for image analysis with high precision. However, the individual being scanned is exposed to modest radiation, and depending on the resolution, an increased radiation dose is often required. Results from the study by Pickhardt et al. suggest that both QCT and simple non-angled region-of-interest (ROI) attenuation measurements (measures employed in colonography CT, CTC) of the lumbar spine are effective for BMD screening [36]. Data also suggests that single-level ROI vertebral attenuation measurement at CTC is reproducible, requires little effort, and adds no additional radiation or costs, but can provide valuable BMD data for osteoporosis screening [37]. Furthermore, by applying either QCT analysis to non-contrast-enhanced CT studies, individuals at risk for osteoporosis can be identified. However, a DEXA scan is still needed if an individual at risk for osteoporosis is identified, even though it has been suggested that QCT may be better for BMD assessment [38].

Magnetic resonance imaging (MRI)

Conventional proton magnetic resonance imaging (MRI) is one of the few non-radiative methods used to characterize bone based on mineral and matrix, and produces a negative image of the bone substance [39]. The microarchitectural details of the trabecular network of the bone is geometrically analysed to determine the volume of the bone substance (similar to BMD) if an image is produced in which one can differentiate between the marrow spaces and the trabeculae of the bone, which is most often a difficult task in human subjects [39]. However, if the image has insufficient dimensional resolution, textural information can be obtained about the trabecular network of the bone which may be related to bone mass [40, 41]. It is this ability of MRI to reflect the micro physiology of tissues that makes it such a powerful tool allowing it to better differentiate patients with and without osteoporotic fractures compared to normal BMD. More specifically, the ability to use MRI for vBMD calculations without losing soft tissue signals makes it more clinically attractive even though using MRI to quantify BMD is somewhat difficult due to the low proton signals in mineral [42].

Several improvements have been made to MRI to overcome the problem of low proton signals. Solid state P31 nuclear magnetic resonance projection MRI have been developed which enhances the phosphorus signals to determine BMD more accurately [42], as well as the more recent development of ultra-short echo MRI [43]. Furthermore, high-resolution MRI has been developed in order to quantify the trabecular architecture at the micro-meter level [44, 45], a difficult process which requires standardization at each stage (high resolution MR images consists of several stages) in order to ensure a high degree of reproducibility [46]. Although various studies have been performed in order to optimize image acquisition, post processing, calibration and validation of measurements using MRI, these methods remain technically challenging if not performed by a trained professional.

Quantitative ultrasound (QUS)

Recent developments in densitometry technology have provided alternative methods, among which heel quantitative ultrasound (QUS) appears to be the most widely used. According to the ISCD, calcaneal QUS is the only recognized measurement of QUS to determine bone health status due to the abundance of research done on this particular bone compared to other bone segments [47]. QUS, albeit inexpensive, portable, ionizing-radiation-free and proven to predict hip fractures and all osteoporotic fractures in Caucasian postmenopausal women and elderly men, also requires a trained technician to interpret the results obtained [48, 49]. QUS of the calcaneus has also been shown to accurately predict osteoporotic fractures in elderly female populations [49]. Furthermore, it has the potential to separate osteoporotic individuals from healthy bone individuals [28].

Some of the key features of QUS are its ability to measure the speed of a sound wave (SOS in meter per second—m/s) and its attenuation as it travels through bone. The latter is termed broadband ultrasound attenuation (BUA, dB/mHz), which occurs as a result of the energy that is absorbed by the soft tissue and bone when the sound waves travel through them. It has also been shown that SOS correlates well with BMD [50, 51], whereas BUA is influenced by certain structural characteristics of trabecular bone, such as porosity [50, 52]. A more complex parameter has also been developed from the combination of SOS and BUA, and is used to measure stiffness. This is termed the stiffness index (SI) and has been shown to be more useful in identifying subjects with low BMD and thus high fracture risk [53]. Studies by Gonnelli et al. and Mészáros et al. indicated that both SOS and BUA can be used to distinguish between individuals with and without fractures, however, SOS seem to be somewhat more useful in men [54, 55]. In contrast, according to a study by Ndongo et al., BUA was the most useful measure for identifying factors associated with bone status, such as age, weight and physical activity in urban Sengalese women [56].

Due to the fact that the principles behind QUS and DEXA's ability to determine bone health differs, the same cut-off points may not be useful for both QUS and DEXA [47], as DEXA's cut-offs may over/underestimate the true incidence of osteoporosis [57]. Although DEXA is the standard reference method for diagnosing osteoporosis, a recent study in Dakar, Senegal have employed ultrasound to determine BMD and have found it a useful tool for assessing BMD especially in areas where DEXA is unavailable as is often the case in SA [58]. In this particular study, human immunodeficiency virus (HIV)-infected patients have reduced QUS BMD in comparison with subjects from the general population. However, there was no association between QUS BMD and duration of treatment—at least 5 years on highly active antiretroviral therapy (HAART). Since the validated reference method for bone density assessment couldn't be used, the clinical significance of these results in terms of osteoporosis remains unknown.

It is evident from the studies mentioned above that QUS has the potential to not only predict fracture risk, but also to determine BMD. To complement the results obtained with QUS, specific biochemical markers can be used in conjunction with BMD testing to determine bone health status.

Biochemical-specific markers

Bone turnover markers Bone turnover is the main contributor to both quality and quantity of bone. An imbalance between bone resorption and formation leads to a net loss or gain of bone tissue. High bone turnover results in bone loss and abnormal bone microarchitecture, whereas, low bone turnover results in increased bone mass, accumulation of microdamage, and bone fragility [59].

Surrogate markers of fracture risk—bone turnover markers (BTMs) and BMD—can be used to monitor a specific treatment response. High levels of bone BTMs were shown to correlate well with increased fracture risk in postmenopausal women [60]. In various studies regarding therapeutic agents, BMD and BTMs were shown to respond differently, a change in BMD only observed after about 1–2 years [61], whereas changes in urinary levels of BTMs were observed within a couple of months [62, 63]. In a study by Bjarnason et al., short-term changes (3–6 months) in BTM was associated with long-term changes (1–2 years) in BMD, therefore both BTM and BMD can be used, albeit at different times [64].

Although several studies have investigated numerous biochemical markers of bone turnover to determine fracture risk, it was recommended by Vasikaran et al. to use serum carboxy terminal telopeptide of collagen type I (s-CTX) as the standard bone resorption marker and serum procollagen type I N-terminal propeptide (s-PINP) as the standard bone formation marker [65]. Serum CTX is shown to be specifically influenced by renal function, diurnal rhythm and food intake, peaking early in the morning and is at its lowest in the afternoon. Food intake also tends to decrease these levels; therefore, it is imperative that sampling time be in the morning and in a fasted state. Serum PINP on the other hand is not influenced that greatly by diurnal rhythm, food intake or temperature.

Biochemical and nutritional markers Several biochemical markers can also be assessed to determine the contributing factors associated with osteoporosis. These include serum total calcium, albumin (to correct for calcium if data is skewed by abnormal albumin) and phosphate amongst others to detect conditions associated with hypercalcemia, such as primary hyperparathyroidism or hypocalcemia and consequent secondary hyperparathyroidism causing bone loss [66]. Serum creatinine measurements and estimations of the glomerular filtration rate are also useful to detect renal failure which can affect bone health [66]. Although serum alkaline phosphatase (ALP) is a useful marker to detect certain disease conditions regarding bone, it is not sensitive enough to detect changes in bone remodelling [66].

Adequate supply of vitamin D is considered essential for bone health as it aids calcium absorption in order to maintain the calcium concentration in the physiologically-relevant range [67, 68]. Vitamin D levels are directly related to BMD irrespective of ethnicity and gender, maximum density achieved with levels of 40 ng/mL (99.8 nmol/L) or higher [69]. Since vitamin D is vital to the regulation of calcium and phosphorous metabolism, bone formation and mineralization, it is documented as one of the key factors associated with bone mass and therefore important in the management of osteoporosis [70]. Although the optimum level of serum 25(OH)D (the inactive form of vitamin D) in a healthy population is not uniformly accepted, a concentration of at least 30 ng/mL

(75 nmol/L) is recognised as the endpoint (lowest) for skeletal health outcomes by most [70–72], whereas 20 up to 30 ng/mL (50–75 nmol/L) is considered acceptable and desirable [73].

Exposure of the skin to sunlight, the melanin concentration, clothing style when exposed to sunlight and the season all play important roles in vitamin D production [74, 75]. Age, BMI, vitamin D supplementation and physical activity also influence the concentration of serum 25(OH)D [72, 75]. Furthermore, serum 25(OH)D concentration also positively correlates with BMD and negatively with parathyroid hormone (PTH) [76–79], and it was determined that serum PTH tended to be higher in individuals with serum 25(OH)D between 50 and 75 nmol/L (20 up to 30 ng/mL), a concentration sufficient to prevent secondary hyperparathyroidism. PTH is primarily responsible for converting 25(OH)D in the kidney to the hormonal, active form of 1,25(OH)2D. However, many other tissues in the body are also able to instigate this conversion in order to act locally as a paracrine or autocrine hormone [80].

Directly linked to vitamin D's role in calcium homeostasis, is the relationship between calcium and PTH (Fig. 3). When calcium absorption is sub-optimal, serum calcium levels decrease which in turn stimulates the production of PTH from the parathyroid glands [81]. This increases the reabsorption of calcium and enhances the expression of the receptor activator of nuclear factor kappa B (NFκB) ligand (RANKL) on osteoblasts to increase the production of mature osteoclasts which mobilizes calcium to bone, restoring serum calcium concentrations to normal [82]. PTH also mobilizes phosphorous from bone, as well as decreases kidney phosphorous reabsorption which causes phosphaturia [82]. Since PTH is regulated by calcium intake, it has been suggested that serum PTH measurements be taken if serum calcium is abnormal to determine the cause of abnormality [66].

Therefore, calcium and vitamin D deficiency are particularly important role players in bone health, because reduced calcium absorption increases PTH concentration and accelerates the rate of bone loss, which raises the number and activity of osteoclasts that release calcium from bone. Though this is an appropriate short-term homeostatic response, the long-term effects are detrimental to the skeleton because of the ongoing imbalance at the remodelling sites.

Additionally, locally produced growth factors such as insulin-like growth factor (IGF)-1 and -2, transforming growth factor (TGF)-β, interleukins (IL)s, prostaglandins, tumour necrosis factor (TNF)-α and osteoprotegrin ligand (OPG-L) have also been implicated as regulators of bone remodelling, together with the hormones oestrogen and androgens. These factors will be discussed at a later stage in this review.

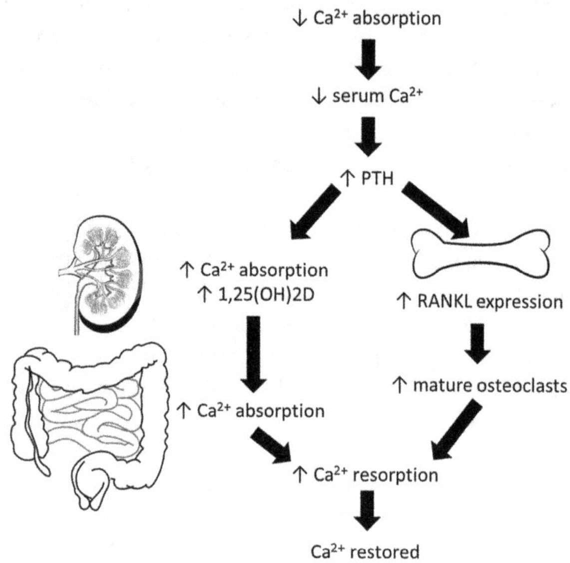

Fig. 3 The restoration of suboptimal calcium levels

Clinical significance of BMD measurements

Bone status is largely absent in SA due to lack and cost of specific equipment for assessing BMD. A few studies suggested that BMD in Africa may be similar to northern world observations, however, the prevalence of fractures appears to be much lower [83–85].

With the use of alternative measuring techniques that are readily available for BMD, the cost will decrease; however, the precision of other bone density measuring techniques compared to DEXA is still not agreed upon. Nevertheless, the potential of diagnosing a person with the predisposition of developing osteoporosis, using easy to use equipment and markers associated with BMD is warranted as proper and earlier treatment may prevent or even delay the onset of osteoporosis. Confirmation however is still necessary with the use of a DEXA scan. HIV specifically has a negative impact on BMD and will be the focus of the next section.

HIV

HIV disease profile

With HIV infections, various complications arise which affect different systems of the body. These include cardiac, metabolic, endocrine, renal and inflammatory/immune systems to name but a few. Apart from these complications, changes in lipid and glucose metabolism, adipose tissue disorders and abnormal bone metabolism are also prevalent. One of the major focuses of research has been the association between HIV, HAART, metabolic disorders and vascular disease. However, the specific effects of HIV on the metabolic, endocrine and renal systems, as well as the bone, and the interactions between these systems have not been that extensively studied. Furthermore, although the use of HAART has improved the prognosis of HIV-infected patients dramatically, long-term HAART is associated with several cardio-metabolic, endocrine, renal and bone perturbations, which will be discussed in the next section.

HIV and the metabolic system

Insulin resistance, impaired glucose tolerance, impaired fasting glucose and diabetes mellitus (DM) are a spectrum of glucose metabolism disorders reported in persons with HIV infection both with and without HAART. In a HIV-positive population, approximately 25–35% of patients have impaired glucose tolerance, whereas 2–7% have DM [86, 87]. Genetic susceptibility and lifestyle seem to be some of the factors that most often cause variation in the prevalence of HIV from one population to another [87].

There is a strong association between insulin resistance and lipid accumulation in muscle and liver tissue in HIV-positive patients with lipodystrophy—increased VAT is associated with excess free fatty acids, increased intramyocellular fat content and reduced adiponectin [88]. Glucose uptake into abdominal subcutaneous adipose tissue (SAT) is increased in HIV-infected patients, whereas glucose uptake in VAT and muscle cells does not differ [88].

With specific reference to BMD, inconsistencies exist regarding the relationship between VAT and BMD. Whilst some studies suggest an inverse relationship [89, 90], a study by Yamaguchi et al. suggests a potential protective effect of VAT especially in patients with DM [91]. A study by Bredella et al. confirmed the findings of an inverse relationship between VAT and BMD in pre-menopausal obese women [92]. They further go on to suggest that this effect may at least by partially mediated by IGF-1, since IGF-1 and muscle mass are positive predictors of BMD. The growth hormone (GH)/IGF-1 axis is a major determinant of BMD [93, 94] and seems to be dysregulated in females specifically in proportion to the degree of VAT [95]. Other potential explanations could include the release of proinflammatory cytokines secreted by adipocytes, such as IL-6, TNF-α, and adipokines, such as E-selectin and adiponectin, stimulating osteoclast activity [90, 96, 97].

A previous study also found that lean body mass is an important predictor of BMD in premenopausal women, whereas fat mass correlated positively with BMD of the hip [98]. The adipokine, leptin, is responsible for regulating several hypothalamic pituitary adrenal (HPA) axes which are involved in mediating the connection between leptin and bone by means of direct and indirect mechanisms. Since the leptin receptor can be found in adult primary osteoblasts, it is suggested that leptin has a direct effect on bone growth through its inhibitory action against bone resorption (osteoblastic activity) [99]. It regulates osteocalcin which in turn regulates bone metabolism [100]. Furthermore, bone marrow adipocytes also secrete leptin which may mediate leptins' local effect on bone. On the other hand, indirect mechanisms are more complex and involve cortisol, thyroid and parathyroid hormones, as well as growth hormones and IGF-1 [101].

HIV and the endocrine system

A wide spectrum of endocrine complications is associated with HIV infection and acquired immunodeficiency syndrome (AIDS). However, these disorders may also be as a consequence of systemic illness, opportunistic infections, body composition and/or HIV-related therapies [102]. The pituitary, thyroid, adrenal gland, gonadal, pancreas and bone are all involved.

Although HIV brings about secondary issues such as endocrine dysregulation, hormonal imbalances are not a common occurrence. HIV does however involve almost all of the hormonal systems and axes. One of the most common endocrine axes to be affected by HIV is the HPA axis [103]. During a condition such as HIV, viral proteins and cytokines activate or inhibit the hormonal system, further contributing to HPA dysregulation, a condition which is exacerbated with HAART [103]. The adrenal gland malfunctions as a result of adrenal insufficiency. Furthermore, due to a glucocorticoid resistant state, impaired adrenal and pituitary reserves cannot react to increased cortisol levels. Various different thyroid hormone disorders also occur which is associated with altered metabolism, poor oral intake and increased prevalence of weight loss and wasting syndrome [103].

Oestrogens and androgens have also been implicated to contribute to changes in BMD, not only during adulthood, but also during the growth of the skeleton. Oestrogen specifically has been shown to inhibit osteoclast function, and stimulate osteoblasts to produce growth factors and cytokines that mediate oestrogen' action, some of which regulate the osteoblasts indirectly [104]. More importantly, oestrogen may play a role in determining the life span of bone cells by controlling the rate of apoptosis, thus decreasing the lifespan of osteoblasts and increasing the longevity of osteoclasts [104]. Two specific and complementing mechanisms have been implicated to explain the effect of oestrogen on bone. Firstly, oestrogen deficiency (most commonly as a result of menopause) causes bone loss through its activation of new bone remodelling sites and through exaggeration of the imbalance between bone formation and resorption [104]. Oestrogen deficiency stimulates osteoblast production of IL-1 and -6 and TNF-α and inhibits apoptosis, thus extending the life span of osteoclasts. Oestrogen deficiency decreases IL-1ra leading to enhanced osteoclast sensitivity to IL-1. These actions mainly occur via oestrogen receptor (ER)α, which then elicits a prominent effect on the regulation of bone turnover and the maintenance of bone mass [105]. Although osteoblast numbers are also elevated, the increase in bone formation is not sufficient to replace the bone matrix removed by osteoclasts, resulting in net bone loss.

One has to take into consideration that HIV-infected subjects already have low BMD, and even more so when treated with HAART. Given the vast proportion of women living with HIV, who are and will be transitioning through menopause, one also needs to consider the additional burden that low oestrogen levels will place on a BMD level that is already compromised by HIV and HAART. Statistics in the USA are largely alarming, as it is anticipated that by 2020, more than 50% of HIV infection will be in patients over the age of 50 years [106]. In women living with HIV, an intricate relationship between HIV and menopause appears to exist in that HIV may influence the natural history, experience, and complications of menopause, while menopause itself could potentially influence the course of HIV infection [107]. This relationship between HIV and menopause further complicates the management of HIV infection in women as they age and challenges clinicians, since lymphocyte subsets, including CD4 counts have been found to decrease with increasing age in non-HIV-infected adults [108]. Considering that older individuals are usually diagnosed later with a more advanced stage of HIV, CD4 counts will be even lower. Therefore, the combination of all of these factors predisposes women to an earlier and even more severe bone loss compared to those individuals without HIV.

In males, testosterone affects BMD through its direct effect on the androgen receptors in trabecular and cortical bone [109, 110]. Testosterone's effect is more complex than that of oestrogen as it is converted to estradiol in adipose tissue or bone, with subsequent stimulation of the oestrogen receptors [110–112]. When androgen levels are low, it is associated with bone loss and increased bone remodelling in men [113, 114]; however, a reduction in oestrogen seems to play a key role in the age-related decrease of BMD [115, 116]. With advancing age, testosterone is also considered the major source of circulating estradiol in women (menopause), and testosterone can regulate local production of cytokines and growth factors in bone, including IL-6, IL-1β, TGFβ and IGFs [109]. The anabolic effects of testosterone on muscle mass and strength can also indirectly affect bone mass.

Data on the effect of low testosterone levels on BMD are not in agreement. One specific study suggests that serum total estradiol, but not testosterone is associated with reduced BMD in HIV-infected men [117]. This study showed that among men with low testosterone, it is only those men that develop an oestrogen deficiency that will have lower BMD, a result which was also evident in other studies [118, 119], although some studies found the opposite to be true [120, 121].

It is therefore evident that older age, and therefore the decrease in sex hormones, impacts BMD even more negatively when associated with HIV and HAART treatment.

HIV and the renal system

Patients with HIV usually show signs of proteinuria which progress rapidly to end-stage renal disease, commonly referred to as HIV-associated nephropathy (HIVAN) [122]. The nucleoside reverse transcriptase inhibitor (NRTI), tenofovir (TDF), has been linked to proximal renal dysfunction (PRTD), which can result in excessive renal phosphate, uric acid and bicarbonate loss. Furthermore, it can also result in proteinuria and glucosuria especially in patients with pre-existing nephropathy [123]. A study by Fux et al. showed that PRTD may promote BMD loss through renal phosphate wasting [124]. Studies originally reported on nephrotoxic effects as a result of TDF, but the incidence of adverse renal effects were low in initial randomized trials [125, 126]. A small but significant loss in renal function was observed in patients on TDF-containing regimens compared to abacavir (ABC)-containing regimens [127]; however, studies are not conclusive regarding renal endpoints and more patients developed clinical renal impairment [128, 129]. Additionally, although both the STEAL and ASSERT study indicated no difference in estimated glomerular filtration rate (eGFR) between patients [130, 131], increases in markers of proximal tubule dysfunction were evident as a result of TDF treatment in the ASSERT study [130]. This is comparable to results obtained by Rasmussen et al. In this particular study, although no difference in renal function was evident when plasma cystatin C (cysC) and estimated creatine clearance (CrCl) were measured (indicative of stable GFR), a minor increase in urinary neutrophil gelatinase-associated lipocalin (NGAL)/creatinine ratio (as a marker of renal dysfunction) was observed in the TDF-containing regimen compared to the ABC-containing regimen [132]. CrCl is however dependent on factors other than plasma creatinine and GFR, such as changes in muscle mass and tubular secretion of creatinine.

A different formulation of TDF was approved by the FDA in order to try and overcome the side effects associated with TDF. Patients that switched to tenofovir alafenamide (TAF) seemed to be more likely to keep their viral load low, whilst kidney function and bone density was improved [133, 134]. Even after 2–3 years, TAF was better at suppressing viral load and safer for the bones and kidneys [135, 136]. A similar study by Brown et al., also showed that participants who switched from TDF to TAF showed improved bone health, including a reduction in osteoporosis [137].

HIV and bone mineral density

A reduction in BMD is a common complication of HIV and its treatment, with low BMD, osteopenia and osteoporosis more commonly associated with both male and female HIV-infected subjects [138, 139], compared to non-infected subjects [140, 141].

The rates of osteopenia and osteoporosis were found to be as high as 67 and 15% respectively, whilst the magnitude of BMD reduction was 6.4-fold higher, and that of osteoporosis 3.7-fold higher in HIV-positive patients, as reported in a meta-analysis [142]. Cazavane et al. indicated that more than half the HIV-infected patients had osteopenia, and approximately a third had osteoporosis [138], results which were verified by a study from McComsey et al. [143]. Triant et al. also reported a higher prevalence of fracture risk in HIV-positive patients compared to HIV-negative patients [144]. A more recent study reported the rates for osteopenia and osteoporosis to be 47.5 and 23% respectively, whilst BMD decreased in about 28% of subjects in a follow-up study of 2.5 years [145]. Sharma et al. found similar results, where rates of 42 and 12% were reported for osteopenia and osteoporosis respectively—the degree of osteopenia was three times higher in the HIV-infected subjects with 12% of patients progressing to osteoporosis [146]. These studies highlighted the existence of high prevalence of osteopenia and osteoporosis in the HIV-positive population.

HIV-positive patients have reduced bone size, mass and strength due to altered metabolism and the infection of bone cells [147]. It has been suggested by Duvivier et al. and Borderi et al. that HIV infection of osteoblasts may be related to a negative balance of bone remodelling [148, 149]. Since osteopenia and osteoporosis is highly prevalent in HAART-naïve patients, it suggests that if viremia is not controlled properly, it might impact BMD via its effects on persistent systemic inflammation and bone remodelling. Not only do the HIV proteins increase osteoclast activity, but they promote osteoblast apoptosis, thereby decreasing bone formation [150].

Under normal conditions, both vitamin D and phosphate metabolism are important for skeletal integrity; however, in HIV, vitamin D and phosphate contributes to low BMD due to impaired mineralization [148]. Approximately 60–75% of patients in a HIV-infected population have low vitamin D levels [151]. Furthermore, hypogonadism may also play a role [152], and lipoatrophy seems to mediate bone loss through adipocyte hormone signalling [89].

Since persistent systemic inflammation can impact bone density, the involvement of various cytokines involved in this process are of great importance. T-cells (specifically targeted by HIV infection), B-cells and monocytes are responsible for the production and regulation of key osteoclastogenic cytokines such as RANKL and OPG [153]. It is speculated that HIV infection results in the alteration of B cell function and subsequently a switch from bone sparing OPG production to the production of bone destroying RANKL, thus leading to increased osteclastogenesis [154]. This data is consistent with the fact that B-cells are mainly regulated by interactions with T-cells, as well as the fact that severe perturbations of the B-cell linage are mediated by HIV infection (through direct effects of viral infection and/or indirectly though disruption of co-stimulatory signals from T-cells and other disrupted immune components) [155, 156]. Along with upregulation of RANKL by HIV gp120 protein, there is further activation of RANKL by TNF-α that is represented in higher numbers in advanced HIV disease [157].

A dramatic increase in the number of osteoclast precursors (defined as monocytes expressing the RANKL receptor, RANK) were also evident, whilst OPG expression was significantly diminished [156]. Data from animal studies showed that HIV infection results in alterations in the immuno-skeletal interface favourable to accelerated bone resorption and loss of bone mass. Low serum OPG concentrations have been reported in HIV/AIDS patients [158], verifying some of the data seen from animal studies. Furthermore, peripheral blood T-cells have been implicated as a potential source of OPG [158]. Other studies have shown that HIV-infected women have higher levels of both RANKL and OPG than their HIV-negative counterparts, suggesting increased overall bone turnover in HIV-infected patients [159], while HAART initiation has been associated with increases in both, again suggesting increased bone turnover [160, 161].

One of the most recent studies performed were able to show that the combination of all B cells were responsible for the increase in RANKL, whilst the decrease in OPG was due to changes in the distribution of B cell subsets [162]. Therefore it is crucial to distinguish between the different B cells and to include naïve and resting memory B cells (decreased number with high expression of OPG), and tissue-like B cells (increased number with low expression of OPG). When the relationship between these markers and BMD in HIV-positive participants was investigated, RANKL/OPG correlated significantly with BMD and T- and/or Z-scores in the femur neck and hip region, which was not evident in the HIV-negative participants. The data therefore supports the concept of B cell alterations in RANKL and OPG production which may contribute to the decline in BMD in the context of HIV. Interestingly, although a decrease in OPG expression in the B cells was observed overall, serum OPG levels were elevated whilst RANKL was decreased, which was also shown in other studies [163, 164]. However, whereas some of the studies showed a decrease in RANKL, the study by Gibellini et al. indicated an increase in RANKL suggesting that relying only on circulating markers is not a true reflection of what happens in bone.

Interferon (IFN-γ) has also been shown to interfere with the RANKL receptor through its action on the adapter protein, (tumour necrosis factor receptor-associated factor-6; TRAF-6) that links RANK to its downstream transcription factors, ultimately inhibiting osteoclast formation [165, 166]. These alterations in the immune-skeletal interface may therefore account for much of the loss of BMD observed in HIV patients.

Even though there are growing concerns regarding osteoporosis, the impact of HIV and its treatment on bones in resource-limited countries is poorly documented.

HAART and bone mineral density

Various studies have reported on low BMD in HIV-infected adults; however, the prevalence of osteoporosis seems to be approximately three times higher in HIV-infected patients receiving HAART treatment than uninfected patients [142]. Although studies reported a 2–6% decrease in BMD (within the first 2 years) with HAART treatment [149, 167], this decline in BMD only pertains to patients starting a new HAART regimen (within 24–48 weeks) [149, 168], and not continuing on a currently established regimen. This decrease seems to be similar to that observed within the first 2 years of menopause [169].

From the literature it is evident that the specific type of treatment can have a significant effect on bone loss. The use of NRTIs has been associated with low BMD [160, 168, 170]. TDF-based treatment patients had a much lower BMD after 96 weeks of treatment compared to other regimens such as lamivudine (3TC) and emtricitabine (FTC) patients, although no higher incidence of fracture were evident [160, 168, 170]. Similar results were obtained in a study using ABC as alternative [160].

Results from the study of Cotter et al. showed no significant alteration in phosphate metabolism that often accompanies bone loss [171], although some studies have shown TDF is able to decrease BMD through persistent urinary loss of phosphates [170, 172]. Instead, higher serum phosphorus among patients with low bone density was evident, although it is not exactly clear why. Furthermore, time on TDF showed a trend to correlate with low BMD Z-scores, which is in direct contrast to other studies which have failed to show any correlation between TDF and low bone mass, even after long-term exposure to the drug [173, 174]. NRTIs can further reduce BMD by elevating lactic acidemia, a mechanism related to calcium hydroxyapatite loss, especially in the trabecular bone, due to the lability of calcium storage [175]. Several studies have directly highlighted HIV factors associated with low BMD: duration of infection, HIV viral burden, and a more advanced HIV disease [171].

Studies regarding PIs remain unclear due to conflicting results. PI use has been shown to result in increased bone turnover, accelerated bone loss, and a higher prevalence of reduced BMD [142, 149, 170, 176], whilst other studies failed to show such a difference [167, 177–179]. A recent study conducted in Asia by Kinai et al. indicated that PI use, but not specific type of PI, was the most significant cause of low BMD at both spine and femoral neck [180]. This finding is consistent with an in vitro study evaluating the effect of different PIs on osteoblast activity [181]. Kinai et al. also observed a large difference in BMD between PI-discontinued and continued patients—PI discontinued patients displayed BMD levels in the lumber spine and not femoral neck [180], consistent with other studies [149, 170]. This is likely due to the fact that the femur contains cortical substance with few osteoclasts, whilst the vertebrae contain osteoclast-rich trabecular substance. Interestingly, discontinuation of ritonavir (RTV), an osteoclast-activating agent, resulted in slower decrease in BMD in vertebrae compared to the femoral neck [180]. Furthermore, RTV was able to cause bone mineral loss in a time dependent manner irrespective of dosage [180]. RTV was also shown to promote the proliferation and activation of osteoclasts in both in vitro [182, 183] and ex vivo studies [184], causing increased bone absorption.

In a study by Duvivier et al., a four percent decline in BMD were evident after 48 weeks on HAART in the lumbar spine and a three percent decline in hip BMD [149]. Although BMD loss occurred with PIs, NNRTIs alone, as well as a combination of PIs and NNRTIs, could not worsen the BMD loss in the spine [149]. In contrast, a significant loss in BMD (5–6%) at the femoral neck by week 48 were evident irrespective of NRTI or PIs [185].

Specific BMD measurements with DEXA showed that immune suppression before starting HIV therapy was a risk factor for loss of BMD during treatment. However, there was no evidence that the extent of immune reconstitution was associated with BMD change after controlling for baseline $CD4^+$ count even with HAART initiation—loss of bone continues after HIV therapy is initiated (up to 2 years) [186]. Data therefore suggests that low pre-treatment CD4 count, but not early change with HAART was a strong and independent risk factor for bone loss after HAART initiation—providing further evidence for the benefits of early initiation of HAART [186].

Although HAART may be associated with the occurrence of fractures, none of the studies thus far were able to show any changes in fracture rates. This is possibly due to the limited number of cohort studies exploring this phenomenon, as well as a too short follow-up period.

The mechanisms of action of HAART-induced bone loss

The specific mechanisms by which HAART induces bone loss remain debatable, but it has been thought to be either due to a direct effect on bone cells (most likely), realignment of HIV-associated pathologies resulting from disease reversal, or a combination of these factors. In vitro and in vivo studies involving animal models have shown that HAART do act on osteoclasts and osteoblasts; however, these effects could not be verified in humans due to the different effects the different HAART classes have on bone. One such example was found in a study by Wang et al. in which the PI, RTV, suppressed osteoclastogenesis and osteoclast function in vitro and in vivo by impairing RANKL-induced signalling, but the PI indinavir (IDV) had no effect on osteoclastogenesis [187]. The PI fosamprenavir (FPV) significantly increased OPG and decreased RANKL production in vitro, which could suggest protection of bone mass if confirmed in vivo. In contrast, other PIs including atazanavir (ATV), saquinavir (SQV), and IDV failed to impact the OPG/RANKL ratio [181]. Furthermore, preliminary studies in vitro have found no effect of several NRTIs on osteoclastogenesis, but NRTIs were found to suppress osteoblast activity instead [188].

Confounding factors and discrepancies in results

Many confounding factors are assumed to play a role in the pathogenesis of decreased bone mass in HIV-infected patients [189]. Fat-free mass, one of the most important components of body composition was shown to be one of the problems [190]; however, according to Reid et al. [191], low weight appears to be the major component in healthy individuals, which has also been verified in a HIV-positive population [147]. Results from a more recent study are in accordance with the important role of body composition and have indicated that weight, BMI, and body fat were all associated with BMD, especially in females [192], which also highlights the importance of nutrition on BMD, especially because low calcium and vitamin D intake reduces BMD [193]. A study in Brazil indicated that HIV-positive populations have calcium and vitamin D deficiencies, even though their dietary intake is similar to that described in other young Brazilian populations [194, 195]. Limitations in studies regarding nutrition and BMD are often due to the fact that participants need to recall what they have consumed and errors might slip in as it is self-reported. Low BMD have been linked to low body weight, testosterone or oestrogen deficiency, glucocorticoids, malabsorption, tobacco use, alcohol and opiate abuse, nadir CD4 cell count, duration of HIV infection, lipodystrophy, insulin resistance and hyperlactatemia, all of which could contribute to the discrepancies in results [196].

Conclusions

Although bone loss is a common complication of HIV, HAART initiation further worsens, rather than ameliorates, bone loss. This effect of HAART on BMD is rather alarming in a population whose skeletal integrity is already seriously compromised due to HIV infection. The interaction between bone and the endocrine, metabolic and renal system in this population complicates bone dynamics even further. Opinions still differ widely among investigators as to the direct effects of HAART or their components on bone cells, or their mechanisms of action on the skeleton. Consequently, it is rather thought that all HAART formulations may be inherently detrimental to the skeleton as bone loss appears to be a general phenomenon observed following HAART initiation, regardless of the regimen type, although PIs and specifically TDF may be the main causes.

Various studies found that continuous exposure to HAART results in a further decline in BMD compared with intermittent HAART exposure. Although most of the important questions regarding HAART-related bone loss are now answered, such as: (1) Are certain HAART regimens more detrimental than others? (2) How soon after HAART initiation does bone loss begin? and (3) Does it occur in a specific timeframe or is it a long-term effect? the fact still remains that HAART treatment has a negative influence on BMD.

The NRTI, TDF has been associated with bone loss in various studies compared to other regimens. PIs on the other hand have also been associated with skeletal deterioration in most studies. While the degree of bone loss may vary somewhat between regimens, almost all HAART regimens resulted in a significant loss of BMD between 2 and 6% over time. The biggest loss following HAART initiation appears to occur within 24–48 weeks. Furthermore, once lost, BMD never recovers to pre-treatment baseline levels, let alone to normal BMD levels characteristic of uninfected individuals of similar age. Therefore, it is imperative that BMD be monitored and treatment started if a patient is diagnosed with low BMD.

Determining BMD in a specific population also appears to be somewhat of a concern, since the gold standard method to determine BMD, the DEXA, is not readily available in all clinics and areas. The ability to use other assessment tools such as QUS in resource limited settings will have to be investigated, but validation of the method needs to first take place before being able to use it as a diagnostic and research tool for a specific population.

Take home message to clinicians The primary goal for any clinician in treating people with osteoporosis is preventing fractures. However, when the patient is faced with HIV or even the additional burden of HAART treatment, the strategies should probably have to be altered. With respect to BMD management, those individuals with HIV should undergo the same treatment process as HIV-negative people, and should also include lifestyle modifications and pharmacological interventions. This will be of great benefit not only when BMD is low, but will also benefit those individuals with HIV. One should always bear in mind that certain pharmacological interventions for other conditions, may have interactions with HAART medication in HIV subjects and might not be safe to use. Some of the medications taken for osteoporosis have also not been tested in combination with the various HAART treatment options. These patients should therefore be carefully monitored for a couple of months to establish whether any side effects arose as a consequence of treatment. For the most part, the benefits of HAART with respect to virologic control are considered to outweigh the risk of potentially exacerbating bone loss. However, in those patients who are at high risk of a fracture, clinicians may want to consider avoiding TDF or PIs if alternatives are available. When also faced with the additional burden of menopause, one has to take into consideration that oestrogen is also now low, and that if oestrogen is given additionally, it might have an effect or even interfere with the other medications already prescribed.

Usage of FRAX is recommended, and secondary causes of osteoporosis other than HIV or menopause should be evaluated. Patients at high risk for fractures should be encouraged to make lifestyle changes, to avoid tobacco and alcohol, and to prevent falls. Once osteoporosis has been diagnosed and therapy started, DEXA should be repeated every 1–2 years as follow-up.

Authors' contributions

MK was in charge of writing the review, whilst both authors approved the review. Both authors read and approved the final manuscript.

Acknowledgements

Not applicable.

Competing interests

The authors declare that they have no competing interests.

Funding

No funding was used for the write-up of this review article.

References

1. Hough S, Ascott-Evans BH, Brown SL, Cassim B, de Villiers TJ, Lipschitz S, et al. NOFSA guideline for the diagnosis and management of osteoporosis. J Endocrinol Metab Diabetes S Afr. 2010;15(3):1–188.
2. Thomas PA. Racial and ethnic differences in osteoporosis. J Am Acad Ortho Surg. 2007;15:S26–30.
3. Kanis JA, Oden A, Johansson H, Borgström F, Ström O, Mccloskey E. FRAX and its application in clinical practice. Bone. 2009;44:734–43.
4. Cooper C, Cole ZA, Holroyd CR, Earl SC, Harvey NC, Dennison EM, et al. Secular trends in the incidence of hip and other osteoporotic fractures. Osteoporos Int. 2011;22:1277–88.
5. National Osteoporosis Foundation. America's bone health: the state of osteoporosis and low bone mass in our nation. Washington DC: National Osteoporosis Foundation; 2002.
6. Cooper C, Campion G, Melton LJ. Hip fractures in the eldery: a world-wide projection. Osteoporos Int. 1992;2:287–9.
7. Chantler S, Dickie K, Goedecke JH, Levitt NS, Lambert EV, Evans J, et al. Site-specific differences in bone mineral density in black and white premenopausal South African women. Osteopor Int. 2012;23:533–42.
8. Goedecke JH, Levitt NS, Lambert EV, Utzschneider KM, Faulenbach MV, Dave JA, et al. Differential effects of abdominal adipose tissue distribution on insulin sensitivity in black and white South African women. Obesity. 2009;17:1506–12.
9. Sumner AE, Micklesfield LK, Ricks M, Tambay AV, Avila NA, Thomas F, et al. Waist circumference, BMI, and visceral adipose tissue in white women and women of African descent. Obesity (Silver Spring). 2011;19(3):671–4.
10. Sanchez-Riera L, Carnahan E, Vos T, Veerman L, Norman R, Lim SS, et al. The global burden attributable to low bone mineral density. Ann Rheum Dis. 2014;73(9):1635–45.
11. Stedman's medical dictionary for the health professions and nursing. 7th ed. Huntingdon Valley: Farlex Inc; 2011.
12. Segen's medical dictionary. Huntingdon Valley: Joe Segen and Farlex Inc; 2012.
13. NIH consensus development panel on osteoporosis prevention, diagnosis and therapy. Osteoporosis prevention, diagnosis, and therapy. JAMA. 2001;285 (6):785-95.
14. Hough S, Ascott-Evans BH, Brown SL, Cassim B, de Villiers TJ, Lipschitz S, et al. NOFSA guideline for the diagnosis and management of osteoporosis. Executive summary. J Endocrinol Metab Diabetes S Afr. 2010;15(3):107–8.

15. Bianchi ML. Osteoporosis in children and adolescents. Bone. 2007;41:486–95.
16. Sherman KP. Metabolic bone disease. Orthop Trauma. 2012;26(3):220–5.
17. Bachrach LK. Acquisition of optimal bone mass in childhood and adolescence. Trends Endocrinol Metab. 2001;12(1):22–8.
18. Baxter-Jones AD, Faulkner RA, Forwood MR, Mirwald RL, Bailey DA. Bone mineral accrual from 8 to 30 years of age: an estimation of peak bone mass. J Bone Miner Res. 2011;26(8):1729–39.
19. Lorentzon M, Mellström D, Ohlsson C. Age of attainment of peak bone mass is site specific in Swedish men–the GOOD study. J Bone Miner Res. 2005;20(7):1223–7.
20. Crawford PB, Wang MC, Sabry ZI, Hudes M, Van LM, Bachrach LK. Adolescent diet is predictive of peak bone mass. Am J Clin Nutr. 2002;75:356–9.
21. Walsh IAP, Oishi J, Coury HJCG. Clinical and functional aspects of workrelated musculoskeletal disorders among active workers. Rev Saude Publica. 2008;42:108–16.
22. Parfitt AM, Chir B. Bone remodeling and bone loss: understanding the pathophysiology of osteoporosis. Clin Obstet Gynecol. 1987;30(4):789–811.
23. WHO Study Group. Assessment of fracture risk and its application to screening for postmenopausal osteoporosis. Geneva: World Health Organization; 1994.
24. Kanis JA, Johnell O, Oden A, Johansson H, McCloskey E. FRAX and the assessment of fracture probability in men and women from the UK. Osteopor Int. 2008;19:385–97.
25. Maalouf G, Gannagé-Yared MH, Ezzedine J, Larijani B, Badawi S, Rached A, et al. Lebanese osteoporosis prevention society, Shariati hospital, Iran. Middle East and North Africa consensus on osteoporosis. J Musculoskelet Neuronal Interact. 2007;7:131–43.
26. Rouzi AA, Al Sibiani SA, Al Senani NS, Radaddi RM, Aradawi MS. Independent predictors of all osteoporosis related fractures among healthy Saudi postmenopausal women: the CEOR study. Bone. 2012;50:713–22.
27. Moyad MA. Osteoporosis: a rapid review of risk factors and screening methods. Urol Oncol. 2003;21:375–9.
28. Sani FM, Sarji SA, Bilgen M. Quantitative ultrasound: measurement of the calcaneus in Southeast Asian children with thalassemia: comparison with dual-energy X-ray absorptiometry. J Ultrasound Med. 2011;30:883–94.
29. Clinician's guide to prevention and treatment of osteoporosis. 2008. http://www.nof.org/professionals/cliniciansguide_form.asp. Accessed 22 Dec 2016.
30. Dawson-Hughes B, Tosteson AN, Melton L, Baim S, Favus MJ, Khosla S, et al. Implications of absolute fracture risk assessment for osteoporosis practice guidelines in the USA. Osteoporos Int. 2008;19(4):449–58.
31. Chatterton B, Schultz C, Roberts T, Need A. Bone densitometry. A user's guide with notes on investigation and management of osteoporosis. http://www.rah.sa.gov.au/nucmed/BMD/bmd_docguide.htm. 2009.
32. Riggs BL, Melton LJ, Robb RA, Camp JJ, Atkinson EJ, Peterson JM, et al. Population-based study of age and sex differences in bone volumetric density, size, geometry, and structure at different skeletal sites. J Bone Miner Res. 2004;19:1945–54.
33. Blake GM, Fogelman I. The clinical role of dual energy X-ray absorptiometry. Eur J Radiol. 2009;71:406–14.
34. Adams JE. Advances in bone imaging for osteoporosis. Nat Rev Endocrinol. 2013;9(1):28–42.
35. Goodpaster BH, Thaete FL, Kelley DE. Composition of skeletal muscle evaluated with computed tomography. Ann NY Acad Sci. 2000;904:18–24.
36. Pickhardt PJ, Lee LJ, Munoz del Rio A, Lauder T, Bruce RJ, Summers RM, et al. Simultaneous screening for osteoporosis at CT colonography: bone mineral density assessment using MDCT attenuation techniques compared with the DXA reference standard. J Bone Miner Res. 2011;26(9):2194–203.
37. Summers RM, Baecher N, Yao J, Liu J, Pickhardt PJ, Choi JR, et al. Feasibility of simultaneous computed tomographic colonography and fully automated bone mineral densitometry in a single examination. J Comput Assist Tomogr. 2011;35:212–6.
38. Rehman Q, Lang T, Modin G, Lane NE. Quantitative computed tomography of the lumbar spine, not dual X-ray absorptiometry, is an independent predictor of prevalent vertebral fractures in postmenopausal women with osteopenia receiving long-term glucocorticoid and hormone-replacement therapy. Arthritis Rheum. 2002;46:1292–7.
39. Jara H, Wehrli FW, Chung H-W, Ford JC. High resolution variable flip angle 3D MR imaging of trabecular microstructure in vivo. Magn Reson Med. 1993;29:528–39.
40. Majumdar S, Thomasson D, Shimakawa A, Genant HK. Quantitation of the susceptibility difference between trabecular bone and bone marrow: experimental studies. Magn Reson Med. 1991;22:111–27.
41. Ford JC, Wehrli FW, Chung H-W. Magnetic field distribution in models of trabecular bone. Magn Reson Med. 1993;30:373–9.
42. Wu Y, Ackerman JL, Chesler DA, Li J, Neer RM, Wang J, et al. Evaluation of bone mineral density using three-dimensional solid state phosphorus-31 NMR projection imaging. Calcif Tissue Int. 1998;62:512–8.
43. Anumula S, Wehrli SL, Magland J, Wright AC, Wehrli FW. Ultrashort echo-time MRI detects changes in bone mineralization and water content in OVX rat bone in response to alendronate treatment. Bone. 2010;46:1391–9.
44. Majumdar S, Kothari M, Augat P, Newitt DC, Link TM, Lin JC, et al. High-resolution magnetic resonance imaging: three-dimensional trabecular bone architecture and biomechanical properties. Bone. 1998;22:445–54.
45. Wehrli FW, Song HK, Saha PK, Wright AC. Quantitative MRI for the assessment of bone structure and function. NMR Biomed. 2006;19:731–64.
46. Newitt DC, van Rietbergen B, Majumdar S. Processing and analysis of in vivo high-resolution MR images of trabecular bone for longitudinal studies: reproducibility of structural measures and micro-finite element analysis derived mechanical properties. Osteoporos Int. 2002;13(4):278–87.
47. Krieg MA, Barkmann R, Gonnelli S, Stewart A, Bauer DC, Del Rio Barquero L, et al. Quantitiative ultrasound in the management of osteoporosis: the 2007 ISCD official positions. J Clin Densitom. 2008;11:163–87.
48. Hans D, Dargent-Molina P, Schott AM, Serbert JL, Cormier C, Kotzki PO, et al. Ultrasonographic heel measurements to predict hip fracture in eldery women: the EPIDOS prospective study. Lancet. 1996;348:511–4.
49. Khaw KT, Reeve J, Luben R, Bingham S, Welch A, Wareham N, et al. Prediction of total and hip fracture risk in men and women by quantitative ultrasound of the calcaneus: EPIC-Norfolk prospective population study. Lancet. 2004;363:197–202.
50. Glüer CC, Wu CY, Jergas M, Goldstein SA, Genant HK. Three quantitative ultrasound parameters reflect bone structure. Calcif Tissue Int. 1994;55:46–52.
51. Vignolo M. Longitudinal assessment of bone quality by quantitative ultrasonography in children and adolescents. Ultrasound Med Biol. 2006;32:1003–10.
52. Sasso M, Haïat G, Yamato Y, Naili S, Matsukawa M. Dependence of ultrasonic attenuation on bone mass and microstructure in bovine cortical bone. J Biomech. 2008;41(2):347–55.
53. Guglielmi G, Njeh CF, de Terlizzi F, De Serio DA, Scillitani A, Cammisa M, et al. Phalangeal quantitative ultrasound, phalangeal morphometric variables, and vertebral fracture discrimination. Calcif Tissue Int. 2003;72(4):469–77.
54. Gonnelli S, Cepollaro C, Gennari L, Montagnani A, Caffarelli C, Merlotti D, et al. Quantitative ultrasound and dual-energy X-ray absorptiometry in the prediction of fragility fracture in men. Osteoporos Int. 2005;16:963–8.
55. Meszaros S, Toth E, Ferencz V, Csupor E, Hosszu E, Horvath C. Calcaneous quantitative ultrasound measurements predicts vertebral fractures in idiopathic male osteoporosis. Joint Bone Spine. 2007;74:79–84.
56. Ndongo S, Sutter B, Ka O, Diouf G, Diongue M, Kemta Lekpa F, et al. Quantitative ultrasound measurements at the calcaneus in a population of urban Senegalese women: least significant difference and T-score. Rheumatology. 2012;2(1):1–4.
57. Rhee Y, Lee J, Jung JY, Lee JE, Park SY, Kim YM, et al. Modifications of T-scores by quantitative ultrasonography for the diagnosis of osteoporosis in Koreans. J Korean Med Sci. 2009;24:232–6.
58. Cournil A, Eymard-Duverna S, Diouf A, Moque C, Coutherut J, Gueye NFN, et al. Reduced quantitative ultrasound bone mineral density in HIV-infected patients on antiretroviral therapy in Senegal. PLoS ONE. 2012;7(2):1–7.

59. Boskey AL, DiCarlo E, Paschalis E, West P, Mendelsohn R. Comparison of mineral quality and quantity in iliac crest biopsies from high- and low-turnover osteoporosis: an FT-IR microspectroscopic investigation. Osteoporos Int. 2005;16(12):2031–8.
60. Szulc P, Delmas PD. Biochemical markers of bone turnover: potential use in the investigation and management of postmenopausal osteoporosis. Osteoporos Int. 2008;19:1683–704.
61. Deal CL. Using bone densitometry to monitor therapy in treating osteoporosis: pros and cons. Curr Rheumatol Rep. 2001;3:233–9.
62. Delmas PD, Eastell R, Garnero P, Seibel MJ, Stepan J. The use of biochemical markers of bone turnover in osteoporosis. Committee of scientific advisors of the international osteoporosis foundation. Osteoporos Int. 2000;11:S2–17.
63. Reginster J, Minne HW, Sorensen OH, Hooper M, Roux C, Brandi ML, et al. Randomized trial of the effects of risedronate on vertebral fractures in women with established postmenopausal osteoporosis. Vertebral efficacy with risedronate therapy (VERT) Study Group. Osteoporos Int. 2000;11:83–91.
64. Bjarnason NH, Christiansen C. Early response in biochemical markers predicts long-term response in bone mass during hormone replacement therapy in early postmenopausal women. Bone. 2000;26:561–9.
65. Vasikaran S, Eastell R, Bruyère O, Foldes AJ, Garnero P, Griesmacher A, et al. Markers of bone turnover for the prediction of fracture risk and monitoring of osteoporosis treatment: a need for international reference standards. Osteoporos Int. 2011;22:391–420.
66. Lee J, Vasikaran S. Current recommendations for laboratory testing and use of bone turnover markers in management of osteoporosis. Ann Lab Med. 2012;32(2):105–12.
67. Holick MF. Vitamin D status: measurement, interpretation and clinical application. Am Epidemil. 2009;19:73–8.
68. Holick MF, Binkley NC, Bischoff-Ferrari HA, Gordon CM, Hanley DA, Heaney RP, et al. Evaluation, treatment, and prevention of vitamin D deficiency: an Endocrine Society clinical practice guideline. J Clin Endocrinol Metab. 2011;96(7):1911–30.
69. Bischoff-Ferrari HA, Giovannucci E, Willett WC, Dietrich T, Dawson-Hughes B. Estimation of optimal serum concentrations of 25-hydroxyvitamin D for multiple health outcomes. Am J Clin Nutr. 2006;84:18–28.
70. Bishoff-Ferrari HA. How to select the doses of vitamin D in the management of osteoporosis. Osteoporos Int. 2007;18:401–7.
71. Holick MF, Chen TC. Vitamin D deficiency: a worldwide problem with health consequences. Am J Clin Nutr. 2008;87:1080S–6S.
72. Unger MD, Cuppari L, Titan SM, Magalhaes MCT, Sassaki AL, Reis LM, et al. Vitamin D status in a sunny country: where has the sun gone? Clin Nutr. 2010;29(6):784–8.
73. Ross AC, Manson JE, Abrams SA, Aloia JF, Brannon PM, Clinton SK, et al. The 2011 report on dietary reference intakes for calcium and vitamin D from the institute of medicine: what clinicians need to know. J Clin Endocrinol Metab. 2011;96:53–8.
74. Holick MF. The vitamin D epidemic and its health consequences. J Nutr. 2005;135:2739S–48S.
75. Maeda SS, Kunii IS, Hayashi LF, Lazaretti-Castro M. Increases in summer serum 25-hydroxyvitamin D (25(OH)D) concentrations in elderly subjects in Sao Paulo, Brazil vary with age, gender and ethnicity. BMC Endocr Disord. 2010;10:12.
76. Bandeira F, Griz L, Freese E, Lima DC, The AC, Diniz ET, et al. Vitamin D deficiency and its relationship with bone mineral density among postmenopausal women living in the tropics. Arq Bras Endocrinol Metab. 2010;54(2):227–32.
77. Camargo MBR, Kunii IS, Fukusima Hayashi L, Muszkat P, Gusman Anelli C, Villa Marin-Mio R, et al. Modifiable factors of vitamin D status among a Brazilian osteoporotic population attended a public outpatient clinic. Arq Bras Endocrinol Metab. 2014;58(5):572–85.
78. Fuleihan GE, Nabulsi M, Tamin H, Maalouf J, Salamoun M, Khalife H, et al. Effect of vitamin D replacement on musculoskeletal parameters in school children: a randomized controlled trial. J Clin Endocrinol Metab. 2006;91(2):405–12.
79. Scalco R, Preamor MO, Froehlich PE, Furlanetto TW. High prevalence of hypovitaminosis and secondary hyperparathyroidism in elders living in nonprofit homes in South Brazil. Endocrine. 2008;33:95–100.
80. Kamen DL, Tangpricha V. Vitamin D and molecular actions on the immune system: modulation of innate and autoimmunity. J Mol Med. 2010;88(5):441–50.
81. Murray TM, Rao LG, Divieti P, Bringhurst FR. Parathyroid hormone secretion and action: evidence for discrete receptors for the carboxyl-terminal region and related biological actions of carboxyl-terminal ligands. Endocr Rev. 2005;26:78–113.
82. Eckard AR, McComsey GA. Vitamin D deficiency and altered bone mineral metabolism in HIV-infected individuals. Curr HIV/AIDS Rep. 2014;11:263–70.
83. Aspray TJ, Prentice A, Cole TJ, Sawo Y, Reeve J, Francis RM. Low bone mineral content is common but osteoporotic fractures are rare in eldery rural Gambian women. J Bone Miner Res. 1996;11:1019–25.
84. Vanderjagt DJ, Bond B, Dulai R, Pickel A, Ujah IO, Wadinga WW, et al. Assessment of the bone status of Nigerian women by ultrasound and biochemical markers. Calcif Tissue Int. 2001;68:277–84.
85. Zebaze RM, Seeman E. Epidemiollogy of hip and wrist fractures in Cameroon, Africa. Ostopor Int. 2003;14:301–5.
86. Grinspoon S, Carr A. Cardiovascular risk and body-fat abnormalities in HIV-infected adults. N Eng J Med. 2005;352:48–62.
87. Samaras K. Prevalence and pathogenesis of diabetes mellitus in HIV-1 infection treated with combined antiretroviral therapy. J Acquar Immune Defic Syndr. 2009;50:499–505.
88. Hadigan C, Kamin D, Liebau J, Mazza S, Barrow S, Torriani M, et al. Depot-specific regulation of glucose uptake and insulin sensitivity in HIV-lipodystrophy. Am J Physiol Endocrinol Metab. 2006;290:E289–98.
89. Gilsanz V, Chalfant J, Mo AO, Lee DC, Dorey FJ, Mittelman SD. Reciprocal relations of subcutaneous and visceral fat to bone structure and strength. J Clin Endocrinol Metab. 2009;94(9):3387–93.
90. Russel M, Mendes N, Miller KK, Rosen CJ, Lee H, Klibanski A, et al. Visceral fat is a negative predictor of bone density measures in obese adolescent girls. J Clin Endocrinol Metab. 2010;95:1247–55.
91. Yamaguchi T, Kanazawa I, Yamamoto M, Kurioka S, Yamauchi M, Yano S, et al. Associations between components of the metabolic syndrome versus bone mineral density and vertebral fractures in patients with type 2 diabetes. Bone. 2009;45:174–9.
92. Bredella MA, Tirruabu M, Ghomi RH, Thomas BJ, Brick DJ, Gerweck AV, et al. Determinants of bone mineral density in obese premenopausal women. Bone. 2011;48:748–54.
93. Adami S, Zivelonghi A, Braga V, Fracassi E, Gatti D, Rossini M, et al. Insulin-like growth factor-1 is associated with bone formation markers, PTH and bone mineral density in healthy premenopausal women. Bone. 2010;46:244–7.
94. Giustina A, Mazziotti G, Canalis E. Growth hormone, insulin-like growth factors and the skeleton. Endocr Rev. 2008;29:535–59.
95. Utz AI, Yamamoto A, Hemphill L, Miller KK. Growth hormone deficiency by growth hormone releasing hormone-arginine testing criteria predicts increased cardiovascular risk markers in normal young overweight and obese women. J Clin Endocrinol Metab. 2008;93:2507–14.
96. Cartier A, Lemieux I, Almeras N, Tremblay A, Bergeron J, Despres JP. Visceral obesity and plasma glucose-insulin homeostasis: contributions of interleukin-6 and tumour necrosis factor-alpha in men. J Clin Endocrinol Metab. 2008;93:1931–8.
97. Pou KM, Massaro JM, Hoffmann U, Vasan RS, Maurovich-Horvat P, Larson MG, et al. Visceral and subcutaneous adipose tissue volumes are cross-sectionally related to markers of inflammation and oxidative stress: the Framingham Heart Study. Circ. 2007;116:1234–41.
98. Lu LJ, Nayeem F, Anderson KE, Grady JJ, Nagamani M. Lean body mass, not estrogen or progesterone, predicts peak bone mineral density in premenopausal women. J Nutr. 2009;139:250–6.
99. Do Prado WL, de Piano A, Lazaretti-Castro M, de Mello MT, Stella SG, Tufik S, et al. Relationship between bone mineral density, leptin and insulin concentration in Brazillian obese adolescents. J Bone Miner Metab. 2009;27:613–9.
100. Ferron M, Lacombe J. Regulation of energy metabolism by the skeleton: osteocalcin and beyond. Arch Biochem Biophys. 2014;561:137–46.
101. Upadhyay J, Farr OM, Mantzoros CS. The role of leptin in regulating bone metabolism. Metabolism. 2015;64(1):105–13.
102. Weinberg ME, Lo JC, Grunfeld C, Schambelan M. Endocrine complications of HIV infection. In: Volberding PA, Sande MA, Greene WC, Lange

JMA, Gallant JE, editors. Global HIV/AIDS medicine. New York: Saunders Elsevier; 2008. p. 287–98.
103. Shashidhar PK, Shashikala GV. Low dose adrenocorticotropic hormone test and adrenal insufficiency in critically ill acquired immunodeficiency syndrome patients. Indian J Endocrinol Metab. 2012;16:389–94.
104. Lindsay R, Cosman F. Osteoporosis. In: Braunwald E, Fauci AS, Kasper DL, Hauser SL, Longo DL, Jameson JL, editors. Harrison's 15th edition: principles of internal medicine, vol. 2. USA: McGraw-Hill; 2001. p. 2226–37.
105. Gennari L, Merlotti D, De Paola V, Calabro A, Becherini L, Martini G, et al. Estrogen receptor gene polymorphisms and the genetics of osteoporosis: a huge review. Am J Epidemiol. 2005;161:307–20.
106. Brooks JT, Buchacz K, Gebo KA, Mermin J. HIV infection and older Americans: the public health perspective. Am J Public Health. 2012;102(8):1516–26.
107. Kojic EM, Wang CC, Cu-Uvin S. HIV and menopause: a review. J Womens Health (Larchmt). 2007;16(10):1402–11.
108. Valdiglesias V, Sanchez-Flores M, Maseda A, Marcos-Perez D, Millan-Calenti JC, Pasaro E, et al. Lymphocyte subsets in a population of nonfrail elderly individuals. J Toxicol Environ Health A. 2015;78(13–14):790–804.
109. Clarke BL, Khosla S. Androgens and bone. Steroids. 2009;74:296–305.
110. Ohlsson C, Vandenput LV. The role of estrogens for male bone health. Eur J Endocrin. 2009;160(6):883–9.
111. Burnett-Bowie SA, McKay EA, Lee H, Leder BZ. Effects of aromatase inhibition on bone mineral density and bone turnover in older men with low testosterone levels. J Clin Endocrinol Metab. 2009;94:4785–92.
112. Sorgren K, Lagerquist M, Moverare-Skrtic S, Andersson N, Windahl SH, Swanson C, et al. Elevated aromatase expression in osteoblasts leads to increased bone mass without systemic adverse effects. J Bone Miner Res. 2009;24:1263–70.
113. Katznelson L, Finkelstein JS, Schoenfeld DA, Rosenthal DI, Anderson EJ, Klibanski A. Increase in bone density and lean body mass during testosterone administration in men with acquired hypogonadism. J Clin Endocrinol Metab. 1996;81(12):4358–65.
114. Daniell HW. Osteoporosis after orchiectomy for prostate cancer. J Urol. 1997;157(2):439–44.
115. Falahati-Nini A, Riggs BL, Atkinson EJ, O'Fallon WM, Eastell R, Khosla S. Relative contributions of testosterone and estrogen in regulating bone resorption and formation in normal elderly men. J Clin Invest. 2000;106(12):1553–60.
116. Rochira V, Balestrieri A, Madeo B, Zirilli L, Granata AR, Carani C. Osteoporosis and male age-related hypogonadism: role of sex steroids on bone (patho)physiology. Eur J Endocrinol. 2006;154(2):175–85.
117. Santi D, Madeo B, Carli F, Zona S, Brigante G, Vescini F, et al. Serum total estradiol, but not testosterone is associated with reduced bone mineral density (BMD) in HIV-infected men: a cross-sectional, observational study. Osteopor Int. 2016;27(3):1103–14.
118. Rochira V, Zirilli L, Orlando G, Santi D, Brigante G, Diazzi C, et al. Premature decline of serum total testosterone in HIV-infected men in the HAART-era. PLoS ONE. 2011;6(12):e28512.
119. Short CE, Shaw SG, Fisher MJ, Walker-Bone K, Gilleece YC. Prevalence of and risk factors for osteoporosis and fracture among a male HIV-infected population in the UK. Int J STD AIDS. 2014;25(2):113–21.
120. Pepe J, Isidori AM, Falciano M, Iaiani G, Salotti A, Diacinti D, et al. The combination of FRAX and ageing male symptoms scale better identifies treated HIV males at risk for major fracture. Clin Endocrinol (Oxf). 2012;77(5):672–8.
121. Pepe J, Isidori AM, Falciano M, Iaiani G, Salotti A, Diacinti D, et al. Effect of risedronate in osteoporotic HIV males according to gonadal status: a pilot study. Endodrine. 2014;47(2):456–62.
122. Inrig JK, Szczech LA, Gerntholtz TE, Klotman PE. Renal complications of HIV infection. In: Volberding PA, Sande MA, Greene WC, Lange JMA, editors. Global HIV/AIDS medicine. New York: Saunders Elsevier; 2008. p. 299–307.
123. Nelson MA, Katlama C, Montaner J, Cooper DA, Gazzard B, Clotet B, et al. The safety of tenofovir disoproxil fumarate for the treatment of HIV infection in adults: the first 4 years. AIDS. 2007;21:1273–81.
124. Fux CA, Christen A, Zgaggen S, Mohaupt MG, Furrer H. Effect of tenofovir on renal glomerular and tubular function. AIDS. 2007;21:1483–5.
125. Karras A, Lafaurie M, Furco A, Bourgarit A, Droz D, Sereni D, et al. Tenofovir-related nephrotoxicity in human immunodeficiency virus-infected patients: three cases of renal failure, Fanconi syndrome, and nephrogenic diabetes insioidus. Clin Infect Dis. 2003;36:1070–3.
126. Peyriere H, Reynes J, Rouanet I, Daniel N, De Boever CM, Mauboussin JM, et al. Renal tubular dysfunction associated with tenofovir therapy: report on 7 cases. J Acquar Immune Defic Syndr. 2004;35:269–73.
127. Cooper RD, Wiebe N, Smith N, Keiser P, Naicker S, Tonelli M. Systematic review and meta-analysis: renal safety of tenofovir disoproxil fumurate in HIV-infected patients. Clin Infect Dis. 2010;51:496–505.
128. Smith KY, Patel P, Fine D, Bellos N, Sloan I, Lackey P, et al. Randomized, double-blind, placebo-matched, multicenter trial of abacavir/lamivudine or tenofovir/emiricitabine with lopinavir/ritonavir for initial HIV treatment. AIDS. 2009;23:1547–56.
129. Martinez E, Arranz JA, Podzameczer D, Lonca M, Sanz J, Barragán P, et al. A simplification trial switching from nucleoside reverse transcriptase inhibitors to once-daily fixed-dose abacavir/lamuvidine or tenofovir/emtricitabine in HIV-1-infected patients with virological supression. J Acquir Immune Defic Syndr. 2009;51:290–7.
130. Post FA, Moyle GJ, Stellbrink HJ, Domingo P, Podzameczer D, Fisher M, et al. Randomized comparison of renal effects, efficacy, and safety with once-daily abacavir/lamivudine versus tenofovir/emtricitabine, administered with efavirenz, in antiretroviral-naive, HIV-1-infected adults: 48-week results from the ASSERT study. J Acquir Immune Defic Syndr. 2010;55:49–57.
131. Martin A, Bloch M, Amin J, Baker D, Cooper DA, Emery S, et al. Simplification of antiretroviral therapy with tenofovir-emtricitabine or abacavir-lamivudine: a randomized, 96-week trial. Clin Infect Dis. 2009;49:1591–601.
132. Rasmussen TA, Jensen D, Tolstrup M, Nielsen US, Erlandsen EJ, Birn H, et al. Comparison of bone and renal effects in HIV-infected adults switching to Abacavir or Tenofovir based therapy in a randomized trial. PLoS ONE. 2012;7(3):e32445.
133. DeJesus E, Haas B, Segal-Maurer S, Ramgopal M, Mills A, Liu Y, et al. Superior efficacy and improved renal and bone safety after switching from a tenofovir disoproxil fumarate (TDF) regimen to a tenofovir alafenamide (TAF) based regimen through 96 weeks (W96) of treatment. Paper presented at: Boston: ASM Microbe; 2016.
134. Mills A, Crofoot GJ, McDonald C, Shalit P, Flamm JA, Gathe JJ, et al. Tenofovir alafenamide versus tenofovir disoproxil fumarate in the first protease inhibitor-based single-tablet regimen for initial HIV-1 therapy: a randomized phase 2 study. J Acquir Immune Defic Syndr. 2015;69(4):439–45.
135. Raffi F, Orkin C, Clarke A, Slama L, Gallant J, Daar E, et al. Brief report: long-term (96-week) efficacy and safety after switching from tenofovir disoproxil fumarate (TDF) to tenofovir alafenamide (TAF) in HIV-infected, virologically suppressed adults. J Acquir Immune Defic Syndr. 2017;75:226–31.
136. Arribas JR, Thompson M, Sax P, Haas B, McDonald C, Wohl D, et al. Significant efficacy and long-term safety difference with TAF-based STR in naive adults. Paper presented at: Seattle: Retroviruses and Opportunistic Infections (CROI); 2017.
137. Brown T, Yin MT, Gupta S, Katlama C, Lazzarin A, Melbourne K, et al. Switching from TDF to TAF in HIV-infected adults with low BMD: a pooled analysis. Paper presented at: Seattle: Retroviruses and Opportunistic Infections (CROI); 2017.
138. Cazanave C, Dupon M, Lavignolle-Aurillac V, Barthe N, Lawson-Ayayi S, Mehsen N, et al. Reduced bone mineral density in HIV-infected patients: prevalence and associated factors. AIDS. 2008;22(3):395–402.
139. Rivas P, Górgolas M, García-Delgado R, Díaz-Curiel M, Goyenechea A, Fernández-Guerrero ML. Evolution of bone mineral density in AIDS patients on treatment with zidovudine/lamivudine plus abacavir or lopinavir/ritonavir. HIV Med. 2008;9(2):89–95.
140. Jones S, Restrepo D, Kasowitz A, Korenstein D, Wallenstein S, Schneider A, et al. Risk factors for decreased bone density and effects of HIV on bone in the eldery. Osteopor Int. 2008;19(7):913–8.
141. Dolan SE, Carpenter S, Grinspoon S. Effects of weight, body composition, and testosterone on bone mineral density in HIV-infected women. J Acquir Immune Defic Syndr. 2007;45(2):161–7.
142. Brown TT, Qaqish RB. Antiretroviral therapy and the prevalence of osteopenia and osteoporosis: a meta-analytical review. AIDS. 2006;20:2165–74.

143. McComsey GA, Teba P, Shane E, Yin MT, Overton ET, Huang JS, et al. Bone disease in HIV infection: a practical review and recommendations for HIV care providers. Clin Infect Dis. 2010;51:937–46.
144. Triant VA, Brown TT, Lee H, Grinspoon SK. Fracture prevalence among human immunodeficiency virus (HIV)-infected versus non-HIV-infected patients in a large U.S. healthcare system. J Clin Endocrinol Metab. 2008;93(9):3499–504.
145. Bonjoch A, Figueras M, Estany C, Perez-Alvarez N, Rosales J, del Rio L, et al. High prevalence of and progression to low bone mineral density in HIV-infected patients: a longitudinal cohort study. AIDS. 2010;24:2827–33.
146. Sharma A, Flom PL, Weedon J, Klein RS. Prospective study of bone mineral density changes in aging men with or at risk for HIV infection. AIDS. 2010;24(15):2337–45.
147. Bolland MJ, Grey A. HIV and low bone density: responsible party, or guilty by association? IBMS BoneKEy. 2011;8:7–15.
148. Borderi M, Gibellini D, Vescini F, De Crignis E, Cimatti L, Biagetti C, et al. Metabolic bone disease in HIV infection. AIDS. 2009;23:1297–310.
149. Duvivier C, Kolta S, Assoumou L, Ghosn J, Rozenberg S, Murphy RL, et al. Greater decrease in bone mineral density with protease inhibitor regimens in HIV-1 infected naïve patients. AIDS. 2009;23:817–24.
150. Gibellini D, de Crignis E, Ponti C, Cimatti L, Borderi M, Tschon M, et al. HIV-1 triggers apoptosis in primary osteoblasts and HOBIT cells through TNF-alpha activation. J Med Virol. 2008;80(9):1507–14.
151. Rodriquez M, Daniels B, Gunawardene S, Robbins GK. High frequency of vitamin D deficiency in ambulatory HIV-positive patients. AIDS Res Hum Retroviruses. 2009;25(1):9–14.
152. Teichmann J, Lange U, Discher T, Lohmeyer J, Stracke H, Bretzel RG. Bone mineral density in human immunodeficiency virus-1 infected men with hypogonadism prior to highly-active-antiretroviral-therapy (HAART). Eur J Med Res. 2009;14(2):59–64.
153. Weitzmann MN. The role of inflammatory cytokines, the RANKL/OPG axis, and the immunoskeletal interface in physiological bone turnover and osteoporosis. Scientifica. 2013;2013:29.
154. Vikulina T, Fan X, Yamaguchi M, Roser-Page S, Zayzafoon M, Guidot DM, et al. Alterations in the immuno-skeletal interface drive bone destruction in HIV-1 transgenic rats. Proc Natl Acad Sci USA. 2010;107(31):13848–53.
155. Moir S, Fauci AS. B cells in HIV infection and disease. Nat Rev Immunol. 2009;9(4):235–45.
156. Moir S, Ho J, Malaspina A, Wang W, Dipoto AC, O'Shea MA, et al. Evidence for HIV-associated B cell exhaustion in a dysfunctional memory B cell compartment in HIV-infected viremic individuals. J Exp Med. 2008;205(8):1797–805.
157. Hittinger G, Poggi C, Delbeke E, Pronfizi N, Lafeuillade A. Correlation between plasma levels of cytokines and HIV-1 RNA copy number in HIV-infected patients. Infection. 1998;26:100–3.
158. Chakravarti A, Marceau AA, Flamand L, Poubelle PE. Normal human primary CD^4+ T lymphocytes synthesize and release functional osteoprotegerin in vitro. Lab Invest. 2008;88(2):171–84.
159. Dolan SE, Kanter JR, Grinspoon S. Longitudinal analysis of bone density in human immunodeficiency virus-infected women. J Clin Endocrinol Metab. 2006;91(8):2938–45.
160. Stellbrink HJ, Orkin C, Arribas JR, Compston J, Gerstoft J, Van Wijngaerden E, et al. Comparison of changes in bone density and turnover with abacavir-lamivudine versus tenofovir-emtricitabine in HIV-infected adults: 48-week results from ASSERT study. Clin Infect Dis. 2010;51:963–72.
161. Brown TT, Ross AC, Storer N, Labbato D, McComsey GA. Bone turnover, osteoprotegerin/RANKL and inflammation with antiretroviral initiation: tenofovir versus non-tenofovir regimens. Antivir Ther. 2011;16(7):1063–72.
162. Tijani K, Vunnava A, Sheth AN, Delille C, Lennox JL, Sanford SE, et al. Dysregulated B cell expression of RANKL and OPG correlates with loss of bone mineral density in HIV infection. PLoS Pathog. 2014;10(11):e1004497.
163. Gibellini D, Borderi M, De Crignis E, Cicola R, Vescini F, Caudarella R, et al. RANKL/OPG/TRAIL plasma levels and bone mass loss evaluation in antiretroviral naïve HIV-1-positive men. J Med Virol. 2007;79:1446–54.
164. Ueland T, Bollerslev J, Godang K, Müller F, Frøland SS, Aukrust P. Increased serum osteoprotegerin in disorders characterized by persistent immune activation or glucocorticoid excess-possible role in bone homeostasis. Eur J Endocrinol. 2001;145:685–90.
165. Gao Y, Grassi F, Ryan MR, Terauchi M, Page K, Yang X, et al. IFN-gamma stimulates osteoclast formation and bone loss in vivo via antigen-driven T cell activation. J Clin Invest. 2007;117(1):122–32.
166. Takayanagi H, Ogasawara K, Hida S, Chiba T, Murata S, Satp K, et al. T-cell-mediated regulation of osteoclastogenesis by signalling cross-talk between RANKL and IFN-γ. Nature. 2000;408(6812):600–5.
167. Brown TT, McComsey GA, King MS, Qaqish RB, Bernstein BM, da Silva BA. Loss of bone mineral density after antiretroviral therapy initiation, independent of antiretroviral regimen. J Acquir Immune Defic Syndr. 2009;51:554–61.
168. Gallant JE, Staszewski S, Pozniak AL, DeJesus E, Suleiman JM, Miller MD, et al. Efficacy and safety of tenofovir DF vs stavudine in combination therapy in antiretroviral-naïve patients: a 3-year randomized trial. JAMA. 2004;292:191–201.
169. Finkelstein JS, Brockwell SE, Mehta V, Greendale GA, Sowers MR, Ettinger B, et al. Bone mineral density changes during the menopause transition in a multi-ethnic cohort of women. J Clin Endocrinol Metab. 2008;93(3):861–8.
170. McComsey GA, Kitch D, Daar ES, Tierney C, Jahed NC, Tebas P, et al. Bone mineral density and fractures in antiretroviral-naive persons randomized to receive abacavir-lamivudine or tenofovir disoproxil fumarate-emtricitabine along with efavirenz or atazanavir-ritonavir: aids clinical trials group A5224s, a substudy of ACTG A5202. J Infect Dis. 2011;203:1791–801.
171. Cotter AG, Powderly WG. Endocrine complications of human immunodeficiency virus infection: hypogonadism, bone disease and tenofovir-related toxicity. Best Pract Res Clin Endocrinol Metab. 2011;25:501–15.
172. Moyle GJ, Stellbrink HJ, Compston J, Orkin C, Arribas JR, Domingo P, et al. 96-week results of abacavir/lamivudine versus tenofovir/emtricitabine, plus efavirenz, in antiretroviral-naïve, HIV-1-infected adults: ASSERT study. Antivir Ther. 2013;18(7):905–13.
173. Giacomet V, Mora S, Martelli L, Merlo M, Sciannanblo M, Vigano A. A 12-month treatment with tenofovir does not impair bone mineral accrual in HIV-infected children. J Acquir Immune Defic Syndr. 2005;40:448–50.
174. Vigano A, Zuccotti GV, Puzzovio M, Pivetti V, Zamproni I, Cerini C, et al. Tenofovir disoproxil fumarate and bone mineral density: a 60-month longitudinal study in a cohort of HIV-infected youths. Antivir Ther. 2010;15:1053–8.
175. Carr A, Miller J, Eisman JA, Cooper DA. Osteopenia in HIV-infected men: association with asymptomatic lactic acidemia and lower weight pre-antiretroviral therapy. AIDS. 2001;15:703–9.
176. Calmy A, Fux CA, Norris R, Vallier N, Delhumeau C, Samaras K, et al. Low bone mineral density, renal dysfunction and fracture risk in HIV-infection: a cross-sectional study. J Infect Dis. 2009;200:1746–54.
177. Arnsten JH, Freeman R, Howard AA, Floris-Moore M, Santoro N, Schoenbaum EE. HIV infection and bone mineral density in middle-aged women. J Clin Infect Dis. 2006;42:1014–20.
178. Bruera D, Luna N, David DO, Bergoglio LM, Zamudio J. Decreased bone mineral density in HIV-infected patients is independent of antiretroviral therapy. AIDS. 2003;17:1917–23.
179. Amiel C, Ostertag A, Slama L, Baudoin C, N'Guyen T, Lajeunie E, et al. BMD is reduced in HIV-infected men irrespective of treatment. J Bone Miner Res. 2004;19:402–9.
180. Kinai E, Nishijima T, Mizushima D, Watanabe K, Aoki T, Honda H, et al. Long-term use of protease inhibitors is associated with bone mineral density loss. AIDS Res Hum Retroviruses. 2014;30(6):553–9.
181. Gibellini D, Borderi M, de Crignis E, Clo A, Miserocchi A, Viale P, et al. Analysis of the effects of specific protease inhibitors on OPG/RANKL regulation in an osteoblast-like cell line. New Microbiol. 2010;33:109–15.
182. Modarresi R, Xiang Z, Yin M, Laurence J. WNT/β-catenin signalling is involved in regulation of osteoclast differentiation by human immunodeficiency virus protease inhibitor ritonavir. Am J Pathol. 2009;174:123–35.
183. Santiago F, Oguma J, Brown AMC, Laurence J. Noncanonical Wnt signalling promotes osteoclast differentiation and is facilitated by the human immunodeficiency virus protease inhibitor ritonavir. Biochem Biophys Res Commun. 2012;417:223–30.

184. Yin MT, Modaressi R, Shane E, Santiago F, Ferris DC, McMahon DJ, et al. Efects of HIV-infection and antiretroviral therapy with ritonavir on induction of osteoclast-like cells in postmenopausal women. Osteopor Int. 2011;22:1459–68.
185. Hansen AB, Obel N, Nielsen H, Pedersen C, Gerstoft J. Bone mineral density changes in protease inhibitor-sparing vs. nucleoside reverse transcriptase inhibitor-sparing highly active antiretroviral therapy: data from a randomized trial. HIV Med. 2011;12(3):157–65.
186. Grant PM, Kitch D, McComsey GA, Dube MP, Haubrich R, Huang J, et al. Low baseline CD^4+ cell count is associated with greater bone mineral density loss after ART initiation. Clin Infect Dis. 2013;57(10):1483–8.
187. Wang MW, Wei S, Faccio R, Takeshita S, Tebas P, Powderly WG, et al. The HIV protease inhibitor ritonavir blocks osteoclastogenesis and function by impairing RANKL-induced signaling. J Clin Invest. 2004;114(2):206–13.
188. Taylor A, Rogers M. HIV treatments and the skeleton: do NRTIs directly affect bone cells? Bone. 2010;46(1):S56.
189. Ozçakar L, Guven GS, Unal S, Akinci A. Osteoporosis in Turkish HIV/AIDS patients: comparative analysis by dual energy X-ray absorptiometry and digital X-ray radiogrammetry. Osteoporos Int. 2005;16:1363–7.
190. Bakker I, Twisk JW, Mechelen WV, Kemper HC. Fat-free body mass is the most important body composition determinant of 10-yr longitudinal development of lumbar bone in adult men and women. J Clin Endocrinol Metab. 2003;88:2607–13.
191. Reid IR. Relationships among body mass, its components, and bone. Bone. 2002;31:547–55.
192. Schtscherbyna A, Pinheiro MF, de Mendonça LM, Gouveia C, Luiz RR, Machado ES, de Farias ML, et al. Factors associated with low bone mineral density in a Brazilian cohort of vertically HIV-infected adolescents. Int J Infect Dis. 2012;16:e872–8.
193. Duran AC, Almeida LB, Segurado AA, Jaime PC. Diet quality of persons living with HIV/AIDS on highly active antiretroviral therapy. J Hum Nutr Diet. 2008;21:346–50.
194. Peters BS, Dos Santos LC, Fisberg M, Wood RJ, Martini LA. Prevalence of vitamin D insufficiency in Brazilian adolescents. Ann Nutr Metab. 2009;54:15–21.
195. Silva HG, Tortora RP, Farias ML. Increased bone turnover during the third trimester of pregnancy and decreased bone mineral density after parturition in adolescents as compared to age-matched control patients. Gynecol Endocrinol. 2005;21:174–9.
196. Pollock E, Klotsas AE, Compston J, Gkrania-Klotsas E. Bone health in HIV infection. Br Med Bull. 2009;92:123–33.

13

Effect of *Moringa oleifera* Lam. leaf powder on the pharmacokinetics of nevirapine in HIV-infected adults

Tsitsi G. Monera-Penduka[1*], Charles C. Maponga[1,2], Alan R. Wolfe[3], Lubbe Wiesner[4], Gene D. Morse[2] and Charles F. B. Nhachi[5]

Abstract

Background: *Moringa oleifera* Lam., an herb commonly consumed by HIV-infected people on antiretroviral therapy, inhibits cytochrome P450 3A4, 1A2 and 2D6 activity in vitro; and may alter the pharmacokinetics (PK) of antiretroviral drugs metabolized via the same pathways. However, in vitro drug interaction activity may not translate to a clinically significant effect. Therefore, the effect of moringa leaf powder on the PK of nevirapine in HIV-infected people was investigated.

Methods: Adult patients at steady-state dosing with nevirapine were admitted for 12-h intensive PK sampling following a 21-day herbal medicine washout. Blood sampling was repeated after 14 days of nevirapine and moringa (1.85 g leaf powder/day) co-administration. Nevirapine plasma concentrations were determined by liquid chromatography-tandem mass spectrometry. To assess the effect of moringa on nevirapine PK, the change in nevirapine area under the plasma concentration–time curve (AUC) was determined. The mean difference in pre- and post-moringa nevirapine, maximum concentration (C_{max}) and concentration at 12 h (C_{12h}) were also calculated. The PK parameters were compared by assessing the post/pre geometric mean ratios (GMRs) and associated 90% confidence intervals (CIs).

Results: Pharmacokinetics analyses were performed on the results from 11 participants for whom complete data were obtained. The post/pre GMRs and associated 90% CIs for nevirapine were 1.07 (1.00–1.14) for the AUC; 1.06 (0.98–1.16) for C_{max} and 1.03 (0.92–1.16) for C_{12h}.

Conclusion: Co-administration of *Moringa oleifera* Lam. leaf powder at the traditional dose did not significantly alter the steady-state PK of nevirapine.

Keywords: *Moringa oleifera*, Nevirapine, Pharmacokinetics, HIV

Background

Concomitant use of herbs with drugs may result in herb-drug interactions through various pharmacokinetic and pharmacodynamic mechanisms [1, 2]. The risk of interaction increases with the number of co-administered agents. As a result, HIV patients in developing countries are at high risk of herb-drug interactions because of the widespread self-directed herbal medicine use; and the polypharmacy associated with HIV treatment [3].

A growing number of studies are being conducted to evaluate the pharmacokinetic effects of herbs on drugs when taken together. However, the majority of studies use preclinical in vitro and animal models, which generate data that often do not translate to a clinical effect [4, 5]. In addition, currently available data are skewed towards

*Correspondence: moneratg@yahoo.co.uk
[1] Drug and Toxicology Information Services (DaTIS), School of Pharmacy, University of Zimbabwe College of Health Sciences, Harare, Zimbabwe
Full list of author information is available at the end of the article

Chinese and Western herbs. Given the high prevalence of herbal medicine use and the rapid scaling up of treatment for HIV infection in developing countries, rigorous clinical studies are urgently required to assess the effects of commonly used herbal medicines on antiretroviral drugs. This will provide evidence to accurately guide herbal medicine use among HIV-infected people who choose to take herbs and drugs together.

In developing countries, the leaf powder of *Moringa oleifera* Lam. is commonly used as a medicinal herb, rather than food as is the case in Asian populations. It is often taken as a supplement by HIV-infected people to enhance immunity and manage opportunistic infections [6, 7]. In-vitro data suggest that moringa inhibits cytochrome P450 (CYP) 3A4, 1A2 and 2D6 activity which could potentially lead to metabolic interactions with antiretroviral drugs metabolized via the same pathways [5, 8, 9]. The non-nucleoside reverse transcriptase inhibitor nevirapine (200 mg twice daily) is widely used as a component of first line antiretroviral therapy in many developing countries. It is metabolized mainly by CYP3A4 and CYP2B6 and to a lesser extent CYP3A5, CYP2C9, and CYP2D6 [10, 11]. Previous studies have demonstrated that concomitant administration of fluconazole, a potent inhibitor of CYPs, results in markedly increased trough plasma nevirapine concentrations when compared to the administration of nevirapine alone [12]. Concomitant dosing with the herb St. John's wort, a CYP3A4 and P-glycoprotein inducer, reduced exposure to nevirapine [13]. Such interactions with CYP inhibitors or inducers could potentially increase toxicity [11] or reduce efficacy, respectively. Prior to this study, it was not known whether the in vitro inhibition potential of *Moringa oleifera* Lam. is of clinical significance when co-administered with nevirapine. It was hypothesized that inhibition of CYP3A4 by *M. oleifera* leaf powder may result in a clinically significant increase in nevirapine exposure. This study was conducted to assess the effect of 14 days *Moringa oleifera* leaf powder supplementation on the steady-state pharmacokinetics of nevirapine in HIV-infected patients.

Methods

Study participants and setting

HIV-infected male and female adults reporting for routine HIV clinic visits at a referral hospital in Zimbabwe were identified through an interviewer-administered questionnaire. To be enrolled in the study, participants had to be >18 years old, on an nevirapine based regimen for at least 2 weeks and to have supplemented their antiretroviral therapy with herbal medicine of their own accord in the past. Exclusion criteria included anemia (hemoglobin <10 g/dL), impaired renal function (serum creatinine >300 μmol/L) or abnormal hepatic function (serum alanine transaminase >5 times the upper limit of normal) at enrolment, and current treatment with rifampicin, isoniazid or imidazoles. All concomitant medications were also evaluated on a case by case basis and current literature reviewed to exclude any drugs with potential to interact with nevirapine. In addition, female participants were required to have a negative pregnancy test and not to be breastfeeding.

Preparation and analysis of moringa

Fresh *Moringa oleifera* Lam. leaves positively identified by a botanist from the National Botanical Gardens were harvested from a rural district in Zimbabwe. A voucher specimen was retained and another deposited at the National Herbarium and Botanical Gardens of Zimbabwe (ref. GPS 13504-C). The leaves were then room dried and coarsely ground into powder using a kitchen blender according to the method published by the Moringa Association of Ghana (batch MO001 [14]. The dried leaf powder was assessed for microbial and heavy metal content and a chemical fingerprint of the methanol extract was generated by ultra-performance liquid chromatography (UPLC) coupled to a time of flight mass spectrometer (TOF MS ES+). The fingerprint was archived at the University of Zimbabwe College of Health Sciences.

Dosage regimen and standardization

In the authors' experiences and findings from previous surveys, moringa leaf powder is consumed in a wide range of doses [6, 15]. The dose of moringa for the trial was planned at approximately two teaspoons (10 mL) once a day because it was within the reported range and could also be encapsulated into a reasonable number of capsules that would not be a barrier to adherence. This was equivalent to about 1.85 g of the dry leaf powder. To standardize the dose, each 1.85 g dose was weighed out and filled into hard gelatin capsules. This was equivalent to 4 size '000' capsules. Each participant was supplied with enough capsules for the 2-week period.

Study design and treatments

An open label, two phase, one sequence, cross-over, pharmacokinetic study was conducted over 35 days. The study had a minimum 3-week herbal medication wash out period prior to the first dosing to reduce the possibility of carryover from any type of previously used moringa or other herbal medication, so the participants would have the same baseline. On the first visit (day one), all enrolled participants were instructed not to take any herbal supplements, including moringa. They were also counseled to continue taking their regular antiretroviral drug regimen supplied at the HIV outpatient clinic which included 200 mg nevirapine twice daily. On the second visit (day 22), serial whole blood (5 mL) samples and spot urine sample were collected for determination of baseline plasma nevirapine concentration and urinalysis, respectively. Pre-dose urine and blood samples were collected immediately before an observed nevirapine morning dose. Additional pharmacokinetic blood samples were also collected via cannula at 0.5, 1, 1.5, 2, 3, 4, 6, 8 and 12 h post nevirapine dose. Participants were given further counseling and instructions to continue taking the regular antiretroviral drug regimen supplied at the HIV outpatient clinic together with moringa supplied by the study staff. On the third visit (day 35), a second set of serial whole blood (5 mL) samples and a spot urine sample were collected for determination of post-moringa plasma nevirapine concentration and urinalysis. Pre-dose urine and blood samples were again collected immediately before an observed nevirapine morning dose, and additional pharmacokinetic blood samples collected via cannula at 0.5, 1, 1.5, 2, 3, 4, 6, 8 and 12 h post nevirapine dose. The observed dose of nevirapine was administered in the fed state on both visits. On blood sampling days, a standard diet was provided and participants were required to remain on-site over the course of both 12 h intensive sampling periods.

Documentation of adherence to medication and supplementation restrictions between visits was achieved through the use of a food/herb/medication diary. Exposure to moringa was based on self-reported adherence and assessed through personal interviews, pill counts and evaluation of the food/herb/medication diary.

Assessment of adverse events

All participants were monitored for adverse events throughout the study. The study medical officer documented any adverse events observed from clinical examinations or self-reported by the participants at each visit.

Sample preparation

Blood samples were collected into 10-mL tubes containing ethylenediaminetetraacetic acid (EDTA) for determination of nevirapine concentration. All blood specimens were centrifuged at 2800×*g* for 5 min at 4 °C. The plasma was harvested and stored at −80 °C until time of analysis.

Determination of nevirapine

Nevirapine concentrations were determined by LC–MS/MS in the laboratory of the Division of Clinical Pharmacology, University of Cape Town. The assay method has been reviewed by the AIDS Clinical Trials Group Quality Assurance and Quality Control program (ACTG CPQA). It was validated according to the United States Food and Drug Administration and European Medicines Agency guidelines using externally prepared proficiency testing samples supplied by the ACTG CPQA.

Plasma samples were extracted from 100 µL human plasma by protein precipitation using acetonitrile (Honeywell, Burdick & Jackson®). The extraction procedure was followed by liquid chromatography with MS/MS detection. Chromatographic separation was achieved on a Luna 5 µm PFP (2), 100 A, 50 mm × 2 mm analytical column column (Phenomenex, Torrance, CA, U.S.). An AB Sciex API 4000 mass spectrometer (SCIEX, Framingham, MA, U.S.) was operated at unit resolution in the multiple reaction monitoring (MRM) mode, monitoring the m/z 266.9 (MH^+) → 198.2 transition for nevirapine, and the m/z 270.1 → 229.1 transition for the deuterated nevirapine internal standard. The calibration curve was fitted by quadratic regression (weighted by 1/concentration^2) over the range 0.0195–20.0 µg/mL. The combined accuracy and precision statistics of the low, medium and high quality control samples during sample analysis were between 89.8 and 93.4%, and 4.2 and 9.1%, respectively.

Statistical and pharmacokinetic analysis

In designing the study, a difference in pre- and post-moringa nevirapine area under the plasma concentration–time curve from 0 to 12 h (AUC_{0-12h}) of at least 20% was considered to be clinically relevant for the purpose of establishing sample size. An intra-individual coefficient of variation of 25% was assumed for nevirapine AUC based on previously published data [16]. With $\alpha = 0.05$, it was determined that a total of 12 participants would provide 80% power in the case of an equivalence range 0.8–1.25 [17]. After making adjustments for loss to follow-up (10%) and the cross-over design, a sample size of 13 was targeted.

Statistical analyses were performed using StataMP® version 13 (StataCorp, College Station, TX). Demographic characteristics were summarized as means and standard deviations or frequencies. Nevirapine pharmacokinetic parameters [i.e. AUC_{0-12h}, peak concentration ($C_{max,ss}$) and concentration at 12 h post dose (C_{12h})] were calculated for each individual using a non-compartmental approach by means of the Phoenix WinNonlin software application (Version 6.0; Certara, Princeton, NJ). AUC was calculated using the linear trapezoidal method. The individual differences in the pharmacokinetic parameters were calculated on log transformed data. The confidence interval approach was used to assess the effect of moringa on the pharmacokinetics of nevirapine. To evaluate if pharmacokinetic changes could have clinical relevance, it is recommended to treat pharmacokinetic interactions as equivalence problems [18]. Absence of a moringa effect was assumed if the 90% confidence interval (CI) of the geometric mean ratio (GMR) of AUC_{0-12h},

$C_{max,ss}$ and C_{12h} with and without moringa were contained within the limits 80–125%. The significance of the GMR results were assessed by paired Student *t* test.

Post-moringa/pre-moringa geometric mean ratios (GMRs) and their confidence intervals were calculated as follows: GM[x] = 10^mean[log[x]]; GMR[y/x] = GM[y]/GM[x]. The 90% confidence interval (CI) of GMR[t2/t1] was calculated from the difference in the logs (DL) of the t2 and t1 values: DL[t2,t1] = log[t2]–log[t1], where t2 and t1 are corresponding values for the same subject post-moringa and pre-moringa, for 11 subjects. If m = mean[DL[t2,t1]], sd = standard deviation [DL[t2,t1]], and (a,b) = CI[m,sd,n], then the CI of GMR[t2/t1] = (10^a,10^b) and GMR[t2/t1] = 10^m. The confidence intervals of the DL values were also verified with that obtained by the statistical package.

Results

Participant enrolment

Thirty-three HIV-infected adult patients were screened. Thirteen participants met the eligibility criteria and were enrolled after giving oral and written informed consent. All participants completed the study. Based on pill counts and a review of entries in the food/herb/medication diaries, all participants were fully compliant with medication and supplementation restrictions. The baseline demographic characteristics are summarized in Table 1.

Adverse events

The combination of moringa with nevirapine was well tolerated. Participants were in good health upon physical examination at the post moringa visit. There were no serious adverse events and all participants completed the study. A total of two adverse events were reported by the participants; one complained of transient mild pain at the site of cannula insertion and the other, a headache. During the observation period, only grade 1 Common Terminology Criteria for Adverse Events (CTCAE) toxicities were observed in the clinical assessments. The incidence rate was 5% (n = 202 readings), and there were no significant differences in the number observed pre-moringa compared to post-moringa. The medical officer and consultant physician monitoring adverse events in the study decided these were not related to the moringa.

Table 1 Baseline characteristics of the study population, n = 13

Characteristic	Value
Age (years), mean ± SD	44 ± 8
Sex, female, n (%)	8 (73)
Weight (kg), mean ± SD	63.5 ± 7.5
Drug frequency n (%)	
Nevirapine	13 (100)
Tenofovir/lamivudine	10 (77)
Stavudine/lamivudine	2 (15)
Zidovudine/lamivudine	1 (8)
Cotrimoxazole	9 (69)
Other drugs[a]	3 (23)

[a] Other drugs included pyridoxine, hydrochlorothiazide, indomethacin, diclofenac and enalapril

Pharmacokinetics

Pharmacokinetic analyses were performed on the results from 11 participants who had complete data. Of the two participants that were excluded, one had difficulties with venous access at points during visit 2. The other took the day 35 nevirapine dose at home instead of at the clinic such that only samples for the latter time points could be collected.

Figure 1 shows the mean plasma concentration–time profiles for nevirapine with and without *Moringa oleifera* leaf powder supplementation (Figs. 2, 3, 4).

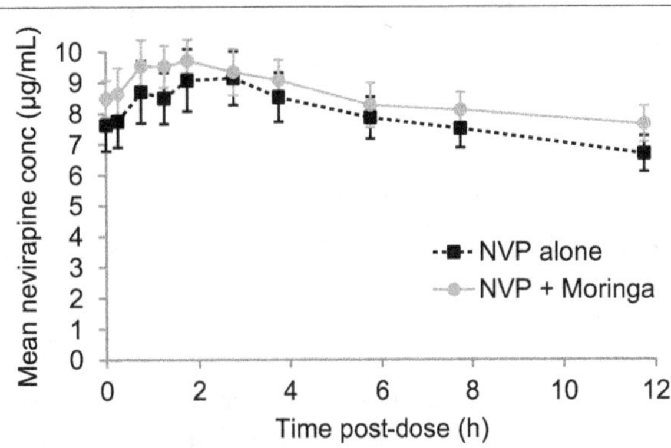

Fig. 1 Mean nevirapine plasma concentration–time profile with and without moringa. The *error bars* represent the standard error of the mean

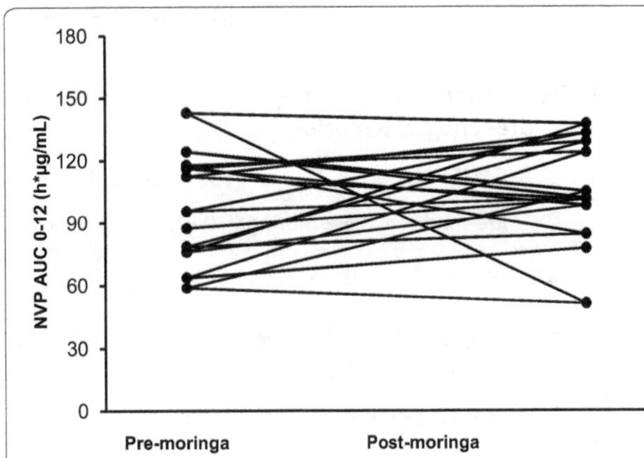

Fig. 2 Individual AUC $_{0-12}$ of nevirapine with and without moringa. All patients maintained therapeutic plasma concentrations (>3.0 μg/mL) 12 h post-dose [19]

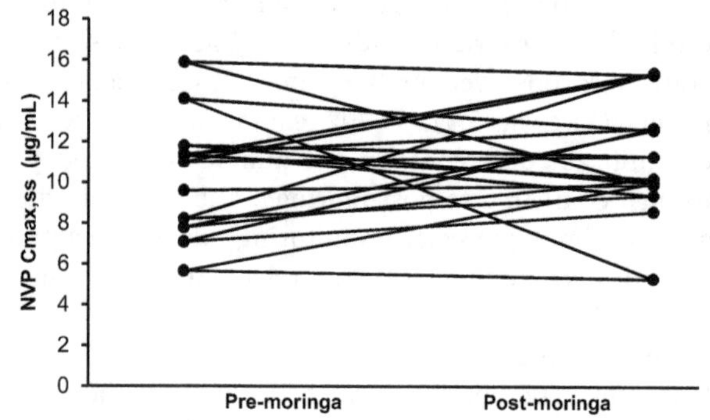

Fig. 3 Individual Cmax,ss of nevirapine with and without moringa. All patients maintained therapeutic plasma concentrations (>3.0 µg/mL) 12 h post-dose [19]

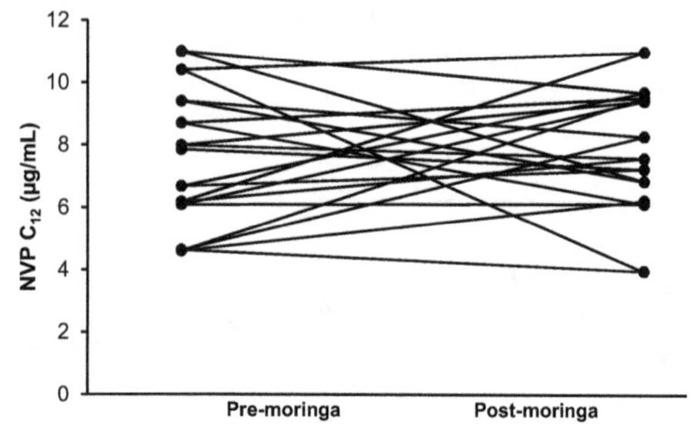

Fig. 4 Individual C_{12} of nevirapine with and without moringa. All patients maintained therapeutic plasma concentrations (>3.0 µg/mL) 12 h post-dose [19]

The plasma pharmacokinetics parameters and comparisons for nevirapine are presented in Table 2.

Discussion

Based on previous in vitro studies that have noted significant inhibitory effects of moringa on the nevirapine-metabolizing CYP3A4 and CYP2D6 isoforms, the effect of *Moringa oleifera* leaf supplementation on nevirapine pharmacokinetics was investigated. While the nevirapine pharmacokinetic profiles from HIV-infected adults at the dosage of moringa used show an inhibitory trend, consistent with that observed in vitro [5, 8, 9], the change in steady-state nevirapine pharmacokinetic parameters is neither clinically nor statistically significant. The 90% confidence intervals for the nevirapine geometric mean ratios for AUC_{0-12h}, $C_{max,ss}$ and C_{12h} following concomitant administration of moringa over 14 days were within the 80–125% limit, indicating lack of a clinically significant interaction.

Table 2 Comparison of nevirapine pharmacokinetic parameters pre- and post- moringa

Parameter	GM (CV %)[a]		GMR (90% CI)[a]	
	Pre-moringa	Post-moringa	Post/Pre	P
AUC_{0-12h} (h*µg/mL)	94.17 (25.24)	100.44 (27.65)	1.07 (1.00–1.14)	0.131
C_{12h} (µg/mL)	7.30 (25.85)	7.55 (28.56)	1.03 (0.92–1.16)	0.702
$C_{max,ss}$ (µg/mL)	9.92 (26.93)	10.57 (29.62)	1.06 (0.98–1.16)	0.261

[a] Post-moringa/pre-moringa geometric mean ratios (GMRs) and their confidence intervals were calculated as follows: GM[x] = 10^{m}ean[log[x]];GMR[y/x] = GM[y]/GM[x]

GMR geometric mean ratio, *CI* confidence interval, AUC_{0-12h} area under the time-concentration curve from 0 to 12 h after dosing, $C_{max,ss}$ maximum concentration, C_{12h} concentration at the end of the dosing interval

The findings are supported by observations from previous studies that demonstrated that the inhibitory effects of moringa on CYP3A4 and CYP2D6 are significantly less as compared to their positive control inhibitors ketoconazole and quinidine [20]. Data from other studies show that nevirapine induces its metabolism by both CYP3A4 and CYP2B6, which may compensate to some degree for CYP3A4 inhibition [21] Any inhibition of CYP3A4 may also have been compensated for by the alternative metabolic pathways (CYP2B6, CYP3A5, CYP2C9, and CYP2D6) reducing the resulting pharmacokinetic changes [22, 23]. This may not be the case for other drugs such as saquinavir, ritonavir, indinavir, darunavir and atazanavir whose main or sole route of elimination is via CYP3A4.

In general, moringa has a good safety profile consistent with its long history of use as food and medicine [24]. The combination of moringa and nevirapine in this study was also well tolerated since moringa did not alter the safety profile of nevirapine when co-administered. A minimum concentration of 3.0 µg/mL is recommended as a therapeutic cut-off for nevirapine trough concentrations [19]. All patients maintained nevirapine 12-h concentrations above 3.0 µg/mL with moringa supplementation. Because the study did not assess clinical outcomes, this observation cannot be discussed in terms viral load.

The toxicity of nevirapine as a function of concentration is not well established. Some studies could not find evidence of a concentration—toxicity relationship while others report an association between hepatotoxicity and higher nevirapine concentrations [25–28]. In this study, no nevirapine related adverse effects were reported despite the C_{12h} and $C_{max,ss}$ values observed being mostly higher than the 6 µg/mL value previously associated with increased toxicity. The findings are consistent with Thai and Ugandan data that did not detect increased toxicity, despite increases in nevirapine C_{trough}.

One limitation of the study is that for operational economy, a single sequence of moringa administration was used; hence, potential period effects cannot be ruled out.

Conclusions

We conclude that co-administration of moringa leaf powder at traditionally used doses has no clinically significant effect on the steady-state pharmacokinetics of nevirapine.

Authors' contributions

TM was responsible for the conception of the study, its design, data collection, drafting of the manuscript and analysis of data. CM supervised the research process, assisted with interpretation of the data, revised the draft critically and gave final approval of the version to be published. GM and AW contributed to the design of the study, analyzed the data, assisted with the interpretation of the data and revised the draft critically. LW analyzed the data and revised the draft critically. CN assisted in the design of the study, supervised the work, contributed to the analysis of data, assisted with the interpretation of the data, revised the draft critically and gave final approval of the version to be published. All authors read and approved the final manuscript.

Author details

[1] Drug and Toxicology Information Services (DaTIS), School of Pharmacy, University of Zimbabwe College of Health Sciences, Harare, Zimbabwe. [2] Center for Integrated Global Biomedical Sciences, University at Buffalo, Buffalo, NY, USA. [3] Department of Bioengineering and Therapeutic Sciences, University of California San Francisco, San Francisco, CA, USA. [4] Division of Clinical Pharmacology, Department of Medicine, University of Cape Town, Cape Town, South Africa. [5] Department of Clinical Pharmacology, University of Zimbabwe College of Health Sciences, Harare, Zimbabwe.

Acknowledgements

The authors thank Emmanuel Chigutsa who provided insight that greatly assisted the research; as well as Alfred Tarumbwa, Tariro Chawana and Noleen Chifamba who assisted with the data collection.

Competing interests

The authors declare that they have no competing interests.

Funding

This publication was made possible by grant numbers 2U2RTW007367, D43TW007991-01A2 and D43TW010313-01 from the Office of Global AIDS Coordinator (U. S. Department of State) and the Fogarty International Centre (National Institutes of Health, U. S. Department of Health and Human Services). The drug assays were also supported in part by the National Institute of Allergy and Infectious Diseases of the National Institutes of Health (UM1 AI068634, UM1 AI068636 and UM1AI106701, U01 AI068632), the Eunice Kennedy Shriver National Institute of Child Health and Human Development, and the National Institute of Mental Health (AI068632). Its contents are solely the responsibility of the authors and do not necessarily represent the official views of the government.

References

1. Meng Q, Liu K. Pharmacokinetic interactions between herbal medicines and prescribed drugs: focus on drug metabolic enzymes and transporters. Curr Drug Metab. 2014;15:791–807.
2. Cho HJ, Yoon IS. Pharmacokinetic interactions of herbs with cytochrome p450 and p-glycoprotein. Evid Based Complement Altern Med. 2015. doi:10.1155/2015/736431.
3. Müller AC, Kanfer I. Potential pharmacokinetic interactions between antiretrovirals and medicinal plants used as complementary and African traditional medicines. Biopharm Drug Dispos. 2011;32:458–70.
4. van den Bout-van den Beukel CJ, Koopmans PP, van der Ven AJ, De Smet PA, Burger DM. Possible drug-metabolism interactions of medicinal herbs with antiretroviral agents. Drug Metab Rev. 2006;38:477–514.
5. Monera TG, Wolfe AR, Maponga CC, Benet LZ, Guglielmo J. *Moringa oleifera* leaf extracts inhibit 6 beta-hydroxylation of testosterone by CYP3A4. J Infect in Dev Ctries. 2008;2:379–83.
6. Monera TG, Maponga CC. Prevalence and patterns of *Moringa oleifera* use among HIV positive patients in Zimbabwe: a cross-sectional survey. J Public Health Afr. 2012;3:22–4.
7. Popoola JO, Obembe OO. Local knowledge, use pattern and geographical distribution of *Moringa oleifera* Lam. (Moringaceae) in Nigeria. J Ethnopharmacol. 2013;150:682–91.
8. Taesotikul T, Navinpipatana V, Tassaneeyakul W. Selective inhibition of human cytochrome P450 1A2 by *Moringa oleifera*. Thai J Pharmacol. 2010;32:256–8.
9. Awortwe C, Bouic PJ, Masimirembwa CM, Rosenkranz B. Inhibition of major drug metabolizing CYPs by common herbal medicines used by HIV/AIDS patients in Africa—implications for herb-drug interactions. Drug Metab Lett. 2014;7:83–95.
10. Riska P, Lamson M, MacGregor T, Sabo J, Hattox S, Pav J, Keirns J. Disposition and biotransformation of the antiretroviral drug nevirapine in humans. Drug Metab Dispos. 1999;27:895–901.
11. Wen B, Chen Y, Fitch WL. Metabolic activation of nevirapine in human liver microsomes: dehydrogenation and inactivation of cytochrome P450 3A4. Drug Metab Dispos. 2009;37:1557–62.
12. Manosuthi W, Athichathanabadi C, Uttayamakul S, Phoorisri T, Sungkanuparph S. Plasma nevirapine levels, adverse events and efficacy of antiretroviral therapy among HIV-infected patients concurrently receiving nevirapine-based antiretroviral therapy and fluconazole. BMC Infect Dis. 2007;7:1–8.
13. de Maat MMR, Hoetelmans RMW, Mathôt RAA, van Gorp ECM, Meenhorst PL, Mulder JW, Beijnen JH. Drug interaction between St John's wort and nevirapine. AIDS. 2001;15:420–1.
14. Sauveur A, Broin M. Growing and processing moringa leaves. Moringa and Plant Resources Network 2010; http://hdl.handle.net/10568/76865.
15. Monera-Penduka TG, Jani ZT, Maponga CC, Mudzengi J, Morse GD, Nhachi CFB. Quality and labeling information of *Moringa oleifera* products marketed for HIV-infected people in Zimbabwe. J Public Health Afr. 2016;7:84–8.
16. Byakika-Tusiime J, Chinn LW, Oyugi JH, Obua C, Bangsberg DR, Kroetz DL. Steady state bioequivalence of generic and innovator formulations of stavudine, lamivudine, and nevirapine in HIV-infected Ugandan adults. PLoS ONE. 2008. doi:10.1371/journal.pone.0003981.
17. Hauschke D, Steinijans VW, Diletti E, Burke M. Sample size determination for bioequivalence assessment using a multiplicative model. J Pharmacokin Biopharm. 1992;20:557–61.
18. Prueksaritanont T, Chu X, Gibson C, Cui D, Yee KL, Ballard J, Cabalu T, Hochman J. Drug-drug interaction studies: regulatory guidance and an industry perspective. AAPS J. 2013;15:629–45.
19. la Porte CJL, Back D, Blaschke T, Boucher CAB, Fletcher CV, Flexner C, et al. Updated guideline to perform therapeutic drug monitoring for antiretroviral agents. Rev Antivir Ther. 2006;3:4–14.
20. Ahmmed SKM, Mukherjee PK, Bahadur S, Kar A, Al-Dhabi NA, Duraipandiyan V. Inhibition potential of *Moringa oleifera* Lam. on drug metabolizing enzymes. Indian J Tradit Know. 2015;14:614–9.
21. Davit B, Reynolds K, Yuan R, Ajayi F, Conner D, Fadiran E, et al. FDA Evaluations using in vitro metabolism to predict and interpret in vivo metabolic drug-drug interactions: impact on labeling. J Clin Pharmacol. 1999;39:899–910.
22. Erickson DA, Mather G, Trager WF, Levy RH, Kearns JJ. Characterization of the in vitro biotransformation of the HIV-1 reverse transcriptase inhibitor nevirapine by human hepatic cytochromes P-450. Drug Metab Dispos. 1999;27:1488–95.
23. Isoherranen N, Lutz JD, Chung SP, Hachad H, Levy RH, Ragueneau-Majlessi I. Importance of multi-P450 inhibition in drug-drug interactions: evaluation of incidence, inhibition magnitude and prediction from in vitro data. Chem Res Toxicol. 2012;25:2285–300.
24. Stohs SJ, Hartman MJ. Review of the safety and efficacy of *Moringa oleifera*. Phytother Res. 2015;29:796–804.
25. Kappelhoff BS, van Leth F, Robinson PA, MacGregor TR, Baraldi E, Montella F, et al. Are adverse events of nevirapine and efavirenz related to plasma concentrations? Antivir Ther. 2005;10:489–98.
26. Wakeham K, Parkes-Ratanshi R, Watson V, Ggayi AB, Khoo S, Lalloo DG. Co-administration of fluconazole increases nevirapine concentrations in HIV-infected Ugandans. J Antimicrob Chemother. 2010;65:316–9.

Immunological outcomes of Tenofovir versus Zidovudine-based regimens among people living with HIV/AIDS

Teshale Ayele[1*], Habtemu Jarso[2] and Girma Mamo[1]

Abstract

Background: Tenofovir (TDF) based regimen was reported to have better immunological outcomes. Unfortunately, there is limited information regarding the immunologic outcome associated with this regimen in Ethiopia, as its routine utilization in this setting begun since 2013.

Methods: A 2 years retrospective cohort study was conducted at Jimma University Specialized Hospital, 346 km Southwest of Addis Ababa, Ethiopia. A total of 280 patients' data from September 2012 to July 2014 was extracted from records from February 10, 2015 to March 10, 2015. Records were selected using a simple random sampling technique. Data on socio-demographic, clinical and drug related variables were collected; entered into EpiData 3.1 and analyzed by STATA 13.1. Mixed effect linear regression was performed to assess difference in CD4+ change between groups adjusting for baseline characteristics. The change in predicted CD4 count attributed to each regimen was also assessed by marginal analysis. $P < 0.05$ for slopes of the random effect linear regression was used as indicators for presence of association.

Results: The mean (SD) duration of cohort follow up was 714.2 (69.6) and 708.8 (78.9) days ($P = 0.753$) for TDF and AZT groups respectively. The minimum follow up duration was 7.4 and 8.9 months for TDF and AZT groups respectively. Most of TDF (93.6%) and AZT (91.4%) groups completed their follow up, 5 (3.6%) TDF and 6 (4.3%) AZT groups died and 4 (2.9%) TDF and 6 (4.3%) AZT groups were lost for follow-up ($P = 0.769$). There was statistically significant difference in immunologic recovery between the groups (B = +34.08, 95% CI [7.8, 60.35], P = 0.027) over time. The predicted CD4+ count for TDF/3TC/EFV was (B = +347.65 cells/mm^3, P < 0.001) whereas that of AZT/3TC/EFV was (B = +281.54 cells/mm^3, P < 0.001).

Conclusions: TDF based regimens have shown more efficacy compared to AZT based regimens though AZT based regimens are more affordable in low income countries like Ethiopia. However, we recommend further study with quality design to assess the prevalence of sub-optimal CD4+ response (net CD4 gain <50 cells/μl/6 month) in this set-up among TDF users.

Keywords: Immunological outcomes, Tenofovir regimen, Zidovudine regimen, Ethiopia

Background

Around 1980s, Acquired immunodeficiency syndrome (AIDS) was globally emerged as a major public health threat. The reaction against it has led to unprecedented attention and commitment from the international community to improve access to human immune virus(HIV) care, antiretroviral treatment (ART) and prevention [1, 2]. The introduction of potent ART has dramatically reduced HIV/AIDS associated crisis—reduced rates of mortality and morbidity, improved quality of life,

*Correspondence: teshale@mtu.edu.et; tesh.ayu2016@gmail.com
[1] Department of Pharmacy, Jimma University Medical Centre, Institute of Health, Jimma University, Jimma, Ethiopia
Full list of author information is available at the end of the article

revitalized communities and transformed perceptions on the disease from a plague to a manageable chronic illness [3–6].

Currently, there are more than 20 ARV compounds approved for use in United States (US) and Europe. Multiple adult HIV treatment guidelines recommend the nucleos(t)ide reverse transcriptase inhibitors; AZT or TDF based regimens and most are in favour of TDF based regimens as the safer regimen for patients with no contraindication due to its proven effectiveness, favourable toxicity profile, and demonstrated regimen durability [1, 7–9].

Safe and efficacious ART regimens improve patient care through rapidly restoring the immune cells, promoting adherence and alleviating the hazards of mortality [1, 10, 11]. TDF is one of the ART drugs that come to be routinely utilized in Ethiopia since the past 2 years. For this drug, the recent WHO report indicated that data on the risk of major clinical events such as mortality, renal failure and, bone fractures were limited, and particularly for our setups there is no immunologic finding as well [11].

Studies from developed regions showed that there were 18.0 and 18.8% immunologic failures in the EFV/FTC/TDF and EFV/3TC/AZT arms, respectively. There were no significant differences in the risk of HIV-1 disease progression or death [12]. In other findings, TDF based regimens has demonstrated a better immunologic outcome only when combined with Efavirenz as compared to AZT based preparations [3, 13, 14]. In contrary, a finding from south Africa concludes that, in population of HIV patients on treatment in resource-limited settings AZT-containing regimens appear to show a slightly protective than TDF-based regimens [15]. Despite, this evidence variation, its immunologic benefits unknown in an Ethiopian setting where patients generally present late, have high rates of TB and other infectious conditions [16]. Hence further investigation, particularly in health setups of the current setting, was warranted. Therefore, this study was aimed to provide additional information by making a head to head comparison of the two regimens in terms of immunologic benefits and associated risk factors in a teaching hospital of Ethiopia, one of the resource constrained settings.

Methods

Study area and period

The study was conducted at Jimma University specialized Hospital which is located in Jimma town; Jimma Zone, 346 km Southwest of Addis Ababa, Ethiopia. The hospital has separate ART clinic with about 7486 clients. The ART clinic provides HIV and TB treatment and care. Patient data from September 2012 to July 2014 was extracted from records from February 10, 2015 to March 10, 2015.

Study design and population

A retrospective hospital based cohort study was conducted on adult patients who were on TDF and AZT based regimens and fulfilled inclusion criteria. The study was conducted by dividing the total sample into two groups: TDF and AZT groups.

Inclusion and exclusion criteria

We included patients who were older than 14 years, have at least 6 months follow-up, whose records were legible and complete, and who have at least baseline and sixth month CD4 count. We excluded pregnant women from the study because there is significant pharmacokinetic change that is enough to impact the treatment outcome in this group of population. Those whose regimen was changed were also excluded from the study.

Sample size and sampling techniques

Sample size determination was guided by the number of patients on TDF/3TC/NVP where only 70 patients fulfilled the inclusion criteria. Patients from other regimens were selected based on the size of this group to satisfy 1:1 ratio of AZT to TDF group. Therefore, frequency matching was used to select a total of 280 subjects (140 TDF group and 140 AZT group). Records were selected by simple random sampling technique using computer generated random numbers.

Data collection

Data on demographic, clinical, laboratory, drug administered, comorbidities and adherence were collected by record review using English version checklist which was prepared after reviewing different relevant literatures. Baseline body mass-index of the subjects was calculated after collection of baseline height and weight of the patient from patients chart. Data from antiretroviral drugs sheet and patient information sheet were collected by pharmacists, while nurses collected data from ART intake and follow up forms.

Data processing and analysis

Data were double entered into Epi-Data 3.1 and exported to STATA 13.1 for cleaning and analysis. Descriptive analyses were performed and results were presented by text, tables and charts. Bi-variate and multivariable mixed effect linear regression for repeated measurements were performed to assess adjusted effect of the ART regimen and identify additional predictors of CD4 recovery. Coefficient of mean CD4 count with 95% confidence intervals was used as measure of strength of association and $P < 0.05$ was considered to declare a statistical significance. Marginal analysis was also conducted to see the difference among specific regimen category.

Results

A total of 1034 patients were on antiretroviral therapy (ART) for at least 6 months during the study period. Nine hundred eighty six had complete CD4+ count at 6 month of treatment. Fourteen records were used for pre-test, 22 and 110 records were excluded because of pregnancy and regimen change respectively. Only 70 patients remained on TDF/3TC/NVP and this governed the sample selection (Fig. 1).

The cohort was followed for 2 years. The overall time the cohort was at risk was 539.39 years. The cohort contributed to a total of 2.74/100 and 2.72/100 person-years of follow-up for TDF and AZT groups respectively. The mean (SD) duration of follow up was 714.2 (69.6) and 708.8 (78.9) days ($P = 0.753$) for TDF and AZT groups respectively. The minimum follow up duration was 7.4 and 8.9 months for TDF and AZT groups respectively. Most of TDF (93.6%) and AZT (91.4%) groups completed their follow up, 5 (3.6%) TDF and 6 (4.3%) AZT groups died and 4 (2.9%) TDF and 6 (4.3%) AZT groups were lost for follow-up ($P = 0.769$).

Baseline socio-demographic and behavioural characteristics

Majority of TDF (64.3%) and AZT (66.4%) groups were females. Majority of TDF (77.1%) and AZT (85.9%) groups were in the age group 25–45 years with mean (SD) of 32.3 (7.4) and 32.3 (9.2) years respectively. Majority of TDF (62.9%) and AZT (73.6%) groups had BMI $\geq$ 18 kg/

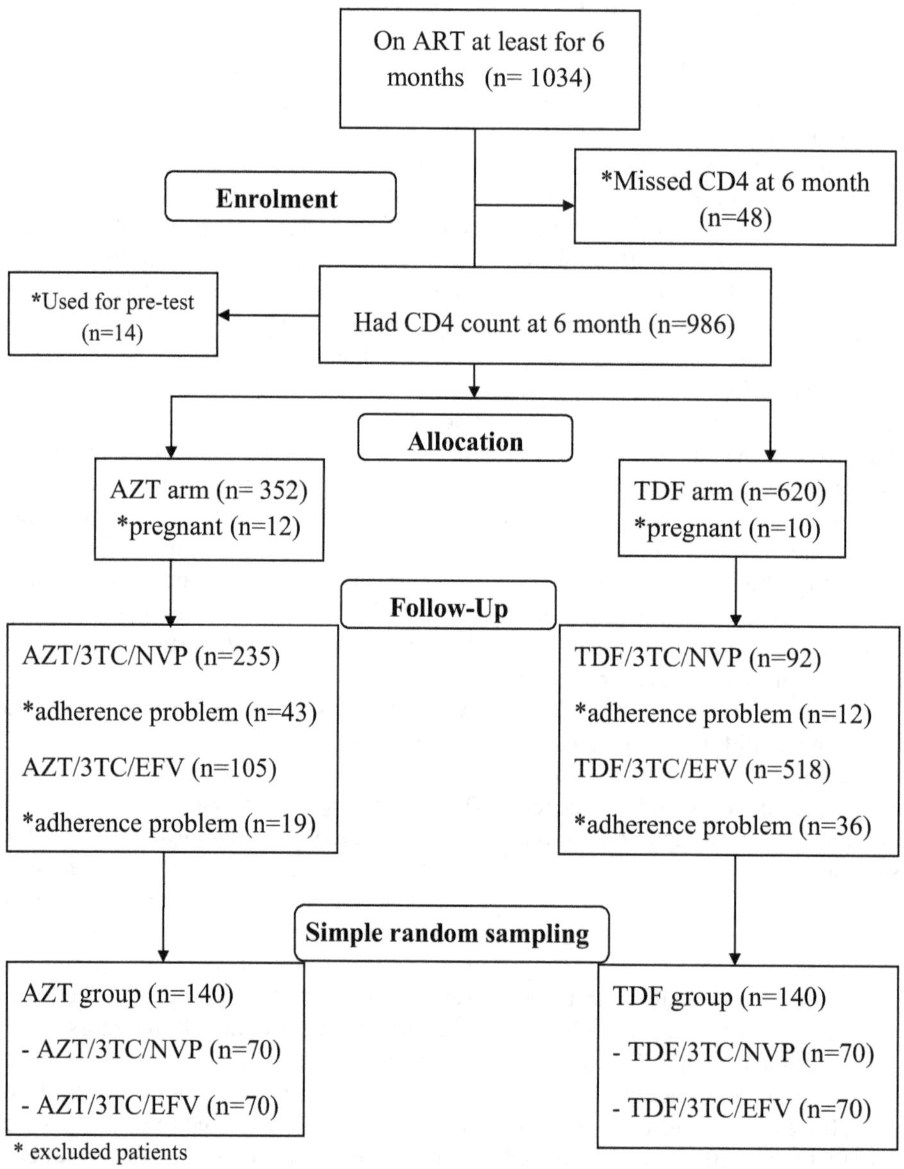

Fig. 1 Sample recruitment diagram from cohort of patients on ART for at least 6 months at JUSH, September, 2012 to July, 2014

m^2 with mean (SD) of 19.7 (3.4) and 20.4 (3.0) respectively. Larger proportion of TDF (48.6%) and AZT (41.5%) groups were employed. Majority of TDF (69.3% and AZT (78.5%) groups were urban. Concerning alcohol use, most of TDF (80.7%) and AZT (72.9%) groups had history of alcohol use. Regarding between groups comparison of distribution of baseline socio-demographic and behavioural characteristics of patients, there was statistically significant difference between groups only in terms of religion (Table 1).

Baseline clinical characteristics

Majority of TDF (65.7%) and AZT (53.9%) groups had baseline CD4+ count <200 cells/mm^3 with mean (SD) of 164.64 (83.36) and 175.21 (89.14) respectively. There was statistically significant difference between groups in terms of baseline CD4 count. Leading percentage (33.6%) both TDF and AZT groups were in WHO clinical stage III and II respectively. Most of TDF (78.6%) and majority of AZT (56.4%) groups had working functional status and there was statistically significant difference between groups. Twenty (15.3%) and 17 (12.1%) of patients were treated for TB from TDF and AZT groups respectively. CPT was prescribed for most of (87.9%) and nearly all of (92.14%) patients in TDF and AZT groups respectively, whereas INH was prescribed for only 26.4 and 21.5% of patients in TDF and AZT groups respectively (Table 2).

Immunologic outcome (CD4+ change)

The mean change in CD4+ over study period is shown by Fig. 2. The overall mean (SD) CD4+ has shown greater improvement among TDF [321.7 (164.8)] than AZT group [299.4 (126.1)]. If each regimen is considered separately, the maximum and minimum mean CD4+ count gain at any given time was attained by TDF/3TC/EFV and AZT/3TC/EFV groups respectively (Fig. 2).

At 6 month, the overall proportion of sub-optimal CD4+ response (net CD4+ gain <50 cells/μl) was 23.95% (30% TDF/EFV, 28.3% AZT/EFV, and 23.8% TDF/NVP). Earlier at the initiation of ART, the CD4+ count showed a linear trend but it becomes more flat after 18th month with a very minimal gain irrespective of the regimen.

Predictors of CD4+ change

Considering consecutive CD4+ count as an outcome variable, multilevel mixed effect linear regression was performed (Table 3). The slope of random-effect multiple linear regression was used to interpret the over-time change in CD4+ count attributed to the predictor variables.

Table 1 Socio-demographic and behavioural characteristics for cohort of patients on ART for a least 6 months at JUSH, September 2012 to July 2014

Baseline socio-demographic and behavioural characteristics	Group		P value
	TDF group no (%)	AZT group no (%)	
Sex			
Male	50 (35.7)	47 (33.6)	0.706
Female	90 (64.3)	93 (66.4)	
Age			
<25	27 (19.3)	32 (25.9)	0.276
25–45	108 (77.1)	98 (85.9)	
>45	5 (3.6)	10 (7.2)	
Mean (SD)	32.3 (7.4)	32.3 (9.2)	0.977**
BMI			
<18.5	52 (37.1)	37 (26.4)	0.130
≥18.5	88 (62.9)	93 (73.6)	
Mean (SD)	19.7 (3.4)	20.4 (3.0)	0.062**
Educational level			
Illiterate	22 (15.8)	30 (21.4)	
Primary	48 (34.2)	58 (41.4)	0.089
Post-primary	70 (50)	52 (37.2)	
Residence			
Urban	97 (69.3)	110 (78.5)	0.077
Rural	43 (30.7)	30 (21.5)	
Occupation			
Employed	68 (48.6)	58 (41.5)	
Unemployed	46 (22.8)	55 (39.2)	0.446
Housewife	26 (18.6)	27 (19.3)	
Religion			
Orthodox	59 (42.1)	80 (57.1)	
Muslim	45 (32.1)	42 (30)	0.010*
Others	36 (25.8)	18 (12.9)	
Marital status			
Married	76 (54.3)	77 (55.0)	
Single	23 (16.5)	29 (20.7)	0.207
Divorced	33 (23.5)	21 (15.1)	
Widowed	8 (5.7)	13 (9.2)	
Alcohol use			
Yes	113 (80.7)	102 (72.9)	
No	27 (19.3)	38 (27.1)	0.120

* Statistically significant at P value 0.05 cut off point

** T test

Accordingly, the average gain in CD4+ count achieved at every visit among the cohort was 38 cells/mm^3 ($B = 38.18$, 95% CI [33.11,43.24], $P < 0.001$) with the conditional correlation coefficient of 64.9%, i.e. 64.9% of the variability in CD4+ count between two visits was explained by unobserved patient specific factors. Among these, 38.99% of the variation in CD4+ change was

Table 2 Baseline and on follow up clinical characteristics for cohort of patients on ART for a least 6 months at JUSH, September 2012 to July 2014

Clinical characteristics	TDF group no (%)	AZT group no (%)	P value
Baseline CD4+ count			
<200	92 (65.7)	74 (53.9)	0.029*
≥200	48 (34.3)	66 (47.1)	
Mean (SD)	164.64 (83.36)	175.21 (89.14)	0.307**
Baseline WHO clinical stage			
I	32 (22.9)	36 (25.7)	
II	46 (32.9)	47 (33.6)	0.928
III	47 (33.6)	43 (30.7)	
IV	15 (10.6)	14 (10)	
Baseline functional status			
W	110 (78.6)	79 (56.4)	
A	24 (17.1)	56 (40.0)	0.000*
B	6 (4.3)	5 (3.6)	
TB Treatment			
No	120 (84.7)	113 (87.9)	0.773
Yes	20 (15.3)	17 (12.1)	
Prophylaxis			
CPT+ INH	37 (26.4)	30 (21.5)	
CPT alone	86 (61.4)	99 (70.7)	0.231
Neither	17 (12.2)	11 (7.8)	

* Statistically significant at P value 0.05 cut off point

** T test

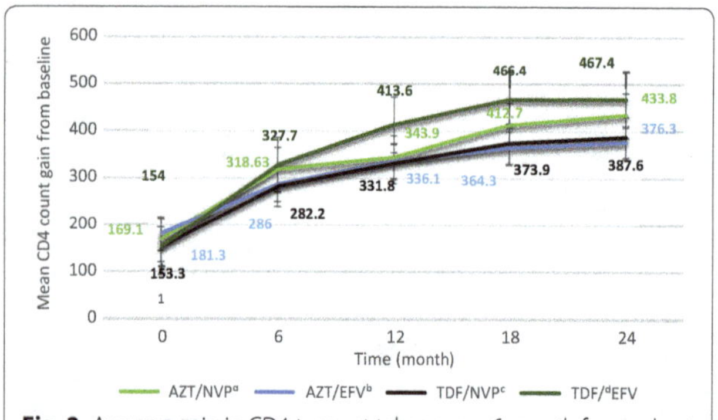

Fig. 2 Average gain in CD4+ count taken every 6 month for a cohort of patients on ART for at least 6 months at JUSH, September, 2012 to July, 2014. Missing values per each regimen at 12, 18 and 24 months respectively: [a](2, 7, 11); [b](11, 3, 2); [c](7, 1, 9); [d](5, 12, 4)

explained by differences in the regimens where as 25.34% of the variation is attributed to other regression variables (P < 0.001), showing an important heterogeneity between patient groups.

In the overall analysis, keeping other factors constant, older age was found to be one of the negative predictors of CD4+ count change. So younger patients (age <25 years) were found to have +66 gain in CD4+ count every 6 months as compared to those aged ≥45 years (B = −66.19 95% CI [−126.68, −5.70], P = 0.032).

Among the predictor variables, female sex was strongly associated with progressive CD4+ count gain at each visit. So, females had +39 CD4+ cells advantage over time (B = 33.86, 95% CI [33.11, 43.24], P = 0.013) as compared to males. Patients with BMI ≥ 18.5 kg/m^2 had a significantly higher CD4+ change (+32 cell/mm^3) over time than those who had BMI < 18.5 kg/m^2 (B = −32, 95% CI [−60.16, −4.27], P = 0.011).

Baseline CD4+ count was also another independent predictor for CD4+ advantage over time (β = 0.879, 95% CI [0.70, 1.06], P < 0.001). More importantly, patients in TDF group had a significant CD4+ count gain per visit compared with their AZT counterparts (B = 34.08, 95% CI [7.80, 60.35], P = 0.027).

In this study, other baseline patient factors such as WHO clinical stage, TB treatment, educational status, place of residence, religion, occupational status, marital status, alcoholic use and prophylaxis had no significant association with CD4+ change.

Marginal analysis

To predict the expected change in CD4+ count in both groups at the end of treatment period, post-estimation marginal analysis was conducted.

In TDF group, the predicted mean CD4+ count changes were 347.65 and 295.73 cells/mm^3 for patients treated with TDF/3TC/EFV and TDF/3TC/NVP respectively. In AZT group, the predicted mean CD4+ count changes were 319.11 and 281.54 cells/mm^3 for patients treated with AZT/3TC/NVP and AZT/3TC/EFV respectively. These figures were exactly the expected increase in CD4+ count associated with each regimen and has a crucial clinical implication in guiding clinicians to choose which regimen to initiate on as the role of good immunologic recovery in treatment of HIV infection is multidimensional. So, this section of analysis (Table 4) clearly showed that the overall outcome was better in TDF than AZT group.

Discussion

Analysis of every 6 month mean CD4+ gain showed that the maximum gain in mean CD4+ count was attained by TDF/3TC/EFV followed by AZT/3TC/NVP and TDF/3TC/EFV at any given time in the course of therapy. AZT/3TC/EFV had the least immunologic recovery over the entire treatment course. The CD4+ count showed a linear trend but became more flat after 18th month with a very minimal gain irrespective of the regimen. The overall prevalence of sub-optimal CD4+ response was found to be 67 (23.95%). At first 6 months, majority of sub-optimal immunologic responders belonged

Table 3 Random-effect linear regression analysis of trend of CD4+ count (slope, cells/mm³/6 month) at JUSH, September 2012 to July 2014

Variable	Unadjusted		Adjusted	
	B [95% CI]	P value	B [95% CI]	P value
Sex				
Male	0		0	
Female	52.373 [21.22, 84.24]	0.001	33.86 [33.11, 43.24]	0.013
Age				
<25	0		0	
25–45	−53.15 [−90.03, −16.27]	0.005	−27.32 [−59.3, 4.66]	0.094
>45	−120.87 [−191.24, −50.49]	0.001	−66.19 [−126.68, −5.70]	0.032
BMI				
<18.5	−48.08 [−80.42, −15.74]	0.004	−32.77 [−60.16, −4.27]	0.011
≥18.5	0		0	
Educ. level				
Illiterate	−0.5 [−42.86, 41.86]	0.982		
Primary	14.42 [−19.59, 48.44]	0.406		
Post-primary	0			
Residence				
Urban	0			
Rural	−12.35 [−47.18, 22.54]	0.488		
Occupation				
Employed	0	0.936	0	0.796
Unemployed	−1.40 [−32.23, 32.44]	0.015	3.96 [−26.04, 33.95]	0.293
House wife	51.50 [10.2, 92.80]		21.35 [−18.42, 61.12]	
Marital status				
Single	30.25 [−11.18, 71.68]	0.152	40.45 [0.52, 80.37]	0.069
Married	0	0.525	0	
Divorced	13.06 [−27.17, 53.29]	0.513	6.42 [−32.27, 45.11]	0.745
Widowed	−19.89 [−79.56, 39.77]		−2.33 [−55.27, 50.6]	0.931
Religion				
Orthodox	0		0	
Muslim	22.91 [−12.00, 57.83]	0.198	20.83 [−8.86, 50.53]	0.166
Other	0.21 [−40.70, 41.13]	0.992	−12.09 [−46.89, 22.71]	0.496
Alcohol				
Yes	−26.1 [−62.15, 9.94]	0.156	8.48 [−22.88, 39.83]	0.596
No	0		0	
ART regimen				
TDF	11.58 [−18.98, 42.15]	0.458	34.08 [7.80, 60.35]	0.027
AZT	0		0	
Baseline CD4+ count	0.97 [0.80, 1.15]	0.000	0.879 [0.70, 1.06]	0.000
WHO stage				
I	0			
II	−16.76 [−57.59, 24.06]	0.421		
III	−23.17 [−64.32, 17.97]	0.270		
IV	−29.27 [−86.35, 27.81]	0.315		
TB (treatment)				
No	0		0	
Yes	−48.18 [−85.37, 5.00]	0.081	−20.74 [−59.05, 17.57]	0.289
Prophylaxis				
CPT+ INH	0		0	
CPT alone	−29.40 [−65.65, 6.85]	0.112	−10.34 [−40.57, 19.88]	0.502
Neither	−40.89 [−97.93, 16.16]	0.160	−22.3 [−70.33, 25.73]	0.363

to TDF/3TC/EFV (30%) and lowest proportion of sub-optimal immunologic responder was observed among AZT/3TC/EFV (17.9%).

Our finding of mean CD4+ recovery was in agreement with a randomized multi-centre open-label study by Gallant et al. [9], where a maximum immunologic response was achieved by TDF/3TC/EFV (270 cells/mm^3) followed by AZT/3TC/EFV (237 cells/mm^3) at 96 weeks. Another finding from Nigeria indicated that TDF/3TC/NVP is much more inferior (208 cells/mm^3) to AZT/3TC/NVP (221.1 cells/mm^3) at 12 months of therapy [17]. The difference in the outcome when TDF/3TC is combined with EFV and NVP may be due to negative pharmacokinetic or pharmacodynamics interaction between this NRTI backbone and NVP. The finding from the marginal analysis also indicated that change in mean CD4+ count is significantly higher in TDF based EFV regimen.

The bi-phasic CD4+ count response shown in our finding was also reported by other findings [18, 19] as a rapid increase of memory CD4+ cells (a high CD4+ count slope) in the first several months after treatment initiation succeeded by a slow increase in naive CD4+ cells (smaller slope compared to the initial several months). The linear trend in CD4+ increment at early phase of of therapy became flat with minimal CD4+ gain latter after 18th month of treatment irrespective of the regimen used. So "when will target CD4+ count (500–800 cells/mm^3) be attained after initiation of ART?" is the question to be addressed by further study.

Immunologic response after 6 months of ART indicates a favourable clinical outcome in HIV-1 infected patients regardless of virologic response [20]. Several studies has reported that as many as 8–40% of patients on ART do not show a significant increase in CD4+ cell count despite viral suppression [18, 21, 22]. Our finding, in general, is almost consistent with these studies.

To these days, studies are unable to justify the impact of ART regimen on sub-optimal immunologic recovery. So, it is not surprising that most of these patients in this study were from TDF based regimens. As the recovery of the CD4+ T-cell count is hindered by several patient and viral factors, including: residual viral replication, impaired thymic function, advanced age, enhanced T-cell activation and apoptosis, genetic variations, baseline anaemia and poor adherence [18, 21, 23, 24], our finding might not quest the efficacy of TDF based regimens in resource limited settings, even though it needs a further workup with adequately powered and methodological high quality study.

Study by Mauro et al. [25] has confirmed older age as a key independent predictor for sub-optimal immunologic response as thymus activity decreases with age [26]. This finding agreed with our result where older age was statistically significant negative predictor of CD4+ gain on multiple regression.

The pre-treatment CD4+ count in relation to sub-optimal immunologic response, however, is controversial as some literatures favour higher baseline CD4+ (>200 cells/mm^3) [26] and explained it as "starting treatment at higher CD4+ cell counts limits the scope for further increases". Other literatures favoured lower baseline CD4+ count (<200 cells/mm^3) and this is biologically plausible given that a low nadir pre-treatment CD4+ cell count is thought to be suggestive of more extensive depletion of CD4+ cells in the gut-associated lymphoid tissue during acute HIV infection, and may be delayed or refractory to reconstitution with ART [27].

As this study has short comings including absence of viral marker measurement to conclude the rate of sub-optimal immunologic recovery among the patients, further study with quality design is needed as lack of knowledge about this subgroup may contribute to inadequate clinical management and current HIV treatment guidelines do not provide specific applicable guidance [18].

The overall random effect linear regression analysis had pointed out that, baseline BMI, sex, age, baseline CD4+ count, and exposure to TDF based regimen were independent predictors for CD4+ change over time. The marginal effects of each regimens confirmed that the immunologic outcome associated with TDF based EFV preparations was more convincing and made it the golden regimen to be utilized in this

Table 4 The predicted mean CD4+ change of patients treated with AZT and TDF based regimens at JUSH, September 2012 to July 2014

Status	Status	Delta-method		t	[95% CI]	P value
		Margins	Standard error			
Unexposed	AZT3TC/NVP	319.11	19.34	16.50	281.02,357.20	P < 0.001
	AZT/3TC/EFV	281.54	18.39	15.31	245.31,317.77	P < 0.001
Exposed	TDF/3TC/NVP	295.73	18.39	16.08	259.50,331.96	P < 0.001
	TDF/3TC/EFV	347.65	18.39	18.90	311.42,383.89	P < *0.001*

setup (margins = 347.65 cells/mm^3/, *P < 0.001*) followed by AZT/3TC/NVP (m = 319.11 cells/mm^3, *P < 0.001)*and TDF/3TC/NVP (m = 295.73, P < 0.001). However, AZT/3TC/EFV had lowest predicted change in CD4+ count (m = 281.54, P < 0.001). This implies that this regimen has minimal immunologic response and its clinical utilization need to be reconsidered.

Females had greater CD4+ improvement over time. Accordingly, every visit of female patients was associated with the average CD4+ count of 39 cells/mm^3 ($\beta = 33.86$ [33.11, 43.24], P = 0.013). Similar study from Lao Democratic Republic strengthen this finding [28]. But it was inconsistent with study from Asia [19] probably due to differences in study setup and sample size (1676 versus 280), where females contribute only 26% of the sample analysed.

The impact of age on immunologic recovery was well described [26] and this study had found concordance with previous findings. Accordingly, the CD4+ gain attained by younger (<25 years) patients was +66 cells/mm^3 as compared to those older than 45 years of age ($\beta = -66.19$, 95% CI [−126.68,−5.70], P = 0.032). The finding is consistent with the studies from Asia [19] and Ghana [29] and which reported the inverse relationship between age and CD4+ gain. This is mainly due to failure of cellular expansion or non-sustained cell survival in the periphery or age related central degeneration of thymus function as patients become older [18].

In the cohort, those with BMI $\geq$ 18.5 kg/m^2 had a better immunologic outcome and each visit was associated with 32 cells/mm^3 of CD4+ count advantage as compared to patients with BMI < 18.5 kg/m^2 ($\beta = -32.22$, 95% CI [17.23,51.85], P < 0.001). This is concurrent with the study by Bastard et al. [[28].] in which BMI > 18 kg/m^2 was reported to have a protective effect for CD4 count increment at 9 months of therapy (HR = 0.39, 95% CI 0.25–0.60). This implies that higher BMI is a sign of good nutritional status and it is fertile ground for better immunologic revival.

The baseline CD4+ count was another positive predictor for successful immunologic revival. So, a patient has a 0.879 CD4+ cell count advantage over time, for every count higher in initial CD4+ count, when compared to his/her counterpart (*B* = 0.879 95% CI [0.70, 1.06], *P* < 0.001). This finding is consistent form study by Lawrence et al. [27] and Mustapha et al. [29] in which higher baseline CD4+ count was associated with good immunologic outcome. This might be due to less extensively depleted immune system will be boosted easily after initiation of ART. The overall clinical and immunological findings were suggestive of better outcome of ART if initiated at higher CD4+ count. This finding also agrees with the recent WHO ART guidelines [30] which described the initiation of ART irrespective of WHO stage and CD4+ count in adolescents and adults.

In contrary, the finding disagrees with some studies showing poor immunologic recovery including discordant responders when ART was commenced at higher CD4+ count [31]. This may be due to the goal CD4+ in HIV patients (500 cells/mm^3) [32] can be attained immediately in those with higher baseline CD4+ and further increment could be impossible. The reason for the deviation might be due to differences in sample size and setup. The multicenterity of the previous study might also contribute for the difference.

From this study, patients randomized to TDF group had a significant CD4+ count advantage per visit relative to patients randomized to AZT group (*B* =+34.08, 95% CI [7.80, 60.35], P = 0.001). This study is consistent with most of the previous findings that described TDF based regimens with better immunologic outcome [9, 14, 31, 32].

Conclusions

The results of this study suggest that TDF based regimens especially, TDF/3TC/EFV had excellent immunologic recovery followed by AZT based NVP. Since aged patients, those with baseline CD4+ count <200 cells/mm^3 and patients with pre-treatment BMI < 18.5 were poor immunologic responders, they need special attention while delivering care and treatment. However, the prevalence of sub-immunologic recovery among the TDF users in the resource constrained settings needs to be assessed further.

Authors' contributions

TA: conceived and led the conduct of study; acquisition of data, analysis and interpretation of data; and drafting of the manuscript. GM: assisted with the design and conduct of study; analysis and interpretation of data; and revision of manuscript for intellectual content. HJ: assisted with the design and conduct of study; analysis and interpretation of data; and revision of manuscript for intellectual content and reviewers' comments. All authors read and approved the final manuscript.

Author details

[1] Department of Pharmacy, Jimma University Medical Centre, Institute of Health, Jimma University, Jimma, Ethiopia. [2] Department of Epidemiology, Public Health Faculty, Institute of Health, Jimma University, Jimma, Ethiopia.

Acknowledgements

We would like to thank pharmacists, nurses and physicians at JUSH ART clinic for their indispensable cooperation during acquisition of data.

Competing interests

The authors declare that they have no competing interests.

References

1. Tirfe ZM, Ahmed TA, Tedla NB, Debere MK, Alamdo AG. Immunological responses of HIV/AIDS patients treated with Nevirapine versus Efavirenz based highly active anti-retroviral therapy in Addis Ababa, Ethiopia. Retrosp Cohort Study. 2013;1508:1502–8.
2. Solomon SS, Ganesh AK, Mehta SH, Yepthomi T, Balaji K, Anand S, et al. Immunologic response among HIV-infected patients enrolled in a graduated cost-recovery programme of antiretroviral therapy delivery in Chennai, India. Indian J Med Res. 2013;6(137):1145–53.
3. Alemayehu L, GizatMollaKassie BAH. Comparative study of the effects of antiretroviral therapy (ART) on the CD4 cell count in the Jimma University specialized hospital. J Pharm Sci Innov. 2014;3(4):310–4.
4. Tang MW, Kanki PJ, Shafer RW. A review of the virological efficacy of the 4 World Health Organization—recommended tenofovir-containing regimens for initial hiv therapy. J Clin Infect Dis. 2012;54(15):862–75.
5. Ruan Y, Xing H, Wang X, Tang H, Wang Z, Liu H, et al. Virologic outcomes of first-line HAART and associated factors among Chinese patients with HIV in three sentinel antiretroviral treatment sites. Trop Med Int Health. 2010;15(11):4–10.
6. Albrecht D, Altfeld M, Behrens G, Bredeek UF, Buhk T, Dickinson L, et al. HIV medicine [Internet]. 2007. www.HIVMedicine.com.
7. Spaulding A, Gw R, Siegfried N. Tenofovir or zidovudine in three-drug combination therapy with one nucleoside reverse transcriptase inhibitor and one non-nucleoside reverse transcriptase inhibitor for initial treatment of HIV infection in antiretroviral-naïve individuals. Cochrane Database Rev 2010;10.
8. Chi BH, Mwango A, Giganti M, Mulenga LB, Tambatamba-chapula B, Reid SE, et al. Early clinical and programmatic outcomes with tenofovir-based antiretroviral therapy in Zambia. J Acquir Immune Defic Syndr. 2010;54(1):63–70.
9. Pozniak AL, Gallant JE, Dejesus E, Arribas JR, Gazzard B, Campo RE, et al. Tenofovir disoproxil fumarate, emtricitabine, and efavirenz versus fixed-dose zidovudine/lattmivudine and efavirenzt in antiretroviral-naive patients virologic, immunologic, and morphologic changes—a 96-week analysis. J Acquir Immune Defic Syndr. 2006;43(5):535–40.
10. Leon Regensberg CW. Aid for AIDS Clinical Guidelines, South Africa; 2010. p. 52.
11. World Health Organization. Monitoring for renal toxicity in people receiving tenofovir and on tenofovir toxicity and how it affects disability-adjusted life-years and quality-adjusted life-years. Systematic review. Basel Univ Hospital, Switzerland; 2014. p. 1–19.
12. Campbell TB, Smeaton LM, Kumarasamy N, Flanigan T, Klingman KL, Firnhaber C, et al. Efficacy and safety of three antiretroviral regimens for initial treatment of HIV-1: a randomized clinical trial in diverse multinational settings. PLoS ONE. 2012;9(8):e1001290.
13. Arribas JR, Pozniak AL, Gallant JE, Dejesus E, Gazzard B, Campo RE, et al. Tenofovir disoproxil fumarate, emtricitabine, and efavirenz compared with zidovudine/lamivudine and efavirenz in treatment-naive patients 144-week analysis. J Acquir Immune Defic Syndr. 2008;47:74–8.
14. Gallant Joel E, DeJesus Edwin, Arribis José R, Pozniak Anton L, Gazzard Brian, Campo Rafael E, Biao Lu, McColl Damian, Chuck Steven, Enejosa Jeffrey, Toole JJ, Tenofovir DF. Emtricitabine, and efavirenz vs. zidovudine, lamivudine, and efavirenz for HIV. N Engl J Med. 2006;354(3):251–60.
15. Babafemi AA. Comparison of clinical and immunological responses to Zidovudine(AZT) and Tenofovir(TDF) containing ARV regimens in patients taking HAART at Roma health service area of Lesetho. J Acquir Immune Defic Syndr. 2010;45(7):8–11.
16. Survey in HIV drug resistance (HIVDR) early warning indicators (EWIs). HIVDR EWI; 2012.
17. Scarsi K, Darin K, Rawizza H, Meloni S, Chang C, Olaitan R, Agbaji O, Gashau W, Murphy R, Kanki P. TDF-3TC-NVP is inferior to AZT-3TC-NVP in a large ART program in Nigeria. J Acquir Immune Defic Syndr. 2010;1:517–21.
18. Muzah BP, Takuva S, Maskew M. Risk factors for discordant immune response among HIV-infected patients initiating antiretroviral therapy: a retrospective cohort study. South Afr J HIV Med. 2012;13(4):168–72.
19. Zhou J, Sirisanthana T, Kiertiburanakul S, Chen YA, Han N, Lim PL. Trends in CD4 counts in HIV-infected patients with HIV viral load monitoring while on combination antiretroviral treatment : results from The TREAT Asia HIV Observational Database. BMC Infect Dis. 2010;10(1):361.
20. Leport C, Grabar S, Lemoing V, Goujard C, Kazatchkine MD, Costagliola D, Weiss L. Clinical outcome of patients with HIV-1 infection according to immunologic and virologic response after. Ann Int Med. 2000;133(6):401–10.
21. Nakanjako D, Kiragga A, Ibrahim F, Castelnuovo B, Kamya MR, Easterbrook PJ. Sub-optimal CD4 reconstitution despite viral suppression in an urban cohort on antiretroviral therapy (ART) in sub-Saharan Africa: frequency and clinical significance. AIDS Res Ther. 2008;5(23):1–9.
22. Casotti JA, Passos LN, Oliveira FJ, Cerutti C. Luciana Neves FJP de O& CCJ. Prevalence of discordant immunologic andvirologic response in patients with AIDS under HAART in specialized care center in Brazil. Rev Inst Med Trop. 2011;53(6):301–7.
23. Kaufmann GR, Furrer H, Ledergerber B, Perrin L, Opravil M, Vernazza P, et al. Characteristics, determinants, and clinical relevance of CD4 T cell recovery to <500 cells/mm3 in HIV type 1—infected individuals receiving potent antiretroviral therapy. Clin Infect Dis. 2005;41(1):361–72.
24. Schechter M, Tuboi SH. Discordant immunological and virological responses to antiretroviral therapy. J Antimicrob Chemother. 2006;58:506–10.
25. Teixeira Â, Valdez H, Mccune JM, Koup RA, Badley AD, Hellerstein MK, et al. Poor CD4 T cell restoration after suppression of HIV-1 replication may reflect lower thymic function. AIDS. 2001;15(14):1749–56.
26. Lubyayi L, Shkedy Z, Mwehire D, Kawuma E, Odiit M, Mukasa B, et al. Evolution of CD4 cell counts over time for HIV/AIDS patients on antiretroviral therapy (ART) in Mildmay. Biometr Biostat Int J. 2015;2(2):00025.
27. Brenchley JM, Schacker TW, Ruff LE, Price DA, Taylor JH, Beilman GJ, et al. CD4+ T Cell Depletion during all stages of HIV disease occurs predominantly in the gastrointestinal tract. J Exp Med. 2004;200(6):749–59.
28. Bastard M, Soulinphumy K, Phimmasone P, Saadani AH, Ciaffi L, Communier A, et al. Women experience a better long-term immune recovery and a better survival on HAART in Lao People' s Democratic Republic. BMC Infect Dis. 2013;13(27):9.
29. Luguterah MA. CD4+ cell counts of HIV-1 patients on antiretroviral therapy(ART) in the Builsa district hospital. Eur Sci J. 2013;9(33):299–309.
30. WHO. Guideline on when to start antiretroviral therapy and on pre-exposure prophylaxis for HIV; 2015.
31. Gallant JE, DeJesus E, Arribas JR, Pozniak AL, Gazzard B, Campo RE, et al. Tenofovir DF, emtricitabine, and efavirenz vs. zidovudine, lamivudine, and efavirenz for HIV. N Engl J Med. 2006;354:251–60.
32. Omeje I, Okwundu CI. Effectiveness and safety of first-line tenofovir + emtricitabine + efavirenz for patients with HIV. Cochrane Libr. 2012;2.

15

Factors associated with loss to follow-up after occupational HIV exposure in Cape Town, South Africa

Nectarios Sophocles Papavarnavas[1], Kathryn Manning[1], Fahd Conrad[2], Milah Govender[3] and Gary Maartens[4*]

Abstract

Background: There is limited data on factors associated with loss to follow-up (LTFU) of health care workers (HCWs) following occupational exposure to HIV, and most studies were conducted in an era when poorly tolerated antiretrovirals like zidovudine were used.

Methods: A retrospective cohort study was conducted of HCWs attending a referral hospital's Occupational Health Clinic in Cape Town, South Africa for post-exposure prophylaxis (PEP) during a period when tenofovir was available. Our primary outcome was LTFU at the 3-month visit. We selected seven variables a priori for our logistic regression model and ensured there were at least 10 outcome events per variable to minimize bias.

Results: Two hundred and ninety-three folders were evaluated for descriptive analysis. LTFU worsened with successive visits: 36% at 6 weeks, 60% at 3 months, and 72% at 6 months. In multivariate analysis at the 3-month visit LTFU was associated with age (adjusted odds ratio (aOR), 0.6 per 10-year increase [95% CI, 0.5–0.9]), HCW category of doctor (aOR 2.7 [95% CI, 1.3–5.5]), and time from exposure to receiving PEP of more than 24 h (aOR 5.9 [95% CI, 1.3–26.9]).

Conclusion: We identified factors associated with LTFU of HCWs after occupational HIV exposure, which could be used to target interventions to improve follow-up.

Keywords: Loss to follow-up, Post exposure prophylaxis, Health care workers, HIV

Background

The World Health Organization (WHO) estimates 3 million occupational human immunodeficiency virus (HIV) percutaneous exposures occur among 35 million healthcare workers (HCWs) annually, with 90% of exposures occurring in resource limited settings [1]. HCWs exposed to potentially infectious material from a source patient with HIV infection, or unknown HIV status, are offered post-exposure prophylaxis (PEP) if this is appropriate, and attend several follow-up visits for PEP toxicity monitoring and exclusion of HIV infection. Although HIV seroconversion following occupational exposure is uncommon, early diagnosis is critical as treatment of early HIV infection reduces the risk of HIV transmission and has direct benefits for the individual by reducing morbidity and mortality [2, 3].

Attendance of HCWs to follow-up visits after occupational exposure to HIV has been highly variable, ranging from 0 to 98.9% in observational studies [4–13]. A literature search yielded three studies that evaluated factors associated with attendance to follow-up [6, 12, 13]. Two studies found that the type of HCW category did not influence attendance to follow-up, [12, 13] but one study found that HCW category did influence attendance to follow-up [6]. One study identified being exposed to an HIV seropositive source increased attendance to follow-up, [13] but another found this had no effect [6]. One study [13] reported that type of exposure and time to reporting did not influence attendance to follow-up; and women had better attendance to follow-up than men [13]. Sample size calculations were not reported in any of these three studies. Furthermore, many of the PEP

*Correspondence: gary.maartens@uct.ac.za
[4] Division of Clinical Pharmacology, Department of Medicine, Groote Schuur Hospital, University of Cape Town, Cape Town 7925, South Africa
Full list of author information is available at the end of the article

regimens used in these studies included poorly tolerated antiretroviral drugs. A recent systematic review reported that tenofovir disoproxil fumarate (TDF) based PEP was better tolerated with higher completion rates than zidovudine based PEP, which used to be the standard of care [14]. The WHO now recommends the use of TDF as part of the backbone for PEP regimens [15].

We aimed to evaluate factors associated with loss to follow-up (LTFU) following occupational exposure to HIV in a referral hospital in Cape Town, South Africa, where the HIV prevalence is 12.7% [16]. We conducted our study in a period when we switched to TDF based PEP, and ensured we had sufficient power to determine variables associated with LTFU.

Methods

Study setting

Data was collected from the Occupational Health Clinic (OHC) of Groote Schuur Hospital, a referral hospital in Cape Town, South Africa. HCWs who have significant occupational HIV exposure are started on PEP if they present within 72 h of the exposure. During the study period the South African national guidelines for PEP recommended the use of TDF and emtricitabine for exposures presenting within 72 h. The policy of adding a 3rd antiretroviral (usually a boosted protease inhibitor) was changed during the study period: initially this was added only for high risk exposures, but subsequently this was added for all exposures. HCWs are counselled about the risks of HIV, the need to document HIV testing for possible compensation, and potential adverse drug reactions to PEP. HIV status of the HCW was determined at baseline using 4th generation Roche COBAS HIV-1/2 Combo automated test with a confirmatory Siemens Integral 4th generation ELISA. PEP was discontinued in HCWs who tested HIV seropositive at baseline. HIV testing was repeated at week 6 (when HCWs were informed that HIV tests may be false negative), and months 3 and 6 after the exposure. Confidentiality of HCWs is protected by keeping all files in the OHC and not in the general records department; only OHC clinic staff are able to access the files.

Study design

We conducted a retrospective cohort review to identify the factors associated with LTFU in HCWs following occupational HIV exposure. The OHC maintains an electronic database of all visits related to HCW occupational HIV exposures. We collected data from the database and additional data from folders between January 2013 and September 2015, with 29 additional folders obtained in 2012.

Outcomes

The primary outcome was the proportion of HCWs LTFU at the 3-month visit, which is the key follow-up date to determine if HIV seroconversion has occurred, in keeping with the WHO guidelines [15]. Secondary outcomes were the proportion of HCWs LTFU at the 6-week and 6-month visits.

Data collection

Data collection at the OHC is collated from an "Occupational Health Clinic Percutaneous Inoculation Report" form. The data are collected each time the HCW presents for follow-up or when contacted by telephone. This form is completed by the occupational health worker on duty, who is either the nurse or doctor. Once 6 months have lapsed since the last visit, the data collected are recorded in an electronic database using Microsoft Excel and HCW folders are then archived in the clinic.

Study population

Inclusion criteria

HCWs were categorized into three groups: 'Doctors', 'Students' and 'Allied Health Professionals' (e.g. nursing, physiotherapists, occupational therapists, administrative clerks, pharmacists, and emergency medical services). HCWs were included if they were exposed to potentially infectious material from patients who are HIV-infected or HIV status unknown and attended the OHC. The following materials were deemed to be potentially infectious: pleural, pericardial, peritoneal, cerebrospinal, synovial fluid, amniotic fluid, and blood [17].

Exclusion criteria

Exclusion criteria were: HCW tested HIV seropositive at baseline; exposed to a HIV seronegative source; those who requested follow-up at a private doctor or who went back to their own training institutions, such as elective students; multiple exposures within the 6-month follow-up period; exposures deemed to be from non-infectious material [17].

Sample size estimation

We selected seven variables a priori for inclusion into our model based on our review of the literature: age at exposure, sex, HCW category, type of exposure, source patient HIV status, dual or triple antiretroviral therapy (ART), and time from exposure to time of receiving PEP. Assuming 25% LTFU at 3 months, [12] we required a sample size of 280 to ensure a minimum of 10 outcome events per variable, which are needed to improve precision and minimize bias in logistic regression models [18].

Statistical analysis

All statistical analysis was performed using Stata (Version 13.1; Stata Corp, College Station, Texas, USA). Descriptive statistics were used to characterize the total sample, and results were expressed as median (interquartile range) for non-normally distributed continuous variables, and frequencies and percentages for categorical variables.

We used separate multivariable logistic regression models for each time point to identify factors associated with LTFU at the 3-month, 6-week, and 6-month follow-up visits. The full model approach was utilized using a priori selected variables in order to ensure decreased risk of selection bias and overfitting [19]. This approach allows multiple epidemiological variables to be assessed independently while controlling effects of other variables [20]. Univariate analysis was used to estimate crude odds ratios (ORs) and 95% confidence intervals (95% CIs), while multivariable logistic regression provided adjusted estimates for odds of LTFU at each time point. Odds ratios were presented with 95% CIs and a level of $P < 0.05$ was considered statically significant.

Results

Two hundred and sixty-four folders were obtained between January 2013 and September 2015, with an additional 29 folders collected according to alphabetical order in 2012. There was incomplete data on 12 HCWs who were included in the descriptive analysis but excluded from the univariate and multivariate analysis as shown in Fig. 1.

The characteristics of the 293 patients from our cohort are shown in Table 1. The dual nucleotide/nucleoside reverse transcriptase inhibitors used in PEP were TDF (97%), zidovudine (2%), and stavudine (1%); all of which were combined with either lamivudine or emtricitabine. The third agent used in 210 HCWs who were given triple ART was lopinavir/ritonavir (82%), atazanavir/ritonavir (13%), raltegravir (4%), and efavirenz (1%).

LTFU at the various visits were: 36% at 6 weeks, 60% at 3 months, and 72% at 6 months (Table 1). The univariate and multivariate analysis of variables associated with LTFU at the 3-month visit are shown in Table 2. In the multivariate analysis, significant risk factors associated with LTFU were: younger age, HCW category of doctor, and time from exposure to receiving PEP of more than 24 h. The multivariate analysis of variables associated with LTFU at the 6-week and 6-month follow-up visits are shown in Table 3. Variables associated with LTFU at the 6-week visit were: male sex and HCW category of doctor. Variables associated with LTFU at the 6-month visit were similar to the 3-month visit: younger age, HCW category of doctor, and time from exposure to receiving PEP of more than 24 h.

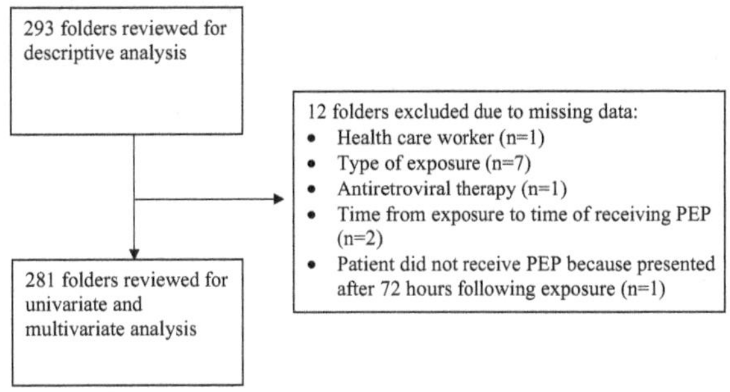

Fig. 1 Flow chart illustrating data set of health care workers chosen for analysis

Table 1 Baseline characteristics and follow-up of 293 health care workers with occupational exposure

Variable	Sample (n)
Age, median (IQR)	28 (24–35)
Sex	
Women	197 (67%)
Men	96 (33%)
Health care worker[a]	
Allied health professional	85 (29%)
Doctor	100 (34%)
Student	107 (37%)
Type of exposure[b]	
Hollow-bore	137 (48%)
Mucocutaneous	86 (30%)
Solid sharp	63 (22%)
Source patient HIV status	
Positive	246 (84%)
Unknown	47 (16%)
Antiretroviral[c,f]	
Dual	81 (28%)
Triple	210 (72%)
Time from exposure to receiving PEP[d] (h)	
<24	268 (92%)
24–48	17 (6%)
48–72	1 (0.3%)
>72	4 (1.4%)
Loss to follow-up[e]	
6 weeks	100 (36%)
3 months	169 (60%)
6 months	203 (72%)

Number with missing data: [a] n = 1, [b] n = 7, [c] n = 1, [d] n = 2, [e] n = 12

[f] One health care worker did not receive PEP because presented too late

LTFU by category of HCW at the various visits is shown in Fig. 2, with doctors having the highest proportion LTFU.

Table 2 Variables associated with loss to follow-up at 3 months

Variables	Unadjusted OR (95% CI)	P value	Adjusted OR (95% CI)	P value
Age (per 10-year increase)	0.7 (0.5–0.9)	0.003	0.6 (0.5–0.9)	0.011
Sex				
Women [a]				
Men	1.4 (0.8–2.4)	0.190	1.4 (0.8–2.5)	0.262
Health care worker				
Allied health professional[a]				
Doctor	2.9 (1.6–5.4)	0.001	2.7 (1.3–5.5)	0.006
Student	2.0 (1.1–3.6)	0.022	1.2 (0.6–2.6)	0.584
Type of exposure				
Hollow-bore[a]				
Mucocutaneous	1.6 (0.9–2.9)	0.095	1.1 (0.6–2.2)	0.707
Solid sharp	1.3 (0.7–2.4)	0.377	1.0 (0.5–1.9)	0.948
Source patient HIV status				
Positive	0.9 (0.4–1.8)	0.742	0.5 (0.2–1.1)	0.074
Unknown[a]				
Antiretroviral				
Dual	1.4 (0.8–2.3)	0.250	1.5 (0.8–2.8)	0.228
Triple[a]				
Time from exposure to receiving PEP (h)				
<24[a]				
>24	3.0 (1.0–9.2)	0.052	5.9 (1.3–26.9)	0.023

[a] Reference category

Discussion

We showed that LFTU of HCWs after occupational HIV exposure was high and increased with successive visits. Younger age, the HCW category doctor, and time from exposure to receiving PEP of more than 24 h were associated with LTFU at the 3-month visit, which was our primary endpoint. Men were more likely to be LTFU at the 6-week visit than women. These findings could be used to target interventions designed to improve follow-up.

Our finding that LTFU increases with successive visits is consistent with other studies [9, 12, 13]. We found that younger age was a significant risk factor for LTFU, which is in keeping with other studies [21–23]. The higher LTFU in younger HCWs may be related to the greater change and instability they experience in their younger years [24]. Men tended to be more likely to be LTFU in our study, which is similar to the findings of Escurdero et al. [13].

The majority (207 out of 281) of HCWs in our study were doctors and students. Doctors and students are often involved in invasive medical procedures, which places them at risk of being exposed to infectious material [7, 9, 11, 25]. Furthermore, students and doctors with less than a year's experience, are prone to occupational exposure because of their inexperience [7, 9, 26]. We found that doctors are more likely to be LTFU than other HCW categories. This could be explained by the ease with which doctors can submit their own blood samples for HIV testing instead of attending the OHC. One study, [27] showed a large proportion of HCWs obtained HIV testing outside of the facility where they worked, which they suggested was due to concern surrounding the confidentiality of HIV testing at the facility. Furthermore, doctors may be making their own assessment of the severity of the exposure and may deem it unnecessary to follow-up [28]. In contrast to our findings of increased LTFU in doctors, Gutierrez et al. [6] showed cleaning personnel were more likely to be LTFU. Two other studies found type of HCW category did not influence attendance to follow-up [12, 13].

Longer time from exposure to receiving PEP at the 3-month visit was positively associated with LTFU. This could be explained by HCWs who present after 24 h having a perceived lower benefit from PEP. However, type of exposure and source patient HIV status, which are associated with risk of HIV acquisition, were not associated with LTFU in our cohort.

Escudero et al. [13] also found that type of exposure was not related to attendance to follow-up. Findings from studies that assessed the effect of the source patient's HIV status on LTFU are contradictory, with one study reporting no effect, [6] while another found positive serological status was associated with improved follow up [13].

Table 3 Variables associated with loss to follow-up at 6 weeks and 6 months

Variables	6-week		6-month	
	Adjusted OR	P value	Adjusted OR	P value
Age (per 10-year increase)	1.0 (0.7–1.3)	0.764	0.6 (0.5–0.9)	0.010
Sex				
Women[a]				
Men	1.8 (1.1–3.2)	0.027	1.8 (0.9–3.4)	0.082
Health care worker				
Allied health professional[a]				
Doctor	2.1 (1.1–4.4)	0.034	2.1 (1.0–4.5)	0.049
Student	1.1 (0.5–2.5)	0.750	1.3 (0.6–2.9)	0.532
Type of exposure				
Hollow-bore[a]				
Mucocutaneous	1.0 (0.5–1.9)	0.988	1.2 (0.6–2.5)	0.659
Solid sharp	1.1 (0.5–2.1)	0.857	1.1 (0.5–2.4)	0.728
Source patient HIV status				
Positive	1.0 (0.5–2.2)	0.952	0.7 (0.3–1.7)	0.489
Unknown[a]				
Antiretroviral				
Dual	1.2 (0.6–2.3)	0.544	0.7 (0.4–1.4)	0.333
Triple[a]				
Time from exposure to receiving PEP (h)				
<24[a]				
>24	1.3 (0.5–3.4)	0.552	7.8 (1.0–61)	0.049

[a] Reference category

There are a number of studies which reported that dual ART regimens are better tolerated than triple regimens [29, 30]. However, many of these studies include ART that are no longer used due to toxicity. Newer studies have shown that completion of PEP is based on the tolerability of ART and not on whether dual or triple therapy are used [31, 32]. This could explain why in our cohort there was no correlation between type of ART used and LTFU.

There were several limitations of our study. First, the retrospective cohort design is inherently prone to bias. However, the data was captured by OHC staff on a standard form and we had very little missing data. Second, although we found that time from exposure to receiving PEP was associated with LTFU, the 95% CIs were wide due to the small sample size of HCWs with delayed presentation. Third, we did not explore associations between years of HCW experience and exposure as we did not have this data. Other researchers have reported an association between years of experience and the incidence of occupational exposures [7, 9, 25]. Finally, Groote Schuur Hospital is a tertiary facility with referrals from other hospitals that fall under the University of Cape Town, so our findings may not be generalizable to other settings such as district hospitals.

We have identified factors associated with LTFU, which could be used to target interventions to decrease LTFU. In one study, [13] contacting HCWs by telephone or mail improved attendance to follow-up from 33 to 54%. Schmid et al. [33] suggested attendance to follow-up could be improved with fewer follow-up visits. The WHO has recently advised the final follow-up visit should be at 3 months rather than 6 months [15]. Furthermore, it has been suggested that the last follow-up visit should be at 6 weeks if laboratory 4th generation HIV ELISA tests are utilized, and 8 weeks if 4th generation rapid HIV tests are utilized [34]. Lastly van der Maaten et al. [9] suggested increasing awareness of the availability of PEP through campaigns.

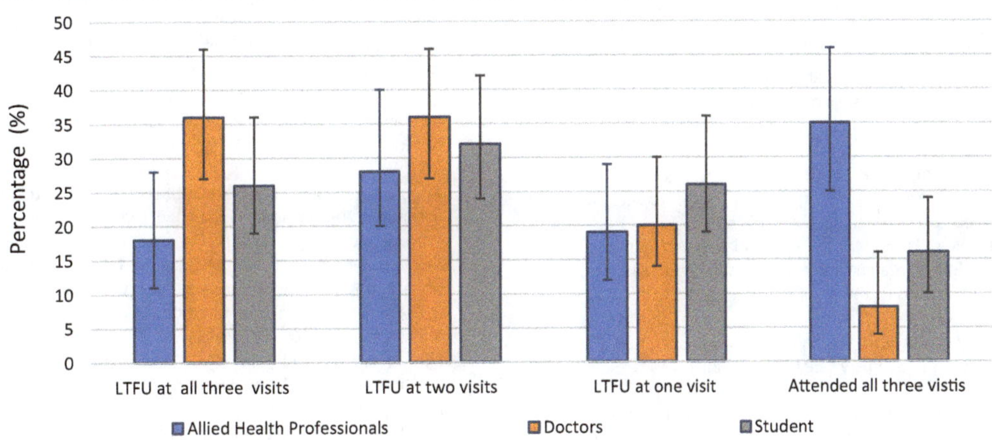

Fig. 2 Percentage loss to follow-up (LTFU) by number of visits of various health care worker categories (visits were scheduled at 6 weeks, 3 months, and 6 months). *Error bars* are shown

Conclusion

We have identified factors associated with LTFU of HCWs after occupational HIV exposure. Future research should identify measures to improve attendance to follow-up, which could be targeted at doctors, younger HCWs, and HCWs with delayed presentation.

Abbreviations

ART: antiretroviral therapy; CIs: confidence intervals; HCW: health care worker; HIV: human immunodeficiency virus; LTFU: loss to follow-up; OHC: Occupational Health Clinic; ORs: odds ratios; PEP: post exposure prophylaxis; TDF: tenofovir disoproxil fumarate; WHO: World Health Organization.

Authors' contributions

NP and GM designed the study, wrote the proposal, analyzed the data, and prepared the manuscript. KM was involved in proposal writing, statistical analysis, and manuscript preparation. NP, FC and MG were involved in data collection. All authors read and approved the final manuscript.

Author details

[1] Department of Medicine, Old Main Building, J-Floor, Groote Schuur Hospital, University of Cape Town, Observatory, Cape Town 7925, South Africa. [2] Trauma and Emergency Unit, Floor E11A, Management Suite, Groote Schuur Hospital, Main Road, Observatory, Cape Town 7925, South Africa. [3] Quality and Safety Unit, Groote Schuur Hospital, Main Road, Observatory, Cape Town 7925, South Africa. [4] Division of Clinical Pharmacology, Department of Medicine, Groote Schuur Hospital, University of Cape Town, Cape Town 7925, South Africa.

Acknowledgements

Not applicable.

Competing interests

The authors declare they have no competing interests.

Funding

GM received partial support from the National Research Foundation of South Africa (Grant Reference Number 85810).

References

1. World Health Organization. The world health report 2002, chapter 4: reducing risks, promoting healthy life. http://www.who.int/whr/2002/chapter4/en/index8.html. Accessed 21 Mar 2016.
2. Cohen MS, Chen YQ, McCauley M, Gamble T, Hosseinipour MC, Kumarasamy N, et al. Prevention of HIV-1 infection with early antiretroviral therapy. N Engl J Med. 2011;365(6):493–505.
3. Lundgren JD, Babiker AG, Gordin F, Emery S, Grund B, Sharma S, et al. Initiation of antiretroviral therapy in early asymptomatic HIV infection. N Engl J Med. 2015;373(9):795–807.
4. de la Tribonniere X, Dufresne MD, Alfandari S, Fontier C, Sobazek A, Valette M, et al. Tolerance, compliance and psychological consequences of post-exposure prophylaxis in health-care workers. Int J STD AIDS. 1998;9(10):591–4.
5. Pungpapong S, Phanuphak P, Pungpapong K, Ruxrungtham K. The risk of occupational HIV exposure among Thai healthcare workers. Southeast Asian J Trop Med Public Health. 1999;30(3):496–503.
6. Gutierrez EB, Heloísa Lopes M, Shikanai Yasuda MA. Accidental exposure to biological material in healthcare workers at a university hospital: evaluation and follow-up of 404 cases. Scand J Infect Dis. 2005;37(4):295–300.
7. Jayanth ST, Kirupakaran H, Brahmadathan KN, Gnanaraj L, Kang G. Needle stick injuries in a tertiary care hospital. Indian J Med Microbiol. 2009;27(1):44–7.
8. Siika AM, Nyandiko WM, Mwangi A, Waxman M, Sidle JE, Kimaiyo SN, et al. The structure and outcomes of a HIV postexposure prophylaxis program in a high HIV prevalence setup in western Kenya. J Acquir Immune Defic Syndr. 2009;51(1):47–53.
9. van der Maaten GC, Nyirenda M, Beadsworth MJ, Chitani A, Allain T, van Oosterhout JJ. Post exposure prophylaxis of HIV transmission after occupational injuries in Queen Elizabeth Central Hospital, Blantyre, Malawi, 2003–2008. Malawi Med J. 2010;22(1):15–9.
10. Olowookere SA, Fatiregun AA. Human immunodeficiency virus postexposure prophylaxis at Ibadan, Nigeria. J Int Assoc Phys AIDS Care (Chic). 2010;9(3):187–90.
11. Onyedum CC, Chukwuka C, Iyoke CA, Omotola OF. HIV postexposure prophylaxis (PEP) in a Nigerian tertiary health institution. J Int Assoc Phys AIDS Care (Chic). 2011;10(3):171–5.
12. Tetteh RA, Nartey ET, Lartey M, Mantel-Teeuwisse AK, Leufkens HG, Nortey PA, et al. Outcomes of a postexposure prophylaxis program at the Korle-Bu Teaching Hospital in Ghana: a retrospective cohort study. J Int Assoc Provid AIDS Care. 2015;14(6):544–52.
13. Escudero DV, Furtado GH, Medeiros EA. Healthcare worker adherence to follow-up after occupational exposure to blood and body fluids at a teaching hospital in Brazil. Ann Occup Hyg. 2015;59(5):566–71.
14. Ford N, Shubber Z, Calmy A, Irvine C, Rapparini C, Ajose O, et al. Choice of antiretroviral drugs for postexposure prophylaxis for adults and adolescents: a systematic review. Clin Infect Dis. 2015;60(Suppl 3):S170–6.
15. World Health Organization. Guidelines on post-exposure prophylaxis for HIV and the use of co-trimoxazole prophylaxis for HIV-related infections among adults, adolescents and children: recommendations for a public health approach: December 2014 supplement to the 2013 consolidated guidelines on the use of antiretroviral drugs for treating and preventing HIV infection. http://www.who.int/hiv/pub/guidelines/arv2013/arvs2013upplement_dec2014/en. Accessed 17 Sep 2016.
16. Statistics South Africa. Statistical release, mid-year population estimates 2016. http://www.statssa.gov.za/?page_id=1854&PPN=P0302. Accessed 22 Jan 2017.
17. Centers for Disease Control. Update: universal precautions for prevention of transmission of human immunodeficiency virus, hepatitis B virus, and other bloodborne pathogens in health-care settings. MMWR Morb Mortal Wkly Rep. 1988;37(24):377.
18. Peduzzi P, Concato J, Kemper E, Holford TR, Feinstein AR. A simulation study of the number of events per variable in logistic regression analysis. J Clin Epidemiol. 1996;49(12):1373–9.
19. Moons KG, Kengne AP, Woodward M, Royston P, Vergouwe Y, Altman DG, et al. Risk prediction models: I. Development, internal validation, and assessing the incremental value of a new (bio)marker. Heart. 2012;98(9):683–90.
20. Stoltzfus JC. Logistic regression: a brief primer. Acad Emerg Med. 2011;18(10):1099–104.
21. Corfield L, Schizas A, Noorani A, Williams A. Non-attendance at the colorectal clinic: a prospective audit. Ann R Coll Surg Engl. 2008;90(5):377–80.
22. Milne V, Kearns R, Harrison A. Patient age, ethnicity and waiting times determine the likelihood of non-attendance at a first specialist rheumatology assessment. Int J Rheum Dis. 2014;17(1):19–25.
23. Hynes L, Byrne M, Dinneen SF, McGuire BE, O'Donnell M, Mc Sharry J. Barriers and facilitators associated with attendance at hospital diabetes clinics among young adults (15–30 years) with type 1 diabetes mellitus: a systematic review. Pediatr Diabetes. 2016;17(7):509–18.
24. Arnett JJ. Emerging adulthood. A theory of development from the late teens through the twenties. Am Psychol. 2000;55(5):469–80.
25. Karstaedt AS, Pantanowitz L. Occupational exposure of interns to blood in an area of high HIV seroprevalence. S Afr Med J. 2001;91(1):57–61.
26. Aggarwal V, Seth A, Chandra J, Gupta R, Kumar P, Dutta AK. Occupational exposure to human immunodeficiency virus in health care providers: a retrospective analysis. Indian J Commun Med. 2012;37(1):45–9.
27. Kassa G, Selenic D, Lahuerta M, Gaolathe T, Liu Y, Letang G, et al. Occupational exposure to bloodborne pathogens among health care workers in Botswana: reporting and utilization of postexposure prophylaxis. Am J Infect Control. 2016;44(8):879–85.
28. Elmiyeh B, Whitaker IS, James MJ, Chahal CA, Galea A, Alshafi K. Needle-stick injuries in the National Health Service: a culture of silence. J R Soc Med. 2004;97(7):326–7.
29. Puro V. Post-exposure prophylaxis for HIV infection. Ital Regist Post Expo Prophyl. Lancet. 2000;355(9214):1556–7.

30. Bassett IV, Freedberg KA, Walensky RP. Two drugs or three? Balancing efficacy, toxicity, and resistance in postexposure prophylaxis for occupational exposure to HIV. Clin Infect Dis. 2004;39(3):395–401.
31. Henderson DK. Management of needlestick injuries: a house officer who has a needlestick. JAMA. 2012;307(1):75–84.
32. McAllister J, Read P, McNulty A, Tong WW, Ingersoll A, Carr A. Raltegravir–emtricitabine–tenofovir as HIV nonoccupational post-exposure prophylaxis in men who have sex with men: safety, tolerability and adherence. HIV Med. 2014;15(1):13–22.
33. Schmid K, Schwager C, Drexler H. Needlestick injuries and other occupational exposures to body fluids amongst employees and medical students of a German university: incidence and follow-up. J Hosp Infect. 2007;65(2):124–30.
34. Gaines H, Albert J, Axelsson M, Berglund T, Gisslen M, Sonnerborg A, et al. Six-week follow-up after HIV-1 exposure: a position statement from the Public Health Agency of Sweden and the Swedish Reference Group for Antiviral Therapy. Infect Dis (Lond). 2016;48(2):93–8.

16

HIV-1 drug-resistant mutations and related risk factors among HIV-1-positive individuals experiencing treatment failure in Hebei Province, China

Xinli Lu, Hongru Zhao, Yuqi Zhang, Wei Wang, Cuiying Zhao, Yan Li, Lin Ma, Ze Cui* and Suliang Chen*

Abstract

Background: To understand HIV-1 drug resistance in 11 prefectures of Hebei Province, China, we implemented a cross-sectional HIV-1 molecular epidemiological survey.

Methods: Blood samples were collected from 122 newly diagnosed drug-naïve HIV-1-positive individuals and 229 antiretroviral therapy (ART)-failure individuals from 11 prefectures in Hebei Province, China. Patient demographic data were obtained via face-to-face interviews using a standardized questionnaire when blood samples were collected. Genotyping of HIV-1 drug resistance (DR) was implemented using an in-house assay.

Results: In this study, the overall prevalence of HIV-1 DR was 35.5%. The prevalence of HIV-1 DR in participants experiencing treatment failure and ART-naïve participants was 51.9 and 5.9%, respectively. Mutations in protease inhibitors, nucleoside reverse transcriptase inhibitors (NRTIs), and non-NRTI (NNRTIs), as well as dual and multiple mutations were extensively seen in participants experiencing treatment failure. The proportions of NNRTI mutations ($\chi^2 = 9.689$, $p = 0.002$) and dual mutations in NRTIs and NNRTIs ($\chi^2 = 39.958$, $p < 0.001$) in participants experiencing treatment failure were significantly higher than those in ART-naïve participants. The distributions of M184V/I and M41L mutations differed significantly among three main HIV-1 genotypes identified. Viral load, symptoms in the past 3 months, CD4 counts, transmission route, and the duration of ART were found to be associated with HIV-1 DR.

Conclusions: Our results suggest that new prevention and control strategies should be formulated according to the epidemic characteristics of HIV-1-resistant strains in Hebei Province, where antiretroviral drugs are widely used.

Keywords: HIV-1, Mutation, Phylogeny, Drug resistance, China

Background

Human immunodeficiency virus (HIV) epidemics can be traced back to the 1920s in Kinshasa, the capital of the Democratic Republic of the Congo [1]. Among the first HIV-1 individuals in China were four hemophiliac patients in 1985 [2]. Some early cases of HIV infection were linked to imported blood products [3]. In 1989, an HIV outbreak occurred among injection drug users (IDUs) in Yunnan Province, China [4]. Since then, individuals with HIV or AIDS have been successively identified in provinces of mainland China [5–7], and an estimated 740,000 individuals in China are currently thought to be infected with HIV/AIDS [8]. Over the past 30 years, the most common route of transmission of HIV-1 infection in China has shifted from blood products to sexual contact [9], and the genetic diversity has rapidly increased because of HIV-1 gene hypermutability [10].

Hebei Province, China comprises 11 prefectures, surrounds the cities of Beijing and Tianjin, and neighbors Henan Province to the south. In 2014, it was inhabited by more than 73 million people [11]. The first case of HIV

*Correspondence: hbcdc888@163.com; hebeicdc2013@sina.com
Hebei Provincial Center for Disease Control and Prevention, 97 Huaian East Road, Yuhua District, Shijiazhuang 050021, China

infection in Hebei Province was detected in Shijiazhuang in 1989 [12]. In the 1990s, local HIV outbreaks occurred in Xingtai and Langfang, and many individuals infected with HIV-1 through blood transmission were identified [13, 14]. More recently, HIV infection has been detected in all 172 counties of Hebei Province, and sexual exposure, especially in men-who-have-sex-with-men population, has gradually replaced blood transmission as the most common transmission route [15]. By the end of 2014, a total of 5315 HIV/AIDS cases had been reported, including 3050 HIV-1-positive individuals and 2265 AIDS patients. The HIV/AIDS infection rate in Hebei was estimated to be 0.011%, which is significantly lower than the 0.059% reported for the whole of China and the 0.8% worldwide [16], representing a low HIV/AIDS epidemic.

Before 2002, it was not practical to use antiretroviral therapy (ART) in China due to a lack of drug access, and HIV-1 drug-resistant strains were rare [17]. Since 2003, the central government has provided free ART to HIV/AIDS patients, and first-line regimens are commonly used in Hebei. By the end of October 2014, 167 of 172 counties in Hebei had carried out the "four free, one care" policy [18], and a total of 2893 HIV/AIDS patients received highly active ART. This represented a large increase in ART coverage, from 9.9% in 2003 to 96.6% in 2014, which coincided with a significant decrease in HIV/AIDS patient mortality from 11.6 to 2.6% [16]. However, with the increase in antiretroviral drug use, the frequency of adaptive mutations in HIV-1 has also increased, generating drug-resistant strains [19]. This has created severe clinical and epidemiological problems [20].

The objective of the present study was to perform a detailed analysis of the prevalence and genetic mechanisms of HIV-1 drug resistance (DR) among participants experiencing treatment failure in Hebei, and to evaluate the underlying influencing factors associated with the development of HIV-1 drug-resistant strains.

Methods

Participants

Between October 2012 and April 2013, 351 whole blood samples were collected from 122 newly diagnosed drug-naïve HIV-1-positive individuals confirmed in 2012 and 229 participants experiencing treatment failure in 11 prefectures of Hebei (Fig. 1). We selected participants experiencing treatment failure according to the following criteria: (1) viral load (VL) $\geq$1000 copies/ml, (2) duration of therapy >6 months, (3) CD4 count lower than the level before ART, and (4) genotyping had not been previously performed. The local centers for disease control and prevention were responsible for the delivery of antiretroviral drugs and sample collection. Controls were 122 newly diagnosed HIV-1-positive individuals who had not received treatment. The study design was cross-sectional.

Demographic data were collected via face-to-face interviews when blood samples were collected, using a standardized questionnaire. A total of 50 μl of whole blood was used to measure the CD4 count using a FACSCount reagent kit (Becton–Dickinson, Franklin Lakes, NJ, USA). Plasma samples were obtained by centrifuging whole blood, and used to detect VL with the COBAS TaqMan 48 analyzer (Roche, Basel, Switzerland).

HIV-1 genotyping and drug resistance

HIV-1 RNA was extracted from 500 μl of blood plasma using the High Pure Viral RNA kit (Qiagen, Valencia, CA, USA). The partial HIV-1 *pol* gene fragment (HXB2:2147–3462) was amplified for HIV-1 genotyping and DR using the One-Step reverse transcription PCR kits (TaKaRa, Dalian, China) with primers MAW26 (5′-TTGGAAATGTGGAAAGGAAGGAC-3′) and RT21 (5′-CTGTATTTCTGCTATTAAGTCTTTTGATGGG-3′) in a 25 μl reaction volume. Cycling conditions were as follows: HIV-1 RNA denaturation at 65 °C for 30 s, addition of the reaction mixtures at 4 °C, incubation at 50 °C for 30 min, 94 °C for 2 min, then 35 cycles of 94 °C for 30 s, 55 °C for 30 s, and 72 °C for 2 min 30 s.

Nested *pol* PCR was implemented using 2× Taq PCR MasterMix (TaKaRa) with primers PRO-1 (5′-CAGAGCCAACAGCCCCACCA-3′) and RT20 (5′-CTGCCAGTTCTAGCTCTGCTTC-3′) in a 50 μl reaction volume. Cycling conditions were: 94 °C for 5 min, then 35 cycles of 94 °C for 30 s, 63 °C for 30 s, and 72 °C for 2 min 30 s. Positive PCR products were analyzed using 1% agarose gel electrophoresis, and sequenced by Biomed (Beijing, China).

All original *pol* sequence fragments were assembled, edited, and aligned as previously described [21], and used to construct an HIV-1 *pol* phylogenetic tree using the neighbor-joining method with 1000 bootstrap replicates, based on the Kimura 2-parameter Model (MEGA5.0). The online jpHMM Program (http://jphmm.gobics.de/submission_hiv.html) and RIP 3.0 (http://www.hiv.lanl.gov/content/sequence/RIP/RIP.html) were used to further analyze the possible intertype mosaicism of unique recombinant forms (URFs). Finally, HIV-1 *pol* sequences were submitted to the HIV DR database (http://hivdb.stanford.edu/) to analyze HIV-1 DR mutations.

Statistical analysis

Statistical analyses were implemented using SPSS software version 21.0 (SPSS Inc., Chicago, IL, USA). Means or frequencies of demographic data (such as age, CD4 counts, and VL) were calculated. Categorical variables were analyzed using the Chi square test. When more

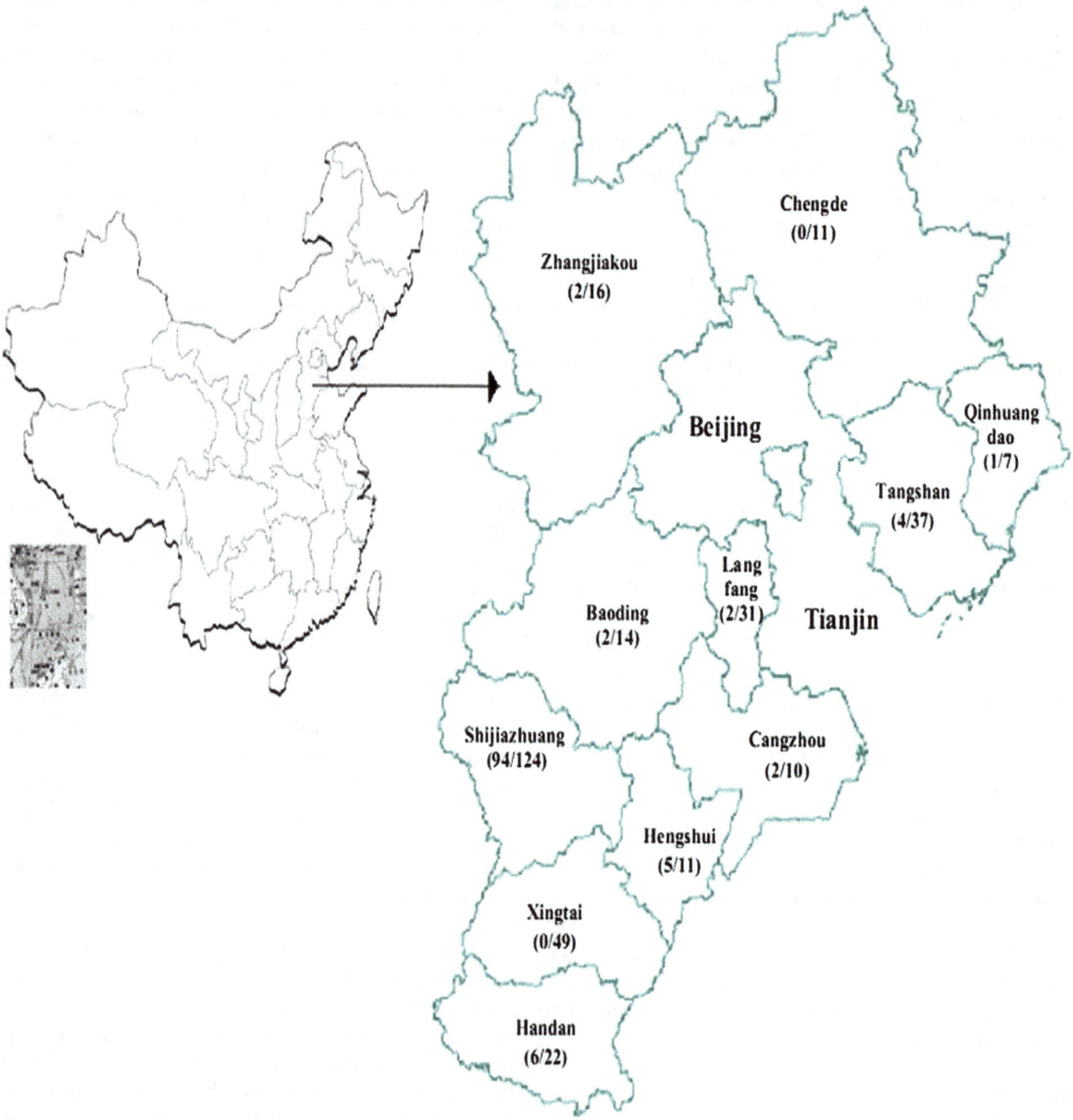

Fig. 1 Geographical distribution of participants collected from 11 prefectures in this study. The *numbers* to the *left* and *right* of the "/" denote the participants genotyped and the total participants, respectively. This figure is adapted from open access map: http://wenku.baidu.com/link?url=u_b5Oe5nC1s_dm7nivfQ1VxQcwj9lDMPsoWfHZHGUNJM5lUiv7JnZo1yAWlVx9KblTt2u5tReJ7qPOtnoxeJw3Ql1VUewd1m9N56eJSxuHm and figure 1 in Ref. [14] with Microsoft PowerPoint 2016

than 20% of cells had an expected count of <5, Fisher's exact test was used. Multivariable logistic regression analysis was used to identify risk factors associated with DR. A stepwise approach was used for variable selection in the multivariate regression model. All tests were two-sided, and a statistical result was considered significant when $p < 0.05$.

Results

Demographic characteristics of participants

Table 1 shows the demographic characteristics of participants. The sex ratio of males to females was 1:0.27. The median values of age, CD4 counts, and VL were 37.0 (range 6–71) years, 220 (range 2–1149) cells/μl, and 4.2 (range 3–6.8) log RNA copies/ml, respectively. Sexual

Table 1 Demographic characteristics of participants in this study

Characteristic	Individuals (%)		
	ART-naïve (n = 122)	ART-failure (n = 229)	Cumulative (n = 351)
Age, median years (IQR)	31.5 (17–71)	39.5 (6–71)	37.0 (6–71)
Gender			
Male	116 (95.1)	160 (69.9)	276 (78.6)
Female	6 (4.9)	69 (30.1)	75 (21.4)
Median CD4+ T cell count, cells/μL (IQR)	432.50 (9–1149)	188 (2–556)	220 (2–1149)
Median VL, RNA (lgcopies/ml) (IQR)	4.6 (3.2–6.8)	4.2 (3.0–6.5)	4.22 (3.0–6.8)
Ethnicity			
Han	121 (99.2)	223 (97.4)	344 (98.0)
Hui	1 (0.8)	2 (0.9)	3 (0.9)
Yi	0 (0.0)	2 (0.9)	2 (0.7)
Uyghur	0 (0.0)	1 (0.4)	1 (0.4)
Man	0 (0.0)	1 (0.4)	1 (0.4)
Transmission routes			
Heterosexual	23 (1.9)	78 (34.1)	101 (28.8)
Homosexual	99 (98.1)	67 (29.3)	166 (47.3)
MTCT	0 (0.0)	19 (8.3)	19 (5.4)
Blood recipient	0 (0.0)	34 (14.9)	34 (9.7)
Paid blood donor	0 (0.0)	29 (12.7)	29 (8.3)
IDU	0 (0.0)	2 (0.9)	2 (0.6)

IQR interquartile range, *IDU* intravenous drug injection, *MTCT* mother-to-child transmission

contact was the most common transmission route in the study participants and accounted for 76.1% of transmission (267/351), including heterosexual contact (28.8%, 101/351) and homosexual contact (47.3%, 166/351), followed by blood (17.9%, 63/351), mother-to-child transmission (MTCT, 5.4%), and IDU (0.6%). In terms of ethnicity, 98.0% (344/351) of participants were Chinese Han, and the remaining seven participants were Hui (0.9%, 3/351), Yi (0.7%, 2/351), Man (0.4%, 2/351), and Uyghur (0.4%, 1/351).

Among all therapy regimens in 214 participants experiencing treatment failure (Fig. 2), the 3TC + AZT + NVP regimen was the most frequent, accounting for 59.3%. The percentage of participants treated with 3TC + D4T + NVP, 3TC + TDF + LPV/r, 3TC + AZT + EFV, 3TC + TDF + EFV, 3TC + D4T + EFV, and 3TC + TDF + NVP was 11.2, 10.3, 9.3, 4.2, 2.8 and 2.8%, respectively.

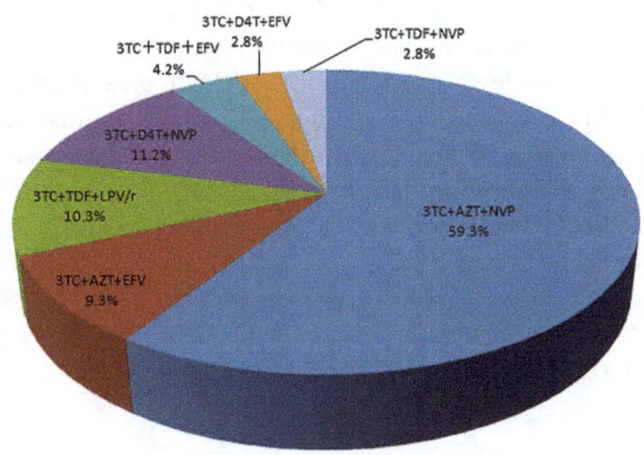

Fig. 2 The therapy regimens of ART participants in this study. *ATV/r* atazanavir/r, *NFV/r* nelfinavir plus ritonavir, *LPV/r* lopinavir plus ritonavir, *3TC* lamivudine, *ABC* abacavir, *AZT* zidovudine, *D4T* stavudine, *DDI* didanosine, *FTC* emtricitabine, *TDF* tenofovir, *EFV* efavirenz, *ETR* etravirine, *NVP* nevirapine

HIV-1 genotype analysis

Viral RNA isolated from 332 out of 351 participants was amplified and sequenced successfully, including 118 from ART-naïve controls (96.7%, 118/122) and 214 from participants experiencing treatment failure (93.4%, 214/229), achieving a positive sequence rate of 94.6% (332/351). As shown in Additional file 1: Table S1 and Figures S1, S2, seven HIV-1 genotypes were identified successfully by the phylogenetic tree analyses of HIV-1 *pol* sequences. HIV-1 subtype B (41.9%, 139/332) was identified as the most frequent genotype, followed by circulating recombinant form (CRF)01_AE (40.1%, 133/332), CRF07_BC (13.6%, 45/332), CRF08_BC (2.1%, 7/332), subtype C (1.2%, 4/332), URFs (0.6%, 2/332), and CRF02_AG (0.6%, 2/332). We identified two URF recombination patterns: CRF01_AE/BC and CRF01_AE/B (Additional file 1: Figure S3). This is the first known identification of CRF02_AG in Hebei.

The prevalent genotypes in the present work were identical to those detected in our previous study [21], with the exception of CRF02_AG. Furthermore, the HIV-1 genotype distribution in 11 prefectures (Additional file 1: Figure S4) was associated with changes of transmission routes (Additional file 1: Table S2), consistent with the geographical distribution characteristics of HIV-1 genotypes reported previously [21]. This suggests that the geographical difference of transmission routes plays a critical role in this distribution.

HIV-1 drug-resistant mutations in ART-naïve controls

In ART-naïve controls, the prevalence of HIV-1 DR was 5.9% (7/118), including protease inhibitor (PI) mutations (2.5%, 3/118), nucleoside reverse transcriptase inhibitor (NRTI) mutations (1.7%, 2/118), non-NRTI (NNRTI) mutations (0.8%, 1/118), and dual mutations in NRTIs and NNRTIs (0.8%, 1/118). One participant infected through heterosexual contact harbored dual mutations in NRTIs (T69N, M184V, and T215Y) and NNRTIs (K103N and M230L), and presented with high-level resistance to lamivudine (3TC) and emtricitabine (FTC) with M184V, intermediate-level resistance to zidovudine (AZT) and stavudine (D4T) with T215Y, and intermediate or high-level resistance to all NNRTIs with K103N and M230L. Two participants harboring M46L and one with M46 V showed low-level resistance to nelfinavir plus ritonavir (NFV/r). Two participants infected through homosexual contact and one participant infected through heterosexual contact harbored NRTI mutations D67N and M184V, and NNRTI mutation K103N. The proportions of resistance to NFV/r, 3TC, FTC, AZT, D4T, EFV, ETR, NVP, and RPV were 2.5% (3/118), 1.7% (2/118), 1.7% (2/118), 1.7% (2/118), 1.7% (2/118), 1.7% (2/118), 0.8% (1/118), 1.7% (2/118), and 0.8% (1/118), respectively.

HIV-1 drug-resistant mutations in participants experiencing treatment failure

Compared with the low prevalence of HIV-1 DR in ART-naïve controls, 51.9% (111/214) of participants experiencing treatment failure showed resistance to at least one antiviral drug. Mutations in PIs, NRTIs, and NNRTIs, and dual and multiple mutations were common in participants experiencing treatment failure. As shown in Table 2, the mutation classes showed significant differences in frequency between ART-naïve participants and participants experiencing treatment failure ($p = 0.014$). The proportions of NNRTIs mutations ($\chi^2 = 9.689$, $p = 0.002$) and dual mutations in NRTIs and NNRTIs ($\chi^2 = 39.958$, $p < 0.001$) in participants experiencing treatment failure were significantly higher than those in ART-naïve participants. Furthermore, dual mutations in NRTIs and NNRTIs were the most common mutation class in participants experiencing treatment failure, accounting for 29.4% (63/214), followed by NNRTI mutations (10.7%, 23/214).

Table 3 lists all mutations that cause different levels of DR to antiviral drugs. In PI coding regions, mutations T74S and M46L were found to cause low-level DR to NFV/r, achieving a resistance rate of 1.8% (4/214). In NRTI coding regions, M184V/I was the most frequent mutation, accounting for 30.4% (65/214), followed by K70R (8.4%, 18/214), D67N (5.6%, 12/214), M41L (5.4%, 11/214), and T215Y (5.4%, 11/214). The percentages of resistance to 3TC, ABC, FTC, AZT, D4T, DDI, and TDF were 30.4% (65/214), 28.5% (61/214), 30.4% (65/214), 22.9% (49/214), 24.3% (52/214), 12.1% (26/214), and 9.8% (21/214), respectively. In NNRTI coding regions, K103 N was the most frequent mutation, accounting for 15.9% (34/214), followed by Y181C (11.7%, 25/214), G190A (5.1%, 11/214), and G190S (3.7%, 8/214). The percentages of resistance to EFV, ETR, NVP, and RPV were 37.4% (80/214), 21.5% (46/214), 37.4% (80/214), and 23.8%

Table 2 Drug resistance in ART-Naïve participants and participants experiencing treatment failure according to drug classes

Drug classes	ART-naïve (%)	ART-failure (%)	χ^2	p
PIs	3 (2.5)	6 (2.8)	0.000	1.000
NRTIs	2 (1.7)	9 (4.2)	0.816	0.366
NNRTIs	1 (0.8)	23 (10.7)	9.689	0.002
Dual resistance to PIs and NRTIs	0 (0.00)	1 (0.5)	F	1.000
Dual resistance to PIs and NNRTIs	0 (0.00)	6 (2.8)	F	0.093
Dual resistance to NRTIs and NNRTIs	1 (0.8)	63 (29.4)	39.958	<0.001
Multiple resistance to PIs, NRTIs and NNRTIs	0 (0.00)	3 (1.4)	F	0.555
Susceptibility	101 (85.6)	103 (48.1)	45.059	<0.001

PIs protease inhibitors, *NRTIs* nucleoside reverse transcriptase inhibitors, *NNRTIs* non-nucleoside reverse transcriptase inhibitors, the mutation classes were exclusive of each other in the study population, *F* Fisher's exact test

Table 3 Prevalence of drug-resistance mutations among ART-naïve participants (n = 118) and participants experiencing treatment failure (n = 214) in Hebei between 2012 and 2013

Mutations	Frequency (%)		HIV-1 drug resistance level							
	Naïve (n = 118)	ART-failure (n = 214)	NFV/r	*ATV/r*	*DRV/r*	FPV/r	IDV/r	*LPV/r*	SQV/r	TPV/r
Protease inhibitors										
L10V	0.85	1.40	S	S	S	S	S	S	S	S
L10I	4.24	0.47	S	S	S	S	S	S	S	S
T74S	0.00	0.93	L	S	S	S	S	S	S	S
A71V/T	11.86	2.80	S	S	S	S	S	S	S	S
K20I	0.85	0.93	P	S	S	S	S	S	S	S
L33I	0.85	1.40	S	S	S	S	S	S	S	S
M46L	1.69	0.93	L	P	S	P	P	P	S	S
M46V	0.85	0.00	L	P	S	P	P	S	S	S
G48W	0.85	0.00	S	S	S	S	S	S	S	S
V11I	0.85	0.00	S	S	S	S	S	S	S	S
K43T	0.85	0.00	S	S	S	S	S	S	S	P
			3TC	*ABC*	*AZT*	*D4T*	*DDI*	*FTC*	*TDF*	
Nucleoside reverse transcriptase inhibitors										
M184V	1.69	27.57	H	L	S	S	P	H	S	
Q151M	0.00	0.47	L	H	H	H	H	L	L	
F116Y	0.00	0.47	S	P	P	P	P	S	S	
M184I	0.00	1.87	H	P	S	S	S	H	S	
T69N	0.85	2.34	S	S	S	S	P	S	S	
T69i	0.00	0.47	M	M	M	M	M	M	M	
A62V	0.00	1.87	S	S	S	S	S	S	S	
M41L	0.00	5.14	S	P	L	L	P	S	P	
D67S	0.00	0.47	S	S	P	P	S	S	S	
V75I	0.85	0.47	S	S	S	P	P	S	S	
V75L	0.00	2.80	S	S	S	P	P	S	S	
T215I	0.00	0.93	S	P	L	L	P	S	S	
T215Y	0.85	5.14	S	L	M	M	L	S	L	
K70T	0.00	0.47	P	P	S	P	P	P	P	
K70E	0.00	0.47	P	L	S	S	L	P	L	
K70R	0.00	8.41	S	P	M	L	P	S	P	
V75M	0.00	0.93	S	S	P	M	L	S	S	
L210W	0.00	0.93	S	P	L	L	P	S	P	
D67N	0.85	5.61	S	S	L	L	S	S	S	
D67G	0.00	0.47	S	S	P	P	S	S	S	
T215F	0.00	2.34	S	L	M	M	L	S	L	
T215N	0.00	0.47	S	P	L	L	P	S	S	
K219E	0.00	3.27	S	S	P	P	S	S	S	
K219Q	0.00	2.34	S	S	P	P	S	S	S	
L74I	0.00	1.40	S	L	S	S	H	S	S	
L74V	0.00	0.93	S	M	S	S	H	S	S	
K65R	0.00	1.87	M	M	S	M	H	M	H	

Table 3 continued

			EFV	*ETR*	*NVP*	RPV
Non-nucleoside reverse transcriptase inhibitors						
A98G	0.00	1.40	P	P	M	L
H221Y	0.00	6.54	P	P	P	P
K101E	0.00	3.27	L	L	M	M
K103N	1.69	15.89	H	S	H	S
K103S	0.00	0.47	M	S	H	S
K103T	0.00	0.47	L	S	H	S
V106A	0.00	0.93	M	P	H	S
V106M	0.00	1.40	H	S	H	S
V106I	7.63	8.88	S	S	S	S
V108I	0.00	3.74	P	S	L	S
E138Q	0.00	2.34	P	P	P	L
E138G	0.85	0.0	P	P	P	L
V179E	4.24	2.80	P	P	P	P
V179D	0.85	0.47	P	P	P	P
Y181C	0.00	11.68	M	M	H	M
Y188L	0.00	1.40	H	L	H	H
Y188C	0.00	0.47	M	S	H	S
Y188W	0.00	0.47	S	S	S	S
G190S	0.00	3.74	H	L	H	L
G190A	0.00	5.14	M	L	H	L
G190R	0.00	0.47	S	S	S	S
P225H	0.00	1.87	M	S	L	S
F227L	0.00	0.93	L	S	M	S
M230L	0.85	0.47	M	M	H	M
M230I	0.00	0.93	L	L	M	M
K238T	0.00	2.34	L	S	M	S
V90I	0.00	5.14	S	S	S	S
E138A	0.00	0.93	S	P	S	L
E138K	0.00	0.47	P	P	P	M

Some (italics) of drugs listed in the Stanford HIV DR database are used in China

S susceptible, *P* potential low-level resistance, *L* low-level resistance, *M* intermediate resistance, *H* high-level resistance, *ATV/r* atazanavir/r, *NFV/r* nelfinavir plus ritonavir, *LPV/r* lopinavir plus ritonavir, *3TC* lamivudine, *ABC* abacavir, *AZT* zidovudine, *D4T* stavudine, *DDI* didanosine, *FTC* emtricitabine, *TDF* tenofovir, *EFV* efavirenz, *ETR* etravirine, *NVP* nevirapine

(51/214), respectively. The overall prevalence of HIV-1 DR was 35.5% (118/332).

Additionally, 5.1% (11/214) of participants experiencing treatment failure harbored thymidine analogue mutations (TAMs; Table 4), accounting for 9.9% (11/111) of participants identified as DR. As shown in Table 4, the mean therapeutic duration of the 11 participants with TAMs was 42.8 (range 10–113) months, the mean VL was 4.3 (range 3.2–5.3) log copies/ml, and the mean CD4 count was 108.9 (range 7–187) cells/μl. Sexual transmission accounted for 90.9% (10/11) of cases, with heterosexual transmission accounting for 81.8% (9/11). TAMs were distributed in five CRF01_AE strains and six subtype B strains.

The distribution of HIV-1 DR mutations among different genotypes

As shown in Table 5, there was no significant difference in the overall distribution of 15 main mutations in the RT coding region in CRF01_AE, subtype B, and CRF07_BC ($p > 0.05$). These 15 mutations largely resided in CRF01_AE and subtype B. Mutations T74S and M46L in the PI coding region were found in CRF01_AE. However, the distributions of M184 V/I ($\chi^2 = 7.289$, $p < 0.05$)

Table 4 Baseline demographic characteristics of 11 participants with TAMs mutation

Sample code	Gender	Age	VL	CD4 counts	Occupation	WB date	ART regimen	Duration of ART	Transmission route	Genotype	NRTIs	NNRTIs
HB0041	Male	29	17,600	181	Worker	2010-7-9	3TC + d4T + NVP	26	Heterosexual	CRF01_AE	D67N, K70R, M184V, K219Q	A98G, K101E, G190A
HB0455	Male	39	51,200	85	Farmer	2010-1-22	3TC + AZT + EFV	34	Heterosexual	B	M41L, D67N, K70R, L74I, M184V, T215F, K219Q	K101E, V106I, V179E, G190S
HB0549	Female	43	50,800	170	Farmer	2011-4-8	3TC + AZT + NVP	20	Heterosexual	CRF01_AE	D67N, T69N, K70R, M184V, T215F, K219E	K103N, Y181C
HB0595	Male	41	195,000	7	Liberal professions	2009-1-9	3TC + AZT + NVP	15	Homosexual	CRF01_AE	D67N, K70R, M184V, T215F, K219E	Y188L
HB0711	Male	31	47,800	175	Jobless	2009-7-20	3TC + AZT + NVP	27	Heterosexual	CRF01_AE	D67N, T69N, K70R, V75M, M184V, T215I, K219Q	Y181C, H221Y
HB0829	Male	49	6360	187	Jobless	2007-5-31	3TC + AZT + NVP	32	Heterosexual	B	D67N, K70R, M184V, K219Q	G190A
HB0869	Male	36	26,500	15	Farmer	2010-6-28	3TC + AZT + NVP	33	Heterosexual	CRF01_AE	D67N, K70R, M184V, K219E	V90I, Y188W, F227L
HB1157	Male	50	10,600	184	Farmer	2003-7-16	3TC + AZT + NVP	10	Heterosexual	B	D67N, K70R, M184V, K219E	V90I, K103N, K238T
HB1160	Female	45	7030	9	Farmer	2003-4-1	3TC + TDF + LPV	133	Heterosexual	B	D67N, K70R, M184V, K219E	V90I, K103N, K238T
HB1161	Female	15	1580	136	Farmer	2004-2-19	3TC + AZT + NVP	80	Mother-to-child	B	D67N, K70R, M184V, K219E	V90I, K103N, K238T
HB1225	Female	71	46,400	59	Farmer	2001-12-14	3TC + d4T + NVP	84	Heterosexual	B	M41L, L74V, M184V, L210W, T215Y	K103N, V108I, Y181C, H221Y

WB western blot, *VL* viral load, *NRTIs* nucleoside reverse transcriptase inhibitors, *NNRTIs* non-nucleoside reverse transcriptase inhibitors

Table 5 The distribution of HIV-1 DR mutations in RTs coding region among different genotypes

Genotypes	Participants	Reverse transcriptase inhibitor mutations														
		M184V/I	M41L	T215Y/F/I/N	K70R	D67N	K65R	T69i	L74I/V	K103N/S/T	Y181C	V106A/M	Y188L/C	G190A/S	M230L/I	P225H
CRF01_AE	133	26	2	8	7	7	0	1	0	15	12	0	2	7	1	1
B	139	35	9	12	11	6	3	0	5	23	14	4	3	12	3	3
07-BC	45	3	0	0	0	0	0	0	0	2	0	1	0	0	0	0
C	4	1	0	0	0	0	1	0	0	0	1	0	0	0	0	0
URFs	2	0	0	0	0	0	0	0	0	0	1	0	0	0	0	0
CRF02-AG	2	0	0	0	0	0	0	0	0	0	0	0	0	0	0	0
08-BC	7	0	0	0	0	0	0	0	0	0	0	0	0	1	0	0
χ^2 test		7.289	F	4.320	4.049	2.398	F	F	6.505	4.889	4.785	F	F	4.714	F	F
P		0.026	0.048	0.115	0.132	0.302	0.367	0.562	0.065	0.087	0.091	0.129	1.000	0.095	0.796	0.796

F Fisher's exact test, *RTs* reverse transcriptase inhibitors

and M41L ($p < 0.05$) were significantly different among CRF01_AE, subtype B, and CRF07_BC, respectively.

Factors associated with HIV-1 drug resistance

As listed in Table 6, 14 potential risk factors were considered in the analysis of univariate logistic regression. Of these factors, VL, symptoms in the last 3 months, CD4 count, transmission route, duration of ART, and genotype were clearly related to HIV-1 DR ($p < 0.05$). To identify risk factors associated with HIV-1 DR, multivariable logistic regression analysis was implemented using stepwise selection. Five factors were found to be significantly associated with the progress of HIV-1 DR in participants experiencing treatment failure: transmission route (compared with sexual contact, blood: odds ratio (OR) 0.1, 95% confidence interval (CI) 0.03–0.24; mother-to-child: OR 1.2, 95% CI 0.3–4.3); CD4 count (>200 vs. ≤200 cells/μl: OR 0.2; 95% CI 0.1–0.5; $p < 0.001$); VL (compared with ≤5000 log copies/ml, 5001–9999: OR 1.7, 95% CI 0.6–5.0; ≥10,000: OR 4.9, 95% CI 2.0–12.0); duration of ART (compared with 0–12 months, 13–54 months: OR 1.7, 95% CI 0.8–3.8; ≥55 months: OR 3.8, 95% CI 1.4–10.1); and symptoms in the last 3 months (yes vs. no: OR 2.4; 95% CI 1.0–5.6; $p < 0.05$).

Discussion

Following the phylogenetic analysis of HIV-1 *pol* sequences in the present study, we successfully identified two HIV-1 subtypes, four CRFs, and two URFs in 11 prefectures of Hebei Province, China. The HIV-1 genotype distribution was shown to be closely related to the route of transmission. Moreover, the prevalence of HIV-1 genotypes in this study differs significantly from that in Sichuan, Yunnan, and Xinjiang provinces, where IDUs are the common high risk group [10], suggesting that the prevalence of HIV-1 genotypes in different provinces of China reflects the geographical difference of HIV-1 high-risk populations.

Traditionally, HIV-1 subtype B was dominant in contaminated blood in the cities of Langfang and Xingtai [14, 22], and our work provides new evidence to support this. CRF01_AE strains in China were identified in IDUs for the first time in Yunnan [4]. Since the first CRF07_BC epidemic in 2002 [23], the prevalence of CRF07_BC has increased significantly, from 4.5% in 2002 to 13.6% in this study, and it has been identified in all transmission routes. From 1989 to 2013, a shift in transmission routes became apparent [15, 21], from which subtype B, CRF01_AE, and CRF07_BC spread out through sexual contact [21, 24] with an increasing diversity of high-risk behaviors and the growing size of the floating population. Currently, sexual transmission is the most common route of transmission in Hebei, accounting for 98.1% of HIV-1-positive cases in 2013 [21]. Subtype B, CRF01_AE, and CRF07_BC are the three main genotypes, and mainly circulate through sexual contact. The co-circulation of these three genotypes has resulted in the occurrence and spread of novel recombinant strains, as evidenced by the detection of recombinant strains CRF01_AE/B and CRF01_AE/BC in this study. To our knowledge, this is the first report of HIV-1 subtype specialty and DR mutations in Hebei.

In our work, the mutation classes of HIV-1 DR showed significant differences between ART-naïve controls and participants experiencing treatment failure. The prevalence of single, dual, and multiple mutations in participants experiencing treatment failure was significantly higher than in ART-naïve participants, which is consistent with previous findings in Yunnan [25]. The dual NRTI and NNRTI DR prevalence (29.4%) was highest, followed by that of NNRTIs (10.7%), NRTIs (4.2%), and PIs (2.8%) in participants experiencing treatment failure. However, in ART-naïve participants, the PI DR prevalence (2.5%) was higher than that of NRTIs (1.7%), NNRTIs (0.8%), and NRTIs and NNRTIs (0.8%), in contrast to an earlier report [26]. Our observed DR rate of 51.9% in participants experiencing treatment failure was higher than that seen in Henan Province (47.1–64.7%) [27, 28] and Switzerland (37–45%) [29], suggesting that the higher prevalence of HIV-1-resistant strains is closely related to the widespread use of antiviral drugs. This has occurred in China since 2003, after which time more HIV-1 drug-resistant variants were identified and have spread.

The prevalence of NNRTI mutations was higher than that of other mutations in this study, which might reflect the replicative fitness of the virus. For example, Y181C can increase HIV-1 subtype B replicative capacity [30]. Moreover, our study also revealed significant differences in the distributions of M184V/I and M41L mutations among three main genotypes, with M46L/V and T74S only found in CRF01_AE. The differences of HIV-1 mutation distribution in three main genotypes provide some clues of replicative fitness of the virus and renewal of the therapeutic regime. By contrast, the distributions of the remaining mutations were not significantly different among three main genotypes, suggesting that they are randomly distributed in these genotypes.

First-line antiretroviral drugs were included in all therapeutic regimens used in this study, and the prevalence of DR did not differ significantly among these regimens. Of all participants using therapeutic regimens containing lopinavir plus ritonavir (LPV/r), 59.1% showed resistance to partial PIs (Table 6). Factors associated with the high prevalence of HIV-1 DR among participants experiencing treatment failure are as follows: first, the higher VL (>5000 copies/ml) and lower CD4 counts (≤200 cells/μl) are closely related to the higher prevalence of HIV-1 DR.

Table 6 Factors associated with HIV-1 DR among participants experiencing treatment failure

Factors	DR rate % (N)	Crude OR (95% CI)	p value	Adjusted OR (95% CI)	p value
Gender					
Male	51.6 (79)	1	0.913		
Female	52.5 (32)	1.034 (0.571, 1.872)			
Age (years)					
0–18	63.2 (12)	1	0.35		
19–49	52.5 (73)	0.646 (0.242, 1.725)			
50–	43.2 (26)	0.444 (0.143, 1.385)			
Marital status					
Married/cohabitation	48.5 (49)	1	0.473		
Unmarried	57.7 (41)	1.45 (0.787, 2.673)			
Divorced/widowed	50 (21)	1.016 (0.517, 2.18)			
Ethnicity					
Han	51 (106)	1	0.118		
Others	83.3 (5)	4.811 (0.553, 41.894)			
VL (copy/ml)					
≤5000	31.4 (16)	1	0.001	1	0.001
5001–9999	45.7 (16)	1.842 (0.756, 4.486)		1.673 (0.558, 5.01)	
≥10,000	61.7 (79)	3.527 (1.768, 7.035)		4.9 (1.996, 12.026)	
CD4 counts (cells/μl)					
≤200	68.4 (78)	1	0.001	1	0.001
>200	33 (33)	0.227 (0.128, 0.404)		0.219 (0.101, 0.474)	
WHO stages					
I	47.3 (71)	1	0.074		
II	76.5 (13)	3.616 (1.127, 11.6)			
III	52.9 (18)	1.252 (0.594, 2.639)			
IV	69.2 (9)	2.54 (0.739, 8.485)			
Symptoms[a] in recent three months					
No	44 (66)	1	0.001	1	0.046
Yes	70.3 (45)	3.014 (1.162, 5.635)		2.386 (1.017, 5.594)	
Education level					
High school or less	51.3 (82)	1	0.755		
College and above	53.7 (29)	1.103 (0.595, 2.048)			
Duration between diagnosis and ART					
0–12	50.4 (66)	1	0.786		
13–54	57.7 (15)	1.343 (0.574, 3.142)			
55–	52.6 (30)	1.094 (0.587, 2.039)			
ART regimens					
3TC + AZT + NVP/EFV	52.8 (67)	1	0.621		
3TC + TDF + LPV/r	59.1 (13)	1.294 (0.516, 3.241)			
Others[b]	47.7 (31)	0.817 (0.449, 1.486)			
Duration of ART (months)					
6–12	36.8 (32)	1	0.001	1	0.025
13–54	57 (45)	2.275 (1.22, 4.242)		1.737 (0.801, 3.766)	
55–	70.8 (34)	4.174 (1.953, 8.923)		3.828 (1.445, 10.14)	
Transmission routes					
Sexual contact	59.9 (91)	1	0.001	1	0.001
Blood	19 (8)	0.158 (0.068, 0.364)		0.082 (0.028, 0.241)	
Mother-to-child	60 (12)	1.005 (0.388, 2.604)		1.156 (0.313, 4.268)	

Table 6 continued

Factors	DR rate % (N)	Crude OR (95% CI)	p value	Adjusted OR (95% CI)	p value
Genotype					
B	55.4 (62)	1	0.035	1	0.484
CRF-1_AE	55.6 (40)	1.008 (0.556, 1.829)		0.765 (0.343, 1.708)	
Others[c]	30.0 (9)	0.346 (0.145, 0.821)		0.543 (0.195, 1.512)	

OR odds ratio, *DR* drug resisitance

[a] Herpes zoster, persistent diarrhea (>1 month), persistent/intermittent fever (>38 °C, >1 month), Brain lymphoma/B-cell non-Hodgkin's lymphoma, tuberculosis or thrush

[b] 3TC + d4T + NVP, 3TC + TDF + EFV, 3TC + D4T + EFV and 3TC + TDF + NVP were included

[c] CRF07_BC (4 cases), CRF08_BC (2 cases), CRF02_AG (1 case), C (1 case) and URF (1 case) were included

Moreover, compared with asymptomatic patients, HIV/AIDS patients who showed symptoms (Herpes zoster, tuberculosis or thrush, etc.) during the past 3 months had a higher prevalence of resistance to antiretroviral drugs. These phenomena provide new evidence for evaluating disease development and monitoring resistant strains using CD4 counts, VL, and clinical symptoms in the course of ART. Second, the duration between diagnosis and ART did not significantly affect the prevalence of DR. However, the ART duration was positively correlated with the prevalence of drug-resistant strains, indicating that following prolonged treatment, HIV-1 strains develop drug-selected mutations adapted to the antiretroviral drug. For example, TAMs resistant to all drugs listed in the HIV DR database were detected after a mean therapeutic duration of 42.8 months, and the long-term use of the first-line regimens may have played a role in the development of TAMs mutations. Additionally, individuals infected with HIV-1 transmitted drug resistance (TDR) strains derived from treated patients were resistant to related drugs. In this study, the most common mutations (M184V/I, K103N, Y181C, etc.) proved HIV-1 fitness to drugs, suggesting that HIV-1 resistant strains would spread out. Lu et al. [31] previously confirmed the existence of HIV-1 TDR strains among men who have sex with men in Hebei. Because the spread of HIV-1-resistant strains through sexual contacts is much faster than through other routes, timely behavioral intervention is particularly important.

Conclusions

In contrast with our previous studies, we observed extensive HIV-1 genetic diversity in the present study. The high prevalence of HIV-1 DR in participants experiencing treatment failure of Hebei appears to have been induced by antiretroviral drug treatment after a longer duration of ART. Moreover, significant differences were observed in the distribution of mutations in different HIV-1 genotypes. Our study results suggest that we should formulate new prevention and control strategies according to geographic characteristics of HIV-1 genotype distribution and the epidemic characteristics of HIV-1-resistant strains in Hebei.

Abbreviations

HIV: human immunodeficiency virus; CRF: circulating recombinant form; SPSS: statistical package for the social sciences; IDU: intravenous drug injection; MTCT: mother-to-child transmission; ART: antiretroviral therapy; URF: unique recombinant form; PIs: protease inhibitors; NRTIs: nucleoside reverse transcriptase inhibitors; NNRTIs: non-nucleoside reverse transcriptase inhibitors; DR: drug resistance; ATV/r: atazanavir/r; NFV/r: nelfinavir plus ritonavir; LPV/r: lopinavir plus ritonavir; 3TC: lamivudine; ABC: abacavir; AZT: zidovudine; D4T: stavudine; DDI: didanosine; FTC: emtricitabine; TDF: tenofovir; EFV: efavirenz; ETR: etravirine; NVP: nevirapine.

Authors' contributions

This study was conceived and designed by ZC, XL, and SC. XL and CZ implemented the study and analyzed results. XL drafted the manuscript. YZ and HZ contributed to the acquisition of data and critical revision, WW and LM carried out statistical analysis. XL and YL completed the sample collection and the CD4 cell count assay. All authors read and approved the final manuscript.

Acknowledgements

The authors thank the staff of local Centers for Disease Control and Prevention in Hebei Province for their assistance, especially with fieldwork.

Competing interests

The authors declare that they have no competing interests.

Funding

Our study was implemented with the support of the Natural Science Fund of Hebei Province (H2016303006).

References

1. Faria NR, Rambaut A, Suchard MA, Baele G, Bedford T, Ward MJ, et al. HIV epidemiology. The early spread and epidemi ignition of HIV-1 in human populations. Science. 2014;346:56–61.
2. Zeng Y, Wang B, Shao Y, Zhao S, Miao X. Isolation of human immunodeficiency virus from AIDS patient. Chung Hua Liu Hsing Ping Hsueh Tsa Chih. 1988;9:135–7.
3. Zeng Y. Serological screening of HIV antibody in China. Chin J Epidemiol. 1988;9:138–40.
4. Zhao SD. AIDS surveillance in Yunnan province in China (1986–1990). Chin J Epidemiol. 1991;12:72–4.
5. Lu L, Jia M, Ma Y, Yang L, Chen Z, Ho David D, et al. The changing face of HIV in China. Nature. 2008;455:609–11.
6. Yu E, Xie Q, Zhang K, Lu P, Chan L. HIV infection and AIDS in China, 1985 through 1994. Am J Pulic Health. 1996;86:1116–22.

7. Wu Z, Sullivan S, Wang Y, Rotheram-Borus M, Detels R. Evolution of China's response to HIV/AIDS. Lancet. 2007;369:679–90.
8. Ministry of Health, People's Republic of China, Joint United Nations Programme on HIV/AIDS, World Health Organization. 2009 estimates for the HIV/AIDS epidemic in China. Beijing: National Center for AIDS/STD Prevention and Control, China CDC; 2010.
9. Wang N, Wang L, Wu Z, Guo W, Sun X, Poundstone K, et al. Estimating the number of people living with HIV/AIDS in China: 2003–09. Int J Epidemiol. 2010;39:21–8.
10. He X, Xing H, Ruan Y, Hong K, Cheng C, Hu Y, et al. A comprehensive mapping of HIV-1 genotypes in various risk groups and regions across China based on a Nationwide Molecular Epidemiologic Survey. PLoS ONE. 2012;7:e47289.
11. Hebei Province's population Database in 2014. http://www.hetj.gov.cn/hetj/tjsj/ndsj/101441506553878.html. Accessed 16 Sept 2015.
12. Liu S, Liu L, Dang J, Liu X, Zhou H, Wang Y. Analysis on the HIV/AIDS epidemic in Shijiazhuang. Modern Prev Med. 2010;37:3153–4.
13. Chen S, Zhang Y, Zhao H, Zhao C, Li B, Bai G, et al. Investigation on status of HIV-1 infection among blood recipients from 1994 to 1998 in certain areas of China. Chin J Epidemiol. 2009;30:998–1000.
14. Chen S, Zhao H, Zhao C, Zhang Y, Li B, Bai G, et al. Eighteen-year follow-up report of the surveillance and prevention of an HIV/AIDS outbreak amongst plasma donors in Hebei Province, China. BMC Infect Dis. 2015;15:316.
15. Guo Z. Analysis on HIV/AIDS epidemic data in Hebei Province during 1989 to 2009. Chin J Derm Venereol. 2010;24:737–8.
16. HIV/AIDS surveillance in Hebei province. http://hebei.hebnews.cn/2014-11/27/content_4348216.htm. Accessed 27 Nov 2014.
17. Li L, Sun G, Liang S, Li J, Li T, Wang Z, et al. Different distribution of HIV-1 subtype and drug resistance were found among treatment naïve individuals in Henan, Guangxi, and Yunnan Province of China. PLoS ONE. 2013;8:e75777.
18. Zhang FJ, Pan J, Yu L, Wen Y, Zhao Y. Current progress of China's free ART program. Cell Res. 2005;15:877–82.
19. Arenas M. Genetic consequences of antiviral therapy on HIV-1. Comput Math Methods Med. 2015;2015:395826. doi:10.1155/2015/395826.
20. Zhang F, Dou Z, Ma Y, Zhao Y, Liu Z, Bulterys M, et al. Five-year outcomes of the China National Free Antiretroviral Treatment Program. Ann Intern Med. 2009;151:241–251, W-252.
21. Lu X, Zhao C, Wang W, Nie C, Zhang Y, Zhao H, et al. HIV-1 genetic diversity and its distribution characteristics among newly diagnosed HIV-1 individuals in Hebei province, China. AIDS Res Ther. 2016;13:3.
22. Zhao C, Zhao H, Li B, Bai G, Xing H, Lu X, et al. Molecular epidemiological study on HIV infection among paid blood donors. Chin J Health Lab Technol. 2010;120:3136–40.
23. Zhao C, Xing H, Zhao H, Huang H, Liu Y, Ma P, et al. Subtyping and sequence analysis of the C2-V3 region of gp120 genes among HIV-1 strains in Hebei province. Chin J Microbiol Immunol. 2005;25:533–5.
24. Li L, Sun G, Zhong P, Han J, Li T, Jia D, et al. HIV-1 Thai B strain has spread out of former plasma donors into general population through sexual contact in Henan. China. J Med Virol. 2016;88:614–21.
25. Li H, Zhong M, Guo W, Zhuang D, Li L, Liu Y, et al. Prevalence and mutation patterns of HIV drug resistance from 2010 to 2011 among ART-failure individuals in the Yunnan Province, China. PLoS ONE. 2013;8:e72630.
26. Avila-Ríos S, García-Morales C, Tapia-Trejo D, Meza RI, Nuñez SM, Parham L, et al. HIV drug resistance surveillance in Honduras after a decade of widespread antiretroviral therapy. PLoS ONE. 2015;10:e0142604.
27. Liu J, Wu Y, Yang W, Xue X, Sun G, Liu C, et al. Population-based human immunodeficiency virus 1 drug resistance profiles among individuals who experienced virological failure to first-line antiretroviral therapy in Henan, China during 2010–2011. AIDS Res Ther. 2015;12:22.
28. Yuan Y, Xing H, Wang X, Liu C, Yang L, Zheng B, et al. The prevalence of HIV-1 drug resistance and associated factors in AIDS patients receiving HAART in Zhecheng county, Henan Province. Zhonghua Yu Fang Yi Xue Za Zhi. 2011;45:619–24.
29. von Wyl V, Yerly S, Bürgisser P, Klimkait T, Battegay M, Bernasconi E, et al. Long-term trends of HIV type 1 drug resistance prevalence among antiretroviral treatment-experienced patients in Switzerland. Clin Infect Dis. 2009;48:979–87.
30. Li J, Li L, Li HP, Zhuang DM, Liu SY, Liu YJ, et al. Competitive capacity of HIV-1 strains carrying M184I or Y181I drug-resistant mutations. Chin Med J (Engl). 2009;122:1081–6.
31. Lu X, Kang X, Chen S, Zhao H, Liu Y, Zhao C, et al. HIV-1 genetic diversity and transmitted drug resistance among recently infected individuals at men who have sex with men sentinel surveillance points in Hebei Province, China. AIDS Res Hum Retroviruses. 2015;31:1038–45.

17

A frailty index predicts post-liver transplant morbidity and mortality in HIV-positive patients

Giovanni Guaraldi[1*], Giovanni Dolci[1], Stefano Zona[1], Giuseppe Tarantino[2], Valentina Serra[2], Roberto Ballarin[2], Erica Franceschini[1], Mauro Codeluppi[1], Thomas D. Brothers[3], Cristina Mussini[1] and Fabrizio Di Benedetto[2]

Abstract

Background: We hypothesized that frailty acts as a measure of health outcomes in the context of LT. The aim of this study was to explore frailty index across LT, as a measure of morbidity and mortality. This was a retrospective observational study including all consecutive 47 HIV+patients who received LT in Modena, Italy from 2003 to June 2015.

Methods: frailty index (FI) was constructed from 30 health variables. It was used both as a continuous score and as a categorical variable, defining 'most frail' a FI > 0.45. FI change across transplant (deltaFI, ΔFI) was calculated as the difference between year 1 FI (FI–Y1) and pre-transplant FI (FI–t0). The outcomes measures were mortality and "otpimal LT" (defined as being alive without multi-morbidity).

Results: Median value of FI–t0 was 0.48 (IQR 0.42–0.52), FI–Y1 was 0.31 (IQR 0.26–0.41). At year five mortality rate was 45%, "optimal transplant" rate at year 1 was 38%. All the patients who died in the post-LT were most frail in the pre-LT. ΔFI was a predictor of mortality after correction for age and MELD (HR = 1.10, p = 0.006) and was inversely associated with optimal transplant after correction for age (HR = 1.04, p = 0.01).

Conclusions: We validated FI as a valuable health measure in HIV transplant. In particular, we found a relevant correlation between FI strata at baseline and mortality and a statistically significant correlation between, ΔFI and survival rate.

Keywords: Frailty, HIV, Transplant

Background

Liver transplantation (LT) is theoretically the best treatment for patients with end stage liver disease (ESLD) but its effectiveness is limited by short-term mortality and morbidity, and by persistent shortage of donors' organs. Specific selection policies have been developed to identify good candidates for this surgical option [1, 2]. In this context, recipients with chronic health conditions, including HIV [3–6], can be admitted to this surgical procedure after appropriate selection.

*Correspondence: giovanni.guaraldi@unimore.it
[1] Department of Medical and Surgical Sciences for Adults and Children, Clinic of Infectious Diseases, University of Modena and Reggio Emilia, Largo del Pozzo, 71, 41124 Modena, Italy
Full list of author information is available at the end of the article

Under the current medical urgency-based selection system, patients with worst outcomes while on the waiting list, are given highest priority for LT [7] using model for end-stage liver disease (MELD) score [8], acting as a predictor of mortality in waiting list period. Unluckily this algorithms fails to depict the extremely relevant heterogeneity of morbidity and quality of life of patients in the post-LT period [9, 10]. In addition, in HIV settings, and in particular in HIV/HCV co-infected patients, the prognostic value of the MELD score is uncertain. Some studies [11, 12] found a significant correlation between MELD and post-LT mortality, whereas in others this model had limited prognostic value [13, 14].

Frailty, conceptualized as frailty phenotype [15] or as an accumulation of deficit measure in a Frailty Index (FI) score [16], has the potential to predict relevant post-LT outcomes and assess the overall health status of the candidates.

Frailty phenotype in the HIV negative solid organ transplant population has been proven to be associated with increased mortality, early hospital readmission, delayed graft function after kidney transplant [17–20] and poor health outcomes in liver disease patients [21–24], including LT waitlist mortality [24].

Derck et al. [23], recently showed that frailty phenotype outperformed MELD in predicting quality of life in the pre-transplant period.

Moreover, Wilson et al. [25] demonstrated the predictive power of pre-transplant FI on post-transplant mortality in the setting of lung transplant.

Finally, Lai et al. [26] showed an association between measures of physical function related to frailty and post-LT mortality.

Frailty Index (FI) describes a multidimensional risk state which summarizes health deficits across a range of symptoms, signs, diseases, disabilities and laboratory abnormalities [16, 27]. This approach is robust across different settings, in different populations, using different numbers and types of health variables, consistently related to age and to adverse outcomes. Notably, this predictive capacity transferred into a scale measure (index) can be used in clinical practice to monitor health transition over time and in relation to medical interventions [28].

Our group have previously validated a FI in HIV-positive patients to measure biological aging, health status and prediction of mortality and multi-morbidity (MM) incidence [29, 30]. We decided to expand this experience in the context of LT in HIV patients. In this peculiar setting patient selection is more stringent due to the higher risk of morbidity and mortality of this vulnerable population [31].

We hypothesized that frailty, conceptualised as a deficit accumulation, acts as a measure of health outcomes that covers the overall LT process.

The aim of this study was to explore frailty index (FI) across LT, as a measure of morbidity and mortality.

Methods

Retrospective observational study including all consecutive HIV infected patients who received cadaveric donor liver transplant at the Liver and Multivisceral Transplant Center of University of Modena and Reggio Emilia from June 2003 to June 2015.

Baseline data included demographics (ethnic origin, gender and age), HIV characteristics (transmission risk factors, duration of HIV infection, HIV CDC classification, nadir CD4 cell count, class type and exposure to antiretroviral therapy, plasma HIV genotypic resistance assay antecedent or concomitant to switching and current HAART) and ESLD history (aetiology, known duration of cirrhosis, HCV genotype, baseline serum HCV–RNA VL, previous cirrhotic decompensation episodes and presence of histologically documented hepatocellular carcinoma).

Donor risk index (DRI), comprising the following variables: donor age, donation after cardiac death, split/partial grafts, African-American race, less height, cerebrovascular accident and 'other' causes of brain death, location and cold time, was retrospectively calculated as a characteristics associated with liver graft failure but was not a graft allocation criteria [32].

Outcomes

Outcome measures considered in this cohort were:

1. Mortality: vital status was regularly updated at Liver and Multivisceral Transplant Center of University of Modena and Reggio Emilia via telephone contact and hospital records.
2. Optimal transplant: per protocol was defined as the post-LT survival of the patient in the absence of multi-morbidity. Multi-morbidity (MM) was described as the presence of three or more of the following six comorbidities: cardiovascular disease (clinical diagnosis with history of myocardial infarction, stroke, revascularization, or peripheral artery disease); hypertension (blood pressure measured twice $\geq$140 mmHg systolic or $\geq$90 mmHg diastolic or taking antihypertensive medicine); type two diabetes mellitus (measured fasting glucose $\geq$126 or oral glucose tolerance test >200 or on treatment); chronic kidney disease (estimated glomerular filtration rate <60 mL/min, via Modification of Diet in Renal Disease study equation [33]); osteopenia (dual-energy X-ray absorptiometry t or z score <−1.5) or osteoporosis (dual-energy X-ray absorptiometry t or z score <−2.5 or fragility fracture); or dyslipidemia (total cholesterol >200 mg/dL or low-density lipoprotein >100 mg/dL or high-density lipoprotein >100 mg/dL or triglycerides >150 mg/dL). COPD was not included as it is an exclusion criteria for liver transplant [34].

Non-optimal transplant was defined as the absence of optimal transplant, due to mortality or MM.

Predictors

Frailty index: was built, as previously described [29] to calculate the proportion of health deficits individuals have accumulated out of a group of 30 relatively nonspecific health variables (Table 1). Each variable included

Table 1 Variables included in the Frailty Index

Nr.	Variable	Deficit description
1	Hypertension	Measured blood pressure or on treatment
2	Diabetes mellitus type II	Fasting glucose >125 mg/dL or on treatment
3	Chronic kidney disease	Two estimated glomerular filtration rate measurements <60 mL/min/1.73 m^2
4	Osteopenia/Osteoporosis	Osteopenia: dual-energy X-ray absorptiometry (DEXA) Tor Z score <−1.5 or Osteoporosis: DEXA Tor Z score <−2.5 or fragility fracture
5	Any cancer	Clinical diagnosis
6	High or low BMI	<18 or >25 kg/m^2
7	High total cholesterol	>200 mg/dL
8	High triglycerides	>150 mg/dL
9	Leucopenia	<4000 cells/μL
10	Anemia	If female: <10 g/dL If male: <12 g/dL
11	Low platelets	<150 billion/L
12	Hyponatremia	<125 mEq/L
13	Abnormal potassium	<3.5 or >5.3 mEq/L
14	Elevated aspartate transaminase	>31 U/L
15	Elevated alanine transaminase	>31 U/L
16	Abnormal alkaline phosphatase	<38 or >126 U/L
17	Elevated γ-glutamyl transphosphatase	>55 U/L
18	Elevated total bilirubin	>1.10 mg/dL
19	Elevated creatinine	If female: >1.0 mg/dL If male: >1.2 mg/dL
20	Elevated INR	>1.2
21	Hepatits C virus viral load	HCV-RNA >12 copies/mL
22	Hepatitis B coinfection	Pre-LT: positive HBeAg Post-LT: HBV-DNA >copies/mL
23	Epstein-Barr virus coinfection	Pre-LT: positive EBV IgG Post-LT: HBV-DNA >copies/mL
24	Cytomegalovirus coinfection	Pre-LT: CMV IgG Post-LT: HBV-DNA >copies/mL
25	HIV viral load	>40 copies/μL
26	Current CD4$^+$ cell count	<500 cells/μL
27	CD4$^+$/CD8$^+$cell ratio	<1
28	Nadir CD4$^+$ cell count	<200 cells/μL
29	History of AIDS	History of CDC category C HIV disease [38]
30	Duration of HIV infection at LT	>20.6 years

was recorded with values of one when a deficit was present, and zero when absent [35]. Missing values were removed from both numerator and denominator of the FI ($FI = \frac{\sum Deficit}{30-\sum Missingvalues}$).

Study visits were applicable for FI evaluation if they had at least 80% of available health variables at that visit.

According to literature [36], we classified as "most frail" in a particular moment patients with FI > 0.45, as "frail" persons with FI between 0.21 and 0.45 and as "fit" or "not frail" people with FI < 0.21.

It must be noticed that in the risk prediction of "optimal/non-optimal transplant" a modified version of FI not listing the 6 comorbidities used to define MM, was used to avoid overlap between predictive variables and study outcome.

Frailty was assessed pre-LT (baseline) and at year 1, 3 and 5. Patients who died or did not reach year 1 post-LT censored FI data at last available assessment.

Pre-transplant FI (FI−t0) was calculated at the last available data before transplant (baseline visit), within 30 days before LT.

Post-LT FI was assessed at a median period of 262 days (IQR = 87–324) at year 1 visit (FI–Y1), at a median period of 1090 days (IQR = 1028–1142) at year 3 visit (FI–Y3) at a median period of 1843 days (IQR = 1800–1877) at year 5 visit (FI–Y5).

FI change across transplant (ΔFI), was calculated as the score difference between FI–Y1 and FI–t0.

$$\Delta FI = FIY1 - FIt0$$

We assessed FI validity using a three part approach that comprehends content, construct, and criterion validity as previously described [29, 37].

Other predictors at transplant time were: donor risk index, gender, age, BMI, MELD HCV antibody and RNA detectability, CD4 nadir and current, history of AIDS conditions and HIV viral load.

Statistical analysis

Descriptive statistics and FI scores at the baseline were calculated and distributions visualized. Cross-sectional relationships between FI scores and years of age were evaluated by linear regression. For prediction models, frailty index score was categorized using 0.1 increment. Each covariate was evaluated in univariate prediction models due to the small sample size and the low rate of events.

Mortality: Kaplan–Meier approach was used to evaluate mortality. Univariate Cox regression analysis was used to assess factors associated with mortality. We also calculated mortality in the 3 categorical frailty strata.

Unsuccessful LT: Multivariate analysis was used to assess the association between FIt0 and non-optimal transplant, FIY1 and non-optimal transplant, correcting for age. A Univariate Poisson analysis was used to assess the association between the 3 frailty strata at the baseline and non-optimal transplant.

Health transition after LT: FI was used to evaluate health transition after LT. LOWESS smoother graphs were drawn to describe FI over time. A linear regression model was used to determine the association between FI–t0 and, ΔFI at the year 1, year 3 and year 5 visit. The same method was used to determine the association between FI–t0 and FI–Y1.

Results

Population characteristics at baseline

Forty-seven HIV-positive patients underwent LT at Liver and Multivisceral Transplant Center of University of Modena and Reggio Emilia since from 2003 to June 2015. Among them, 5 underwent simultaneous transplant of liver and kidney.

Most LT patients were males (80.8%) with a median age of 51.2 years; IQR = 45.91–54.35).

Median pre-transplant $CD4^+$ count was 260 cells/μL (IQR 153–360 cells/μL), with only 9 patients (17%) having a CD4 count above 500 cells/μL. Most of the patients (44; 93.6%) presented undetectable HIV-RNA at transplant time.

Median baseline frailty index was 0.48 (IQR 0.42–0.52).

Liver transplant indications

The most common indication for liver transplant was HCV-induced ESLD (82.9%), followed by hepatocellular carcinoma (HCC; 44.6%). Twenty-eight patients presented multiple indications, in particular, two of them had four indications (association of HCV, HBV, HDV and HCC in both cases), six had three indications and 20 had two indications. Among this latter group, the most prevalent association (60%) was HCV and HCC. Median pre-transplant MELD was 22 (IQR 16.5–29).

Mortality

Mortality at year five post-LT was 45%, while at year 1 and year 3 was respectively 21 and 38%.

A multivariate analysis including all baseline FI variables was performed, but none of them reached statistical significance in predicting post-transplant mortality.

Figure 1 describes how mortality was related to HCV antibody status and HCV RNA detectability at transplantation. Of interest, seven HCV + patients were treated in the pre-LT with HCV directly active agents (DAA) and none of them died in the 1-year follow up.

Optimal transplant/Non-optimal transplant

Prevalence of MM was fairly stable in the post-LT period, respectively prevalent in 39, 46 and 38% at year 1, 3 and 5.

As reported in Additional file 1: Figure S1 the proportion of survivors with no MM, who met the definition of

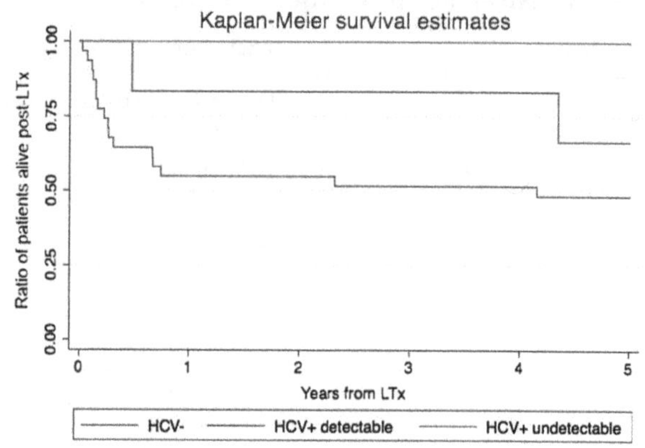

Fig. 1 Kaplan–Meier survival estimate in relation to HCV RNA at the time of transplantation

"Optimal transplant", were respectively 38% (17 patients) at year 1, 29% (10) at year 3 and 26% (8) at year 5.

Frailty index

Construct validity: frailty index description

Pre-transplant frailty index ranged from 0.32 to 0.62, with a median of 0.48 (IQR 0.42–0.52). Consistently with literature [29, 35, 38, 39], its upper limit was close to 0.7. It was significantly associated with age (r = 0.30, p = 0.048) and followed a normal distribution. At baseline 29 patients (61.7%) were classified as "most frail", whilst 18 (38.3%) were "frail" and no one was "not frail".

No significant correlation was observed between baseline FI and pre-transplant MELD (r = 0.14, p = 0.932). Pre-LT frailty index was conversely correlated with donor risk index [32] (DRI) (r = −0.50; p = 0.008).

Criterion validity: DELTA FI ability to predict major outcomes

Baseline FI, analysed into 0.1 increment was not significantly associated with survival (HR = 1.47; p = 0.90). However, all the 10 deceased patients (100%) at year 1 were "most frail" at baseline (HR and p value are not statistically applicable in this situation).

FI at year 1 was associated with mortality after correction for age (HR = 1.12, p = 0.04) or for FIt0 (HR = 1.13, p = 0.03).

Univariate Poisson regression analysis of the association between non-optimal transplant and frailty strata at the baseline showed an IRR = 1.45 (CI 0.7078–2.98; p = 0.3).

Figure 2 shows that ΔFI at multivariate Cox regression was a predictor of mortality after correction for age and MELD (HR = 1.10, p = 0.006) as well as a predictor of non-optimal transplant at multivariate Poisson regression after correction for age (HR = 1.04, p = 0.01).

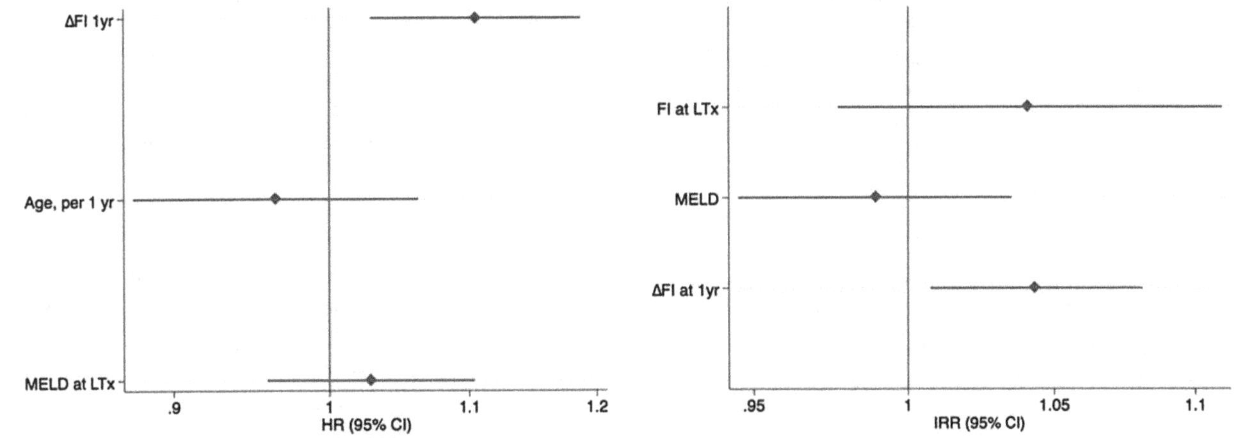

ΔFI Y1 is a predictor of mortality at Cox regression analyses

ΔFI Y1 is a predictor of unsuccessful transplant at Poisson regression analyses

Fig. 2 Independent predictors of survival and successful transplant

Frailty index to describe health transition across liver transplant

Survivors and deceased patients showed a different pattern FI reduction post-LT. This is visually depicted in Fig. 3 by a LOWESS smoother of the FI in function of time and describes a different health transition across LT in the two groups.

Among the 29 most frail patients at the baseline, during the first year post-LT 10 died, three remained stable and 16 improved (reverted from "most frail" to "frail"). In contrast, among the 18 patients who were "frail" at baseline, 6 did not have enough data to calculate the Y1FI, 10 remained stable and two reverted their condition to "non frail". Notably, none of them worsened their "frail" status to "most frail".

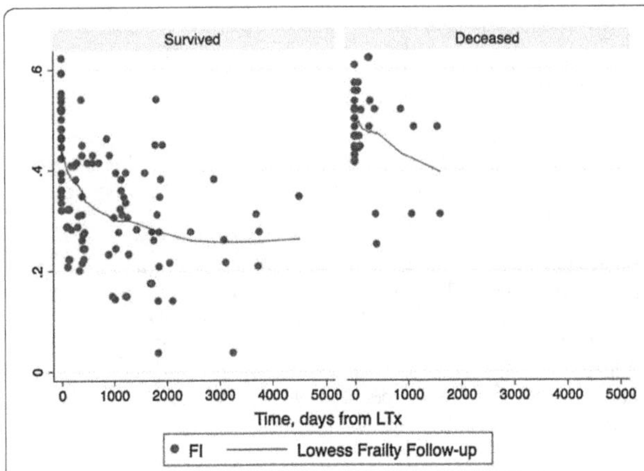

Fig. 3 LOWESS smoother: FI time course in survived and deceased. *Red vertical line* represents transplant date

Baseline frailty index scores strongly influenced transition probabilities at year 1 ($r = 0.37$, $p = 0.027$).

Discussion

This study validates FI in HIV transplant setting and describes health status transition across the overall LT process.

In the pre-transplant assessment FI measurement (baseline FI) exhibited expected characteristics of the general population with regards to normal distribution, association with age and upper limit ceiling effect [29, 40].

Of interest, baseline FI was conversely associated with DRI. This index can be considered a proxy of the "quality of the graft". Thus, in our cohort better livers were allocated to patients with a higher FI, suggesting that baseline FI reflected the clinical judgment of vulnerability that surgeons empirically consider when allocating organs, within the respect of urgency criteria established by MELD score.

With regards to criterion validity, baseline "most frail" condition was able to predict mortality and in the post-LT, with 10 out 29 patients died at year 1 between the "most frail" group vs 0 out of 18 among the "frail" one. Moreover, FI at year 1 was able to independently predict mortality.

It must be noticed that in this cohort pre-LT MELD was not associated with neither post-LT mortality nor baseline FI. The MELD provide a parsimonious measure of liver-related health associated with pre-transplant outcome, whereas FI is a copious measure of overall health throughout the transplant process. Thus, we believe that not only the use of FI in the LT setting has the potential to be clinically useful for candidates selection and targeted rehabilitation therapies, but also that it could be of particular interest in the HIV population, where a higher vulnerability is present, comorbidities are more prevalent and where MELD is often less meaningful.

Unfortunately, even though the IRR of the association between optimal transplant and "most frail" condition at the baseline is consistent with the survival analysis, baseline FI was not significantly able to predict optimal transplant. However, its significant association with Y1FI suggests that this could be explained with a lack of statistical power due to the small sample size of this unique cohort.

In addition, we used our FI the health transition across the LT period. As shown in Fig. 3, frailty reduction was present in both deceased and survived patients, but the slope was more evident in the latter group. This picture is consistent with the FI change observed in HIV-negative elderly population where frailty reduction was associated with improved survival [41, 42].

ΔFI is an interesting clinical conceptualization given that it allows considering a health status measure as the net change of biological events happening across LT, therefore taking in consideration in the same measure patient vulnerability both in the pre and in the post LT period. Applicability of FI in this clinical setting may also offer a measure of intensity of care giving insight in the large variability of health status in the post-LT.

ΔFI beyond year 1 was associated with both mortality and non-optimal transplant outcome, after correction for baseline confounders. Δ *FI* describes health transition across transplant, visually depicted by the LOWESS smoother curve. Mitnitski et al. [16, 43, 44] state that frailty can be considered a proxy of biological age, thus, this findings quantifies the empirical perception of both patients and physicians that LT "puts the biological clock back" to the time before ESLD.

On a clinical standpoint, monitoring FI and delta FI after transplant can be useful. In particular, for patients that experienced less FI improvement more frequent follow-up appointments can be considered or hospital discharge should be delayed.

Some limitations can be acknowledged. The retrospective observational nature of the study avoided the possibility to expand FI variable list, which were close to the minimum number suggested for a FI validation. In particular, our FI lacks of patient-related outcome and geriatric syndrome evaluation usually part of geriatric FI variable lists.

The relatively small sample size of our cohort could be responsible of low statistical power of multivariable analysis not reaching statistical significant value.

Some strength points may also be recognised:

The validation of FI in the transplant setting provide a new biological variable able to capture not only recipient vulnerability and surgical risk but also describe health transition across LT.

Frailty could play a role in a "blended principle model" [1] of organ allocation, as it is able to assess patients' overall health status and at the same time potential to be a predictor of both mortality and quality of life [23].

This approach also allows to link health status with biological age conceptualization: at an individual basis, LT is a turning point, with different perspective in patients and physicians. Patients often describe LT as a "re-birth", meaning the biological and psychological aspect related to a new donated life. Along with the obvious psychological benefit of passing from facing death to a longer life expectancy, the health and liver-related symptoms gain after LT reflects in a well-documented improvement in health [45–48]. Physicians often describe LT as a "reverse time" story, somehow putting back the biological clock to the time before ESLD. Both "re-birth", and "reverse time" refer to the biological age categories, which can be depicted in the frailty assessment. This approach depicting health transition across the transplant period allows interpreting LT as a time reversing event measuring health improvement.

We hope these results may pilot future studies to compare different tools to evaluate frailty in the transplant setting and to expand the validation of FI toward other transplant settings.

Abbreviations

AIDS: acquired immunodeficiency syndrome; DeltaFI: delta frailty index; ESLD: end stage liver disease; FI: frailty index; FIY1: frailty index at year 1; FIt0: frailty index at the baseline; HIV: human immunodeficiency virus; HR: hazard ratio; IQR: inter-quartile range; LT: liver transplant; MELD: model for end stage liver disease; MM: multimorbidity.

Authors' contributions

GG and GD designed the study. GD, GT, VS, RB, EF and MC collected the data. SZ performed the statistical analysis. GG, GD and SZ wrote the first draft of the paper. GG, GD, SZ, TDB, CM and FDB gave key contributions to the interpretation of data. GD formatted the manuscript for publication. All authors read and approved the final manuscript.

Author details

[1] Department of Medical and Surgical Sciences for Adults and Children, Clinic of Infectious Diseases, University of Modena and Reggio Emilia, Largo del Pozzo, 71, 41124 Modena, Italy. [2] Department of Medical and Surgical Sciences for Adults and Children, Liver and Multivisceral Transplant Center, University of Modena and Reggio Emilia, Modena, Italy. [3] Faculty of Medicine, Dalhousie University, Halifax B3H 2E1, Canada.

Acknowledgements

The authors would like to acknowledge Yuval Neeman for the contribution and the suggestions about this paper. Furthermore, they would like to acknowledge Giovanni Bettelli, Andrea Malagoli, Laura Rossi and Antonella Santoro for the contribution in the data collection. Without them this paper would not be possible. Prof. Giovanni Guaraldi confirms that he listed everyone who contributed significantly to the work and has obtained a written consent from all contributors who are not authors and are named in the Acknowledgment section.

Competing interests

GG received research grants from Gilead Sciences, ViiV healthcare and Merck. He received honoraria as speaker and/or advisor from Gilead Sciences, GlaxoSmithKline, Merck, Jansen, BMS. GD received research grants from Gilead Sciences. All other authors declare that they have no competing interests.

Funding

There was no funding support for this paper.

References

1. Cillo U, Burra P, Mazzaferro V, Belli L, Pinna AD, Spada M, et al. A multistep, consensus-based approach to organ allocation in liver transplantation: toward a "Blended Principle Model". Am J Transplant. 2015;15(10):1–10.
2. Vitale A, Volk M, Cillo U. Transplant benefit for patients with hepatocellular carcinoma. World J Gastroenterol China. 2013;19:9183–8.
3. Di Benedetto F, Di Sandro S, De Ruvo N, Berretta M, Montalti R, Guerrini GP, et al. Human immunodeficiency virus and liver transplantation: our point of view. Transplant Proc. 2008;40:1965–71.
4. Di Benedetto F, Tarantino G, De Ruvo N, Cautero N, Montalti R, Guerrini GP, et al. University of Modena experience in HIV-positive patients undergoing liver transplantation. Transplant Proc. 2011;43:1114–8.
5. Mindikoglu AL, Regev A, Magder LS. Impact of human immunodeficiency virus on survival after liver transplantation: analysis of United Network for Organ Sharing database. Transplantation. 2008;85:359–68.
6. Ragni MV, Belle SH, Im K, Neff G, Roland M, Stock P, et al. Survival of human immunodeficiency virus-infected liver transplant recipients. J Infect Dis. 2003;188:1412–20.
7. Schaubel DE, Guidinger MK, Biggins SW, Kalbfleisch JD, Pomfret EA, Sharma P, et al. Survival benefit-based deceased-donor liver allocation. Am J Transplant. 2009;9:970–81.
8. Kamath PS, Wiesner RH, Malinchoc M, Kremers W, Therneau TM, Kosberg CL, et al. A model to predict survival in patients with end-stage liver disease. Hepatology. 2001;33:464–70.
9. Saab S, Ibrahim AB, Shpaner A, Younossi ZM, Lee C, Durazo F, et al. MELD fails to measure quality of life in liver transplant candidates. Liver Transplant. 2005;11:218–23.
10. Heits N, Meer G, Bernsmeier A, Guenther R, Malchow B, Kuechler T, et al. Mode of allocation and social demographic factors correlate with impaired quality of life after liver transplantation. Health Qual Life Outcomes. 2015;13:162.
11. Terrault NA, Roland ME, Schiano T, Dove L, Wong MT, Poordad F, et al. Outcomes of liver transplant recipients with hepatitis C and human immunodeficiency virus coinfection. Liver Transplant. 2012;18:716–26.
12. Subramanian A, Sulkowski M, Barin B, Stablein D, Curry M, Nissen N, et al. MELD score is an important predictor of pretransplantation mortality in HIV-infected liver transplant candidates. Gastroenterology. 2010;138:159–64.
13. Duclos-Vallee J-C, Feray C, Sebagh M, Teicher E, Roque-Afonso A-M, Roche B, et al. Survival and recurrence of hepatitis C after liver transplantation in patients coinfected with human immunodeficiency virus and hepatitis C virus. Hepatology. 2008;47:407–17.
14. Miro JM, Montejo M, Castells L, Rafecas A, Moreno S, Aguero F, et al. Outcome of HCV/HIV-coinfected liver transplant recipients: a prospective and multicenter cohort study. Am J Transplant. 2012;12:1866–76.
15. Fried LP, Tangen CM, Walston J, Newman AB, Hirsch C, Gottdiener J, et al. Frailty in older adults: evidence for a phenotype. J Gerontol. 2001;56:M146–56.
16. Mitnitski AB, Mogilner AJ, Rockwood K. Accumulation of deficits as a proxy measure of aging. Sci World J. 2001;1:323–36.
17. Exterkate L, Slegtenhorst BR, Kelm M, Seyda M, Schuitenmaker JM, Quante M, et al. Frailty and transplantation. Transplantation. 2016;100(4):727–33.
18. McAdams-Demarco MA, Law A, Salter ML, Chow E, Grams M, Walston J, et al. Frailty and early hospital readmission after kidney transplantation. Am J Transplant. 2013;13:2091–5.
19. Garoznik-Wang J, Govindan P, Grinnan JJW, Al E, Garonzik-Wang JM, Govindan P, et al. Frailty and delayed graft function in kidney transplant recipients. Arch Surg. 2012;147:190–3.
20. McAdams-DeMarco MA, Law A, King E, Orandi B, Salter M, Gupta N, et al. Frailty and mortality in kidney transplant recipients. Am J Transplant. 2015;15:149–54.
21. Tapper EB, Finkelstein D, Mittleman MA, Piatkowski G, Lai M. Standard assessments of frailty are validated predictors of mortality in hospitalized patients with cirrhosis. Hepatology. 2015;62:584–90.
22. Cron DC, Friedman JF, Winder GS, Thelen AE, Derck JE, Fakhoury JW, et al. Depression and frailty in patients with end-stage liver disease referred for transplant evaluation. Am J Transplant. 2015;16(6):1805–11.
23. Derck JE, Thelen AE, Cron DC, Friedman JF, Gerebics AD, Englesbe MJ, et al. Quality of life in liver transplant candidates: frailty is a better indicator than severity of liver disease. Transplantation. 2015;99:340–4.
24. Lai JC, Feng S, Terrault NA, Lizaola B, Hayssen H, Covinsky K. Frailty predicts waitlist mortality in liver transplant candidates. Am J Transplant. 2014;14:1870–9.
25. Wilson ME, Vakil AP, Kandel P, Undavalli C, Dunlay SM, Kennedy CC. Pretransplant frailty is associated with decreased survival after lung transplantation. J Heart Lung Transplant. 2015;35(2):173–8.
26. Lai JC, Volk ML, Strasburg D, Alexander N. Performance-based measures associate with frailty in patients with end-stage liver disease. Transplantation. 2016;100(12):2656–60.
27. Whitehead JC, Hildebrand BA, Sun M, Rockwood MR, Rose RA, Rockwood K, et al. A clinical frailty index in aging mice: comparisons with frailty index data in humans. J Gerontol. 2014;69:621–32.
28. Mitnitski A, Fallah N, Rockwood MRH, Rockwood K. Transitions in cognitive status in relation to frailty in older adults: a comparison of three frailty measures. J Nutr Health Aging. 2011;15:863–7.
29. Guaraldi G, Brothers TD, Zona S, Stentarelli C, Carli F, Malagoli A, et al. A frailty index predicts survival and incident multimorbidity independent of markers of HIV disease severity. AIDS. 2015;29:1633–41.
30. Guaraldi G, Malagoli A, Theou O, Brothers TD, Wallace L, Torelli R, et al. Correlates of frailty phenotype and frailty index and their associations with clinical outcomes. HIV Med. 2017. doi:10.1111/hiv.12527.
31. Guaraldi G, Orlando G, Zona S, Menozzi M, Carli F, Garlassi E, et al. Premature age-related comorbidities among HIV-infected persons compared with the general population. Clin Infect Dis. 2011;53:1120–6.
32. Feng S, Goodrich NP, Bragg-Gresham JL, Dykstra DM, Punch JD, DebRoy MA, et al. Characteristics associated with liver graft failure: the concept of a donor risk index. Am J Transplant. 2006;6:783–90.
33. Levey AS, Bosch JP, Lewis JB, Greene T, Rogers N, Roth D. A more accurate method to estimate glomerular filtration rate from serum creatinine: a new prediction equation. Modification of Diet in Renal Disease Study Group. Ann Intern Med. 1999;130:461–70.
34. Associazione Italiana per lo Studio del Fegato (A.I.S.F.). Il trapianto di fegato. Raccomandazioni dell'Associazione Italiana per lo studio del Fegato. 2007. p. 27. http://www.webaisf.org/media/7898/commissione_trapianto_fegato.pdf.
35. Rockwood K, Mitnitski A. Frailty defined by deficit accumulation and geriatric medicine defined by frailty. Clin Geriatr Med. 2011;27:17–26.
36. Hoover M, Rotermann M, Sanmartin C, Bernier J. Validation of an index to estimate the prevalence of frailty among community-dwelling seniors. Health Reports. 2013;24:10–7.
37. Streiner D, Norman G. Health measurement scales: a practical guide to their development and use. 4th ed. Oxford: Oxford University Press; 2008.
38. Mitnitski A, Song X, Skoog I, Broe GA, Cox JL, Grunfeld E, et al. Relative fitness and frailty of elderly men and women in developed countries and their relationship with mortality. J Am Geriatr Soc. 2005;53:2184–9.
39. Theou O, Brothers TD, Pena FG, Mitnitski A, Rockwood K. Identifying common characteristics of frailty across seven scales. J Am Geriatr Soc. 2014;62:901–6.
40. Searle SD, Mitnitski A, Gahbauer EA, Gill TM, Rockwood K. A standard procedure for creating a frailty index. BMC Geriatr. 2008;8:24.
41. Gill TM, Gahbauer EA, Allore HG, Han L. Transitions between frailty states among community-living older persons. Arch Intern Med. 2006;166:418–23.
42. Partridge JSL, Harari D, Dhesi JK. Frailty in the older surgical patient: a review. Age Ageing. 2012;41:142–7.

43. Mitnitski A, Song X, Rockwood K. Assessing biological aging: the origin of deficit accumulation. Biogerontology. 2013;14:709–17.
44. Mitnitski AB, Graham JE, Mogilner AJ, Rockwood K. Frailty, fitness and late-life mortality in relation to chronological and biological age. BMC Geriatr. 2002;2:1.
45. Butt Z, Parikh ND, Skaro AI, Ladner D, Cella D. Quality of life, risk assessment, and safety research in liver transplantation: new frontiers in health services and outcomes research. Curr Opin Organ Transplant. 2012;17:241–7.
46. Grover S, Sarkar S. Liver transplant-psychiatric and psychosocial aspects. J Clin Exp Hepatol. 2012;2:382–92.
47. Yang LS, Shan LL, Saxena A, Morris DL. Liver transplantation: a systematic review of long-term quality of life. Liver Int. 2014;34:1298–313.
48. Perez-San-Gregorio MA, Martin-Rodriguez A, Perez-Bernal J, Maldonado MD. Quality of life in spanish patients with liver transplant. Clin Pract Epidemiol Ment Health. 2010;6:79–85.

Risk factors and outcomes for the Q151M and T69 insertion HIV-1 resistance mutations in historic UK data

Oliver T. Stirrup[1*], David T. Dunn[1], Anna Tostevin[1], Caroline A. Sabin[2], Anton Pozniak[3], David Asboe[3], Alison Cox[4], Chloe Orkin[5], Fabiola Martin[6,7], Patricia Cane[8] on behalf of the UK HIV Drug Resistance Database and the UK Collaborative HIV Cohort

Abstract

Background: The prevalence of HIV-1 resistance to antiretroviral therapies (ART) has declined in high-income countries over recent years, but drug resistance remains a substantial concern in many low and middle-income countries. The Q151M and T69 insertion (T69i) resistance mutations in the viral reverse transcriptase gene can reduce susceptibility to all nucleoside/tide analogue reverse transcriptase inhibitors, motivating the present study to investigate the risk factors and outcomes associated with these mutations.

Methods: We considered all data in the UK HIV Drug Resistance Database for blood samples obtained in the period 1997–2014. Where available, treatment history and patient outcomes were obtained through linkage to the UK Collaborative HIV Cohort study. A matched case–control approach was used to assess risk factors associated with the appearance of each of the mutations in ART-experienced patients, and survival analysis was used to investigate factors associated with viral suppression. A further analysis using matched controls was performed to investigate the impact of each mutation on survival.

Results: A total of 180 patients with Q151M mutation and 85 with T69i mutation were identified, almost entirely from before 2006. Occurrence of both the Q151M and T69i mutations was strongly associated with cumulative period of virological failure while on ART, and for Q151M there was a particular positive association with use of stavudine and negative association with use of boosted-protease inhibitors. Subsequent viral suppression was negatively associated with viral load at sequencing for both mutations, and for Q151M we found a negative association with didanosine use but a positive association with boosted-protease inhibitor use. The results obtained in these analyses were also consistent with potentially large associations with other drugs. Analyses were inconclusive regarding associations between the mutations and mortality, but mortality was high for patients with low CD4 at detection.

Conclusions: The Q151M and T69i resistance mutations are now very rare in the UK. Our results suggest that good outcomes are possible for people with these mutations. However, in this historic sample, viral load and CD4 at detection were important factors in determining prognosis.

Keywords: 151 complex, 69 insertion complex, HIV, Multidrug resistance, Multi-NRTI resistance, NRTI

*Correspondence: oliver.stirrup@ucl.ac.uk
[1] Centre for Clinical Research in Infection and Sexual Health, Institute for Global Health, University College London, London, UK
Full list of author information is available at the end of the article

Background

Highly potent and effective antiretroviral therapies (ART) to treat HIV-1 infection are now available and although drug resistance was a considerable problem in the early years of ART use, its impact has now declined in high-income countries. In the UK HIV Drug Resistance Database (UK-HDRD) only about 30% of treated patients receiving resistance tests following virological failure in 2014 showed any drug resistance, compared with 72% in 2002 [1]. Likewise, a decline in drug resistance in treated patients has been observed in Canada [2] and overall in Western Europe [3]. In Switzerland it is now considered that the emergence of new drug resistance "can be virtually stopped with new potent therapies and close monitoring" [4]. However, drug resistance remains a considerable problem in the successful treatment of HIV infection in many low- and middle-income countries (LMICs) [5–7]. This is in part due to limited drug options, but also to a lack of (or limited) routine viral load (VL) monitoring [8] as patients continuing to use ART while failing to suppress viral replication may develop resistance mutations. This has led to calls for improved provision of VL monitoring and resistance testing [9–11].

HIV mutations that confer resistance to multiple drugs, and hence have the potential to severely limit treatment options, are of particular concern. The T69 insertion (T69i) and associated mutations in reverse transcriptase confer high level resistance to all nucleoside/nucleotide reverse transcriptase inhibitors (NRTIs) [12]. Likewise the Q151M mutation causes intermediate/high-level resistance to zidovudine (ZDV), didanosine (DDI), stavudine (D4T), and abacavir (ABC) and low level resistance to tenofovir (TDF), lamivudine (3TC) and emtricitabine (FTC) [12]. The Stanford University Drug Resistance Database reports that in combination with mutations at associated positions (62, 75, 77 and 116) Q151M confers high-level resistance to ZDV, DDI, D4T and ABC, and intermediate resistance to TDF, 3TC and FTC [13].

The T69i mutation has been linked to DDI use [14] whilst for Q151M an association with D4T has been observed [15], and most reports of the mutations occurring in Europe date to 10 or more years ago when the use of these drugs was still widespread [14, 16, 17]. However, a relatively high prevalence of Q151M has been observed in more recent studies of patients failing ART from LMICs [15, 18–23] (ranging 2–14% in these studies). Whilst a fall in prevalence is to be expected to follow from the complete phase-out of D4T use [24], there is the potential for cases of the mutation to persist for years to come. Although the occurrence of the T69i mutation appears to remain rare even in LMICs (ranging 0–1% in these studies [15, 18–22], with the 1% value based on a single patient in Saravanan et al. [21]), there nonetheless remains a motivation to investigate outcomes in affected patients given the potential impact on future treatment. Some recent studies have found that the presence of NRTI resistance is actually predictive of successful virological suppression on second-line ART [25, 26], so it is of interest to evaluate whether boosted protease inhibitor regimens are effective in those cases with these specific rare mutations.

This paper reports changes in the prevalence of multidrug resistance mutations Q151M and T69i in the UK-HDRD over time and evaluates outcomes in affected patients. Risk factors for the occurrence of the mutations and predictors of subsequent viral suppression are investigated, with the aim of helping to inform clinical management in regions in which the development of drug resistance is an increasing concern.

Methods

Data and general approach

We considered all available data in the UK-HDRD for blood samples obtained in the period 1997–2014. Few data are available before this period, as resistance testing was not widely available, with no recorded observations of either Q151M or T69i mutations. The prevalence of each resistance mutation studied was assessed in relation to calendar time stratified by whether patients were recorded as ART-naïve or -experienced in the UK-HDRD. Where possible, clinical data were obtained through linkage to the UK Collaborative HIV Cohort (UK CHIC) study [27]. Patients without classification recorded were assumed to be ART-experienced for the evaluation of prevalence, but ART-status was available in all UK CHIC-linked patients for the analyses of risk factors and outcomes.

The identification of drug resistance mutations was based on output from the Stanford University HIV Drug Resistance Database program. Following established convention (and software output) [13], the term 'T69i mutation' is used throughout to refer to any insertion in the β3–β4 loop of reverse transcriptase between codons 66 and 70.

A Bayesian approach to statistical analysis was used throughout, with models implemented in the Stan probabilistic programming language [28] using the rstan [29] interface for R. This approach was chosen to guard against the erroneous inferences that can arise from model building based on large numbers of sequential classical hypothesis tests [30]. Continuous variables were standardised for analyses (by subtracting their mean and then dividing by their SD) so that their associated parameters are on a comparable scale. Additional technical details are provided in Additional file 1.

Risk factors for development of mutations

Matched case–control analyses were conducted in order to investigate factors associated with the occurrence of each of the mutations studied. These analyses only included patients for whom resistance test data could be matched to clinical records in the UK CHIC study. ART-experienced patients were defined as 'cases' at time of blood sampling for the first observation of the relevant mutation and were matched in a 1:10 ratio to 'controls', who were randomly sampled (without replacement) from a subset of patients with at least one resistance test available for whom the relevant mutation had never been detected. Matching in each instance was conditional on the control patient having first initiated ART within 6 months (in calendar time) of the case patient doing so, and current and historic treatment variables for both case and control patients were defined with respect to the time of blood sampling for the resistance test in the case patient. Multivariable conditional logistic regression analyses were conducted accounting for the matched case–control groups. This form of analysis was chosen so that key factors associated with the development of the resistance mutations could be investigated whilst controlling for the evolution of ART drug combinations and treatment strategies over time. The complexity of ART histories for each patient and the limited numbers of cases available for analysis precluded more complex modelling of the probability of the development of each resistance mutation conditional on full details of ART history.

Details of variable selection for these models are provided in Additional file 1. For some patients included in the UK-HDRD, the original viral sequence data is not recorded and so it is not possible to obtain a viral subtype. As such, viral subtype was added to the final model in the subset of patients for whom this was possible (using REGA, classified as A, B, C, circulating recombinant form (CRF), or other).

Factors associated with successful viral suppression following detection of resistance

Multivariable Cox regression was used to investigate the factors associated with successful viral suppression following detection of either the Q151M or T69i mutation. Change to ART regimen following detection of a resistance mutation was taken as the zero time point for these analyses, and the survival outcome was defined as the time to the first of two consecutive undetectable VL observations (considering observations <200 copies/mL to be 'undetectable'). Patients in whom there was no change to ART regimen recorded were not included in these analyses. Baseline CD4 cell counts and VL were defined as the most recent observation recorded within 6 months prior to the start of the new ART regimen, and outcomes were censored at any subsequent change to ART regimen.

In the Cox regression analyses, baseline square-root(CD4) and $\log_{10}$(VL) were included as predictors, alongside treatment-naïve or experienced status, sex, patient age and variables representing individual drugs received by $\geq 10\%$ patients. Protease inhibitors (PIs) were grouped into the presence or absence of un-boosted or ritonavir-boosted PI (ubPI/rbPI) and non-nucleoside/nucleotide reverse transcriptase inhibitors (NNRTIs) were also grouped into a single variable. A dummy variable was included to indicate patients receiving an ART regimen containing drugs from only a single class. Presence or absence of the K65R mutation was also included as a predictor, and analyses were also conducted including the respective accessory mutations for Q151M and T69i. Further analyses were conducted to investigate the durability of viral suppression in ART-experienced patients, based on the proposal of McKinnon et al. [31]; briefly, viral suppression and subsequent virological failure are modelled using sequential Weibull time-to-event models so that the proportion of patients with sustained viral suppression can be estimated (Additional file 1).

Factors associated with mortality

To investigate the association between Q151M and 69i and mortality, we carried out a matched cohort analysis of comparable patients in whom ART data were available. Patients were matched from a subset of patients with at least one resistance test available for whom the relevant mutation had never been detected. Matching was conditional on the observation of a resistance test within 12 months of that in the case patient (effectively matching on treatment failure or interruption in ART-experienced patients), date of ART initiation within 12 months of the case patient in those who were ART-experienced at the time of detection (or ART-naïve status in ART-naïve cases), and patient sex and mode of infection. Matching was carried out with up to 10 'controls' for each 'case' (dependent on availability). Survival analyses (for the outcome of any-cause death from date of resistance test) were then conducted using Cox regression including a normally distributed shared frailty term for each matched group and adjusted for CD4 count at time of resistance test, age at resistance test, prior diagnosis of an AIDS-defining illness at resistance test and number of other reverse transcriptase resistance mutations detected at the index resistance test (grouping ≥ 9 mutations).

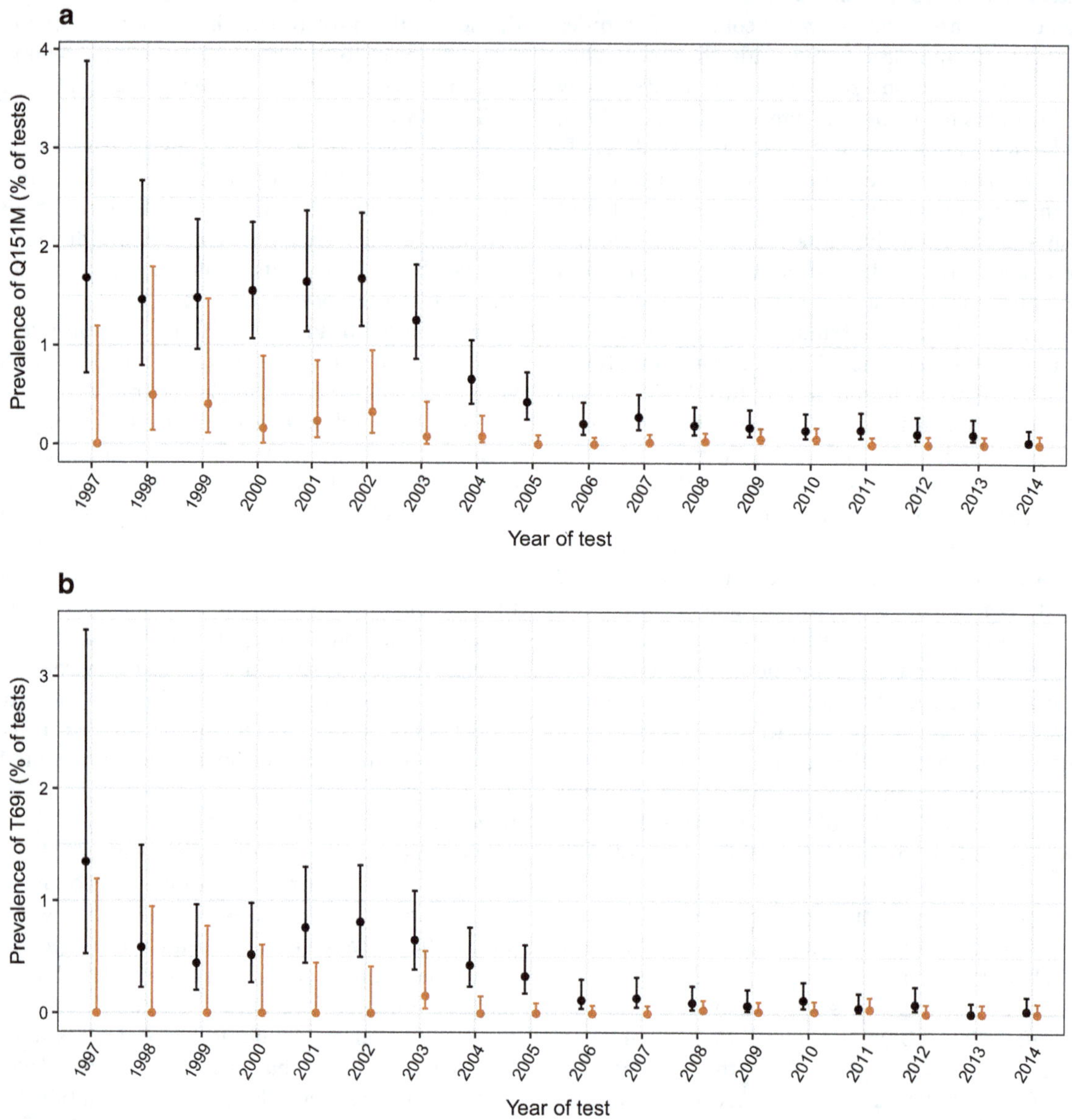

Fig. 1 Prevalence of (**a**) the Q151M mutation and (**b**) the T69i mutation per patient by calendar year of sequencing (patients can be included in multiple calendar years, but are only counted once per year), according to whether the patient was ART experienced (black circle) or naïve (orange circle) at the time of blood sample. The denominator in each year is the total number of patients with at least one reverse transcriptase sequence recorded in that year. Binomial 95% CIs are shown

Results

Q151M

A total of 180 patients with at least one observation of the Q151M mutation were recorded in the UK-HDRD, out of a total of 80,281 patients with at least one resistance test. At first observation of the Q151M mutation, 18 (10%) patients were recorded as being ART-naïve, 139 (77%) as experienced and 23 (13%) as 'not classified'. Figure 1a shows the prevalence of the Q151M mutation by calendar year according to whether the patient was ART experienced or naïve at the time of blood sample. The prevalence of the mutation was consistently low in ART-naïve patients, with a maximum of 0.5% (2/402) of patients in 1998, whilst in ART-experienced patients there was a fall in prevalence from 1.7% (33/1966) in 2002 to 0.2% (8/3376) 2006 and then to 0.027% (1/3733) in 2014.

Table 1 provides a summary of the associated major reverse transcriptase mutations at first observation of the Q151M mutation in each of the affected patients. Only

Table 1 Summary table for associated mutations for Q151M (*n* = 180 patients)

	n (%)
Q151M isolated major RT mutation	5 (3)
Q151M accessory mutations[a]	
0	38 (25)
1	50 (32)
2	14 (9)
3	33 (21)
4	20 (13)
NRTI major mutations other than Q151M	
0	20 (11)
1	44 (24)
2	45 (25)
3	32 (18)
4	24 (13)
5	14 (8)
6	1 (1)
TAMs present[b]	
0	82 (46)
1	40 (22)
2	18 (10)
3	23 (13)
4	15 (8)
5	2 (1)
NNRTI major mutations	
0	35 (19)
1	43 (24)
2	64 (36)
3	24 (13)
4	11 (6)
5	3 (2)
PI major mutations[c]	
0	108 (60)
1	33 (18)
2	14 (8)
3	10 (6)
4	9 (5)
5	1 (1)
6	4 (2)
Number of classes with resistance[d]	
1	17 (9)
2	110 (61)
3	53 (29)

[a] Including A62V, V75I, F77L and F116Y, data available for 155 patients

[b] M41L, D67N, K70R, L210W, T215Y/F and K219Q/E

[c] PI PCR failed in one case.

[d] Of NRTI, NNRTI and PI. A full list of mutations and further information regarding associated K65R mutations are provided in Additional file 1

3% of patients showed no other mutation, and the most common associated major reverse transcriptase mutations were M184V (47%), K103N (35%) and K65R (29%). Data regarding accessory mutations to Q151M [12, 13] were available in 155 (86%) patients: A62V was present in 49 (32%), V75I in 62 (40%), F77L in 47 (30%) and F116Y in 99 (64%), and 75% of patients showed at least one accessory mutation.

Of the patients in whom the Q151M mutation was detected, 96 could be linked to clinical data. Of these patients, 82 (85%) were recorded as ART-experienced and one as 'not classified', with 13 being ART-naïve. Information regarding the ART regimen prior to the resistance test was available in 74/82 (90.2%) of the ART-experienced patients, and these 74 patients were included in the matched case–control analysis to investigate factors associated with the occurrence of the mutation (Fig. 2a). For the final fitted model, the strongest evidence for a positive association was for 'total years of virological failure' (standardised odds ratio (sOR), 95% credibility interval (CrI) 2.39, 1.52–3.82; OR of 2.92 on original scale (years)), followed by 'years of virological failure on D4T' (sOR 1.80, 1.28–2.59; OR of 1.68 on original scale), whilst 'current' treatment using a rbPI showed a negative association (OR 0.28, 0.08–0.79) with occurrence of the mutation (Fig. 2a). There was not strong evidence of any positive or negative association with viral subtype (results in Additional file 1).

In 62/96 (65%) patients, a confirmed undetectable VL was observed (at any point) following the detection of the Q151M mutation at a median of 1.0 (IQR 0.5–2.3) years from the date of the resistance test sample. For a total of 62 patients there were data on change to ART regimen after detection of the Q151M mutation and before viral re-suppression (for patients in whom this occurred), but six of these patients were missing a baseline CD4 cell count (three were also missing baseline VL) and so were dropped from the Cox analysis. Hence, 56 patients were included in the Cox analysis, with a total of 22 events (confirmed viral suppression) observed before censoring. Higher baseline VL (prior to new ART regimen) showed a substantial negative association with the probability of viral suppression (standardised hazard ratio (sHR) 0.32, 0.14–0.64; HR of 0.30 on original scale of $\log_{10}$ copies/mL) as did use of DDI (21/56 patients; HR 0.12, 0.02–0.61), whilst the use of a rbPI showed a positive association (31/57 patients; HR 4.62, 1.03–30.88) (Fig. 2b). The model also indicated that TDF use is likely to be associated with suppression, although this result is not definitive. Information regarding the presence or absence of

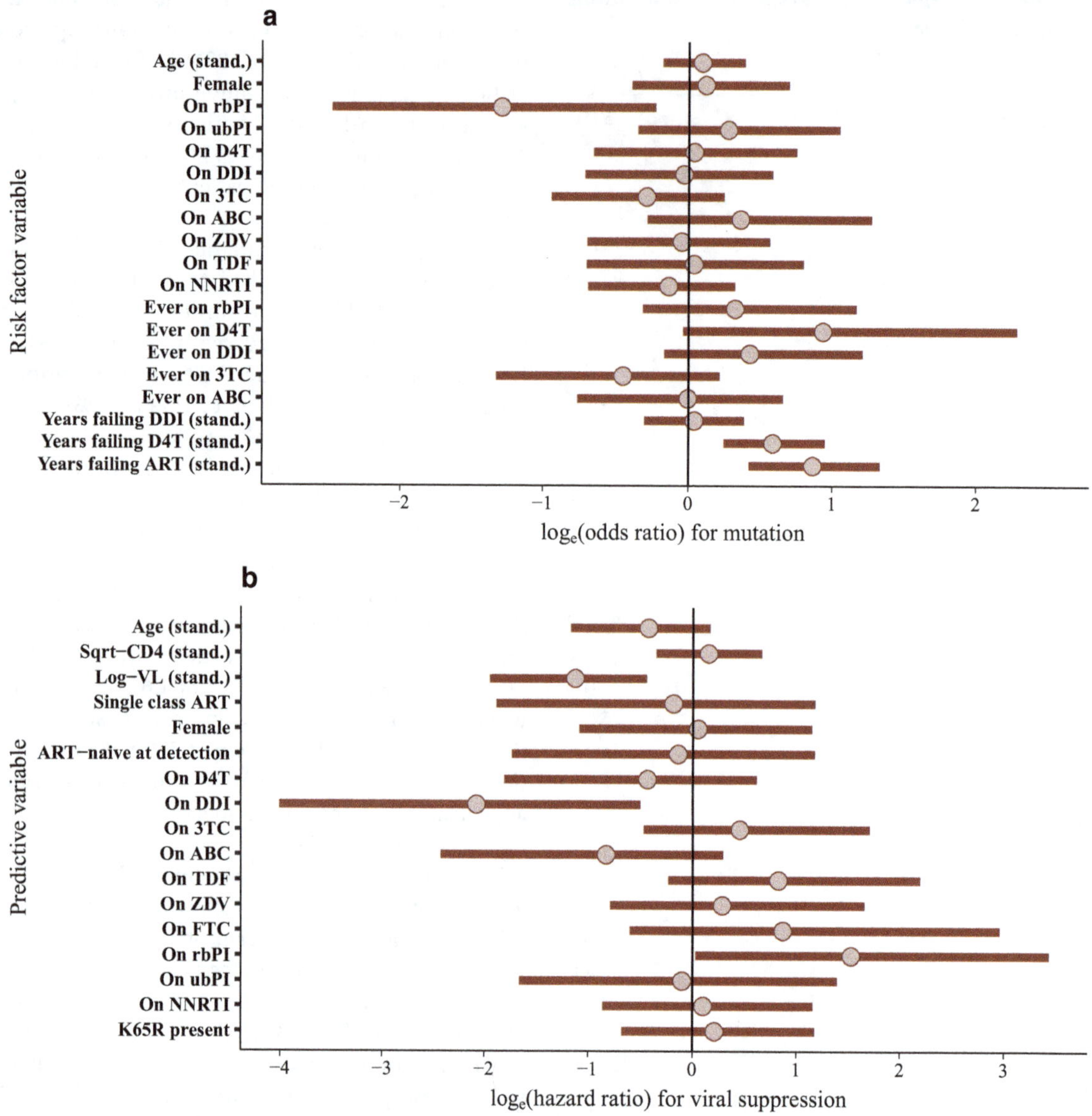

Fig. 2 Posterior mean values and 95% credibility intervals for (**a**) log-odds ratios in the matched case–control analysis investigating factors associated with the occurrence of the Q151M mutation and (**b**) log-hazard ratios in the Cox regression for confirmed viral suppression following treatment change after detection of Q151M mutation. Continuous variables were standardised (stand.), by subtracting the mean and dividing by SD, for these analyses. The results presented are from multivariable models in each case

accessory mutations was available for 46 of these patients, but no strong evidence of an association with success of viral suppression was found. An additional analysis was conducted accounting for resistance to PI drugs used in rbPI regimens, with no notable change in the results obtained and no detected reduction in viral suppression when PI resistance was present (further details in Additional file 1).

A model was fitted to assess the durability of viral suppression that included parameters for baseline VL, rbPI and DDI use. This analysis indicated that the durability of viral suppression was good for patients with low baseline VL, but that the overall probability of suppression was worse for patients with higher baseline VL values (Fig. 3).

For the matched cohort analysis of mortality, 72 patients with and 665 patients without the Q151M mutation were included. Higher age and lower CD4 count were strongly associated with mortality, but no clear association with the number of reverse transcriptase resistance mutations was observed. There was no evidence that presence of the Q151M mutation was associated with increased mortality (HR 1.25, 95% CrI

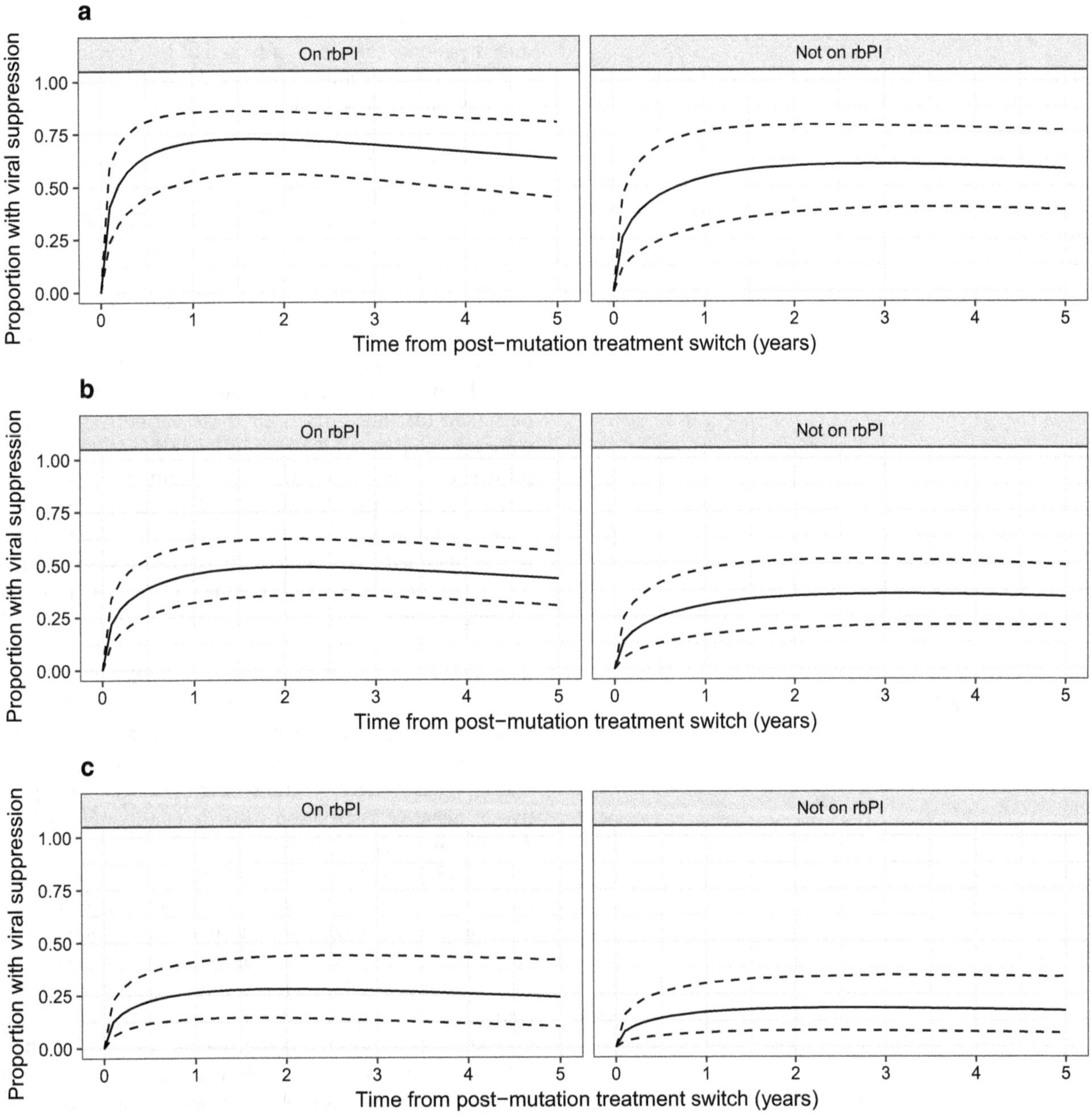

Fig. 3 Modelled probability of viral suppression in ART-experienced patients in terms of time since treatment switch following detection of the Q151M mutation for patients with a baseline viral load of (**a**) 2000 copies/mL (≈10th centile), (**b**) 40,000 copies/mL (≈50th centile) or (**c**) 500,000 copies/mL (≈90th centile). Response is modelled according to presence or absence of a ritonavir-boosted protease inhibitor in the ART regimen at time zero, but patients were not censored at change to drug regimen in this analysis. The expected probability (solid line) and 95% credibility interval (dashed lines) from Bayesian fitting of sequential Weibull models for viral suppression and rebound are shown. DDI use was adjusted for in this analysis, but results are shown for patients not on DDI

0.84–2.1). In patients with Q151M, most deaths occurred amongst those with CD4 count < 100 cells/μL (12 deaths/24 patients vs 6/54 for patients with CD4 ≥ 100 cells/μL, further details in Additional file 1).

T69i

A total of 85 patients with at least one detection of the T69i mutation are present in the UK-HDRD. At first observation of the T69i mutation, seven (8.2%) patients were recorded as being ART-naïve, 69 (81.2%) as

Table 2 Summary table for associated mutations for T69i (*n* = 85 patients)

	n (%)
T69i isolated major RT mutation	2 (2)
T69i associated mutations[a]	
0	16 (19)
1	14 (16)
2	33 (39)
3	22 (26)
NRTI major mutations other than T69i	
0	2 (2)
1	8 (9)
2	19 (22)
3	36 (42)
4	15 (18)
5	2 (2)
6	3 (4)
TAMs present[b]	
0	4 (5)
1	8 (9)
2	37 (44)
3	29 (34)
4	6 (7)
5	1 (1)
NNRTI major mutations	
0	34 (40)
1	10 (12)
2	26 (31)
3	13 (15)
4	2 (2)
PI major mutations	
0	45 (53)
1	10 (12)
2	16 (19)
3	9 (11)
4	4 (45)
5	0 (0)
6	1 (1)
Number of classes with resistance[c]	
1	20 (24)
2	39 (46)
3	26 (31)

[a] TAMs at codons 41, 210 or 215

[b] M41L, D67N, K70R, L210W, T215Y/F and K219Q/E

[c] Of NRTI, NNRTI and PI. A full list of mutations is provided in Additional file 1

experienced and nine (10.6%) as 'not classified'. Figure 1b shows the prevalence of the T69i mutation per patient by calendar year according to whether the patient was ART experienced or naïve at the time of blood sample. Similar to Q151M, the prevalence of the mutation was consistently very low in ART-naïve patients, with a maximum of 0.15% (2/1311) in 2003, whilst in ART-experienced patients there was a large fall in prevalence from 0.8% (16/1966) in 2002 to 0.1% (4/3376) in 2006 and then to 0.03% (1/3734) in 2014.

Table 2 provides a summary of the associated major reverse transcriptase mutations at first observation of the T69i mutation in each of the affected patients. Thymidine analogue mutations (TAMs) were most frequently seen, with TAM1 mutations (M41L, L210W and T215Y) being most common. In combination with the T69i, these mutations have been linked to high level resistance to all NRTIs [12]; 63/85 (74.1%) of the patients were observed to have at least one of these mutations present.

Of the patients with T69i mutation detected, 45 could be linked to clinical data. Of these patients, 39 (86.7%) were recorded as ART-experienced and six as naïve. Full information regarding the ART regimen prior to the resistance test was available in 36/39 (92.3%) of the ART-experienced patients, and these 36 patients were included in the matched case–control analysis to investigate factors associated with the occurrence of the mutation. For the final fitted model, only 'total years of virological failure' showed a substantial positive association with the occurrence of the T69i mutation (standardised odds ratio (sOR), 95% CrI 2.16, 1.34–3.60; OR of 3.48 on original scale (years)), although there was also some evidence for a positive association with 'DDI use ever' (OR 1.73, 0.86–5.16) (Fig. 4a). There was no strong evidence of any positive or negative association with viral subtype (results in Additional file 1).

In 33/45 (73.3%) patients, at least one confirmed undetectable VL was observed (at any point) following the detection of the T69i mutation at a median of 1.5 (IQR 0.5–2.2) years from the date of the resistance test blood sample. For a total of 31 patients there were data on change to ART regimen after detection of the T69i mutation and before viral re-suppression, but five of these patients were missing both baseline CD4 cell count and VL (prior to new ART regimen) and so were dropped from the Cox analysis. Hence, 26 patients were included, with a total of 12 events (confirmed viral suppression) observed before censoring. Higher baseline $\log_{10}$(VL) showed a substantial negative association with the probability of viral suppression (sHR 0.016, 0.00–0.54; HR of 0.024 on original scale of $\log_{10}$ copies/mL), as did the use of D4T (HR 0.010, 0.00–0.88). 3TC (HR 0.021, 0.00–1.02) also showed some evidence of a negative association (Fig. 4b), possibly attributable to the inclusion of two patients on 3TC monotherapy. Very wide credibility intervals were observed for the HR values for several drugs, reflecting the limited data available. There was no strong evidence that linked TAMs were associated

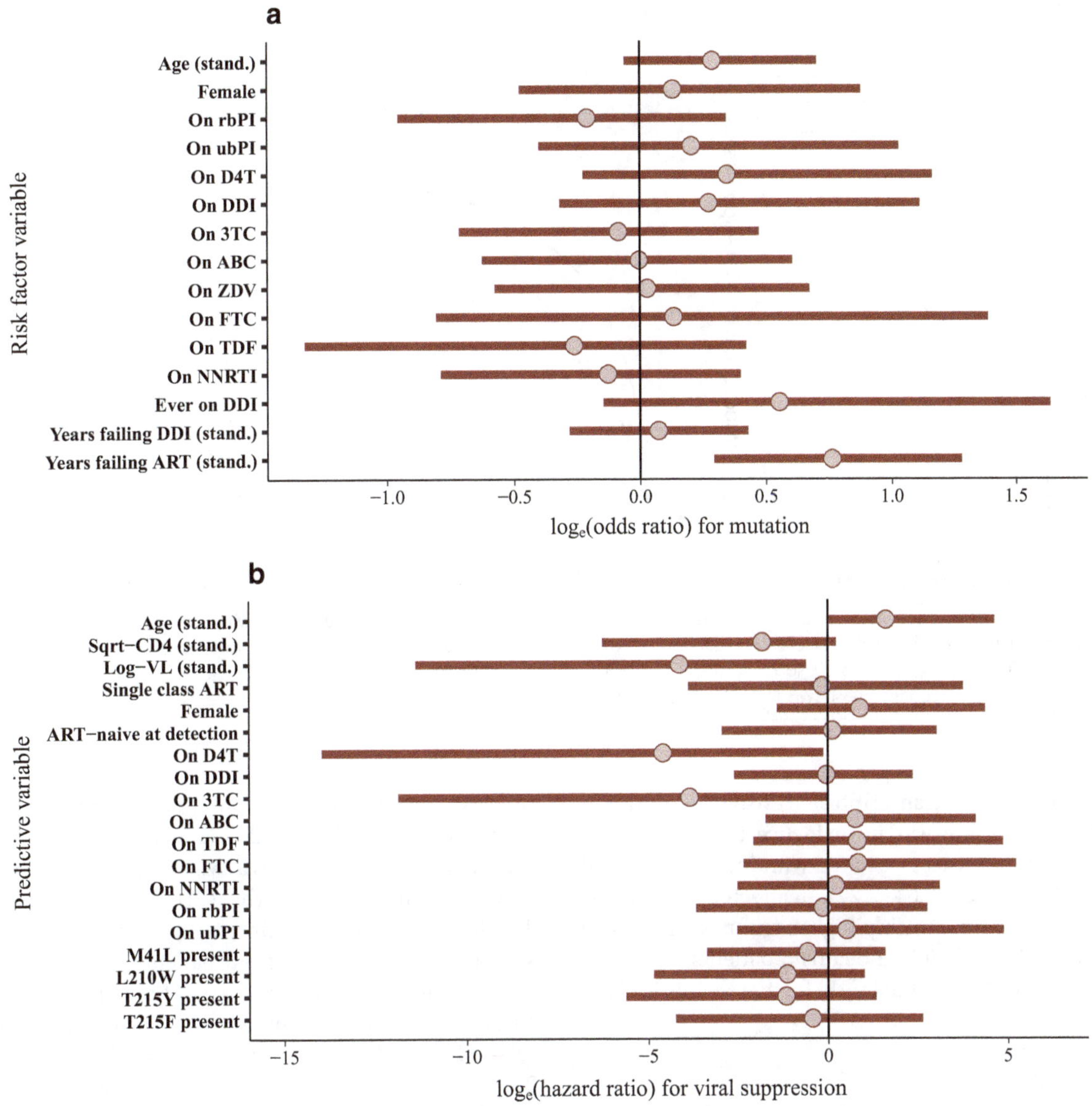

Fig. 4 Posterior mean values and 95% credibility intervals for (**a**) log-odds ratios in the matched case–control analysis investigating factors associated with the occurrence of the T69 insertion mutation and (**b**) log-hazard ratios in the Cox regression for confirmed viral suppression following treatment change after detection of T69 insertion mutation. Continuous variables were standardised (stand.), by subtracting the mean and dividing by SD, for these analyses. The results presented are from multivariable models in each case

with the probability of viral suppression, although negative effects cannot be ruled out, and there were no cases with a K65R mutation included in this analysis. There is some evidence that single amino acid insertions may be associated with a lower level of NRTI resistance [32] and so a sensitivity analysis was conducted only considering multiple amino acid insertions; the results obtained did not show any substantial differences in comparison to the main analysis (details in Additional file 1).

A model was fitted to assess the durability of viral suppression that included parameters for baseline VL and D4T use. This analysis indicated that the durability of viral suppression was good for patients with low baseline VL, but that the overall probability of suppression was worse for patients with higher baseline VL values (Fig. 5). The wide 95% credibility intervals for the modelled probability of viral suppression in each plot reflect the small sample size for this analysis.

For the matched cohort analysis of mortality, 35 patients with and 294 patients without the T69i mutation were included. Lower CD4 count was strongly associated with mortality, but no clear association with the

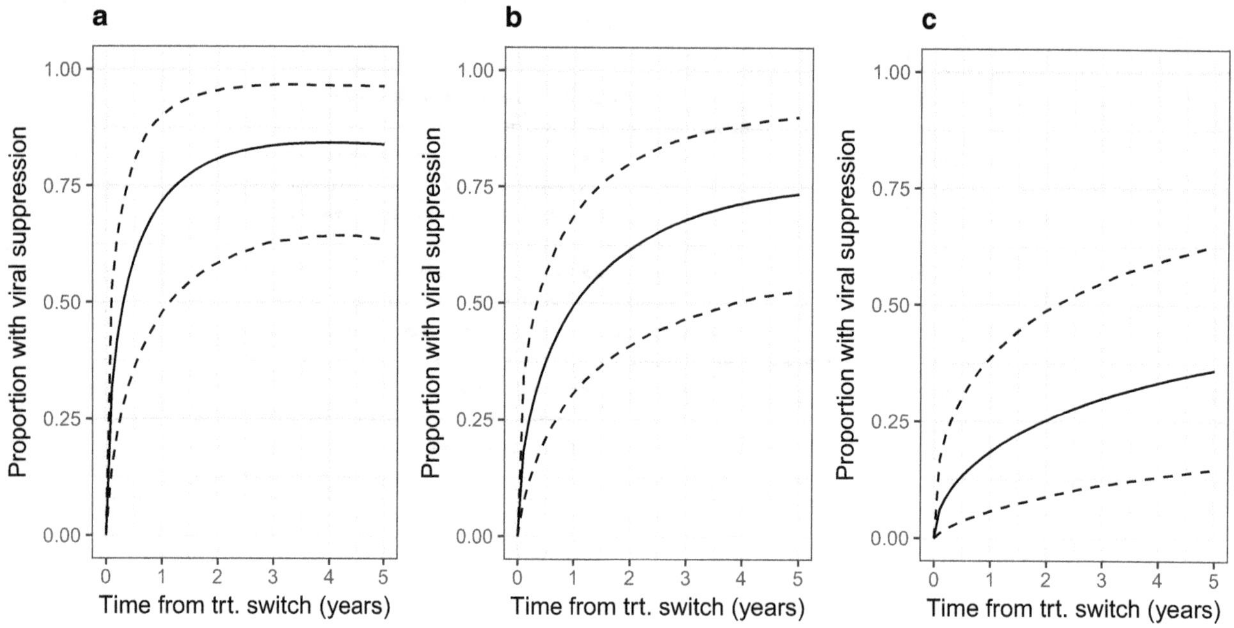

Fig. 5 Modelled probability of viral suppression in ART-experienced patients in terms of time since treatment switch following detection of the T69i mutation for patients with a baseline viral load of (**a**) 2000 copies/mL (≈ 10th centile), (**b**) 10,000 copies/mL (≈50th centile) or (**c**) 225,000 copies/mL (≈90th centile). The expected probability (solid line) and 95% credibility interval (dashed lines) from Bayesian fitting of sequential Weibull models for viral suppression and rebound are shown. D4T use was adjusted for in this analysis, but results are shown for patients not on D4T

number of reverse transcriptase resistance mutations was observed. There was no evidence that presence of the T69i mutation was associated with increased mortality (HR 1.12, 95% CrI 0.64–2.22). In affected patients, the hazard of death was notably higher amongst those with CD4 count < 100 cells/μL (2 deaths/3 patients vs 3/34 for patients with CD4 ≥ 100 cells/μL, further details in Additional file 1).

Discussion

We have found that the prevalence of multi-drug resistance mutations Q151M and T69i has declined to almost zero in the UK and, as such, it is likely that observation of these mutations will now be very rare in any high-income country. However, the more recent introduction of widespread ART in LMICs has been associated with an increase in transmitted drug resistance [33] and whilst it may be expected that the phase-out of older drug regimens [24] and improved access to VL monitoring [11] will lead to an eventual reduction, the overall levels of drug resistance have yet to show such a decline [34]. Our analysis regarding the risk factors and outcomes associated with these mutations may therefore be relevant for drug resistance monitoring and clinical management of any observed cases in such settings.

Marked declines in prevalence were observed for both Q151M and T69i in the period 2003–2006, but even in the years before this these mutations were relatively rare amongst patients failing ART (1.5–1.7% for Q151M and 0.4–1.3% for T69i) and Q151M was even rarer in ART-naïve patients (0–0.5%) whilst T69i was not observed. The levels amongst treatment-experienced patients are similar to those in subtype-B patients in the Swiss HIV Cohort Study, for which Scherrer et al. reported an overall prevalence up to February 2010 of 0.8 and 0.5% for Q151M and T69i, respectively [14]. In the period 2010–2014 the prevalence of Q151M in treatment-experienced patients undergoing viral sequencing stabilised at around 0.1% in the UK cohort, equating to an average of four cases per year, whilst the prevalence of T69i was even lower in this period at 0.04% (an average of 1.5 patients per year).

Patients who received ART in the earlier years of the HIV epidemic in the UK were treated using a wide variety of drug combinations, with changes often implemented as new drugs became available. The very high level of complexity of treatment histories for HIV hampers epidemiological investigation of risk factors for the occurrence of specific resistance mutations, particularly for the analysis of rare mutations such as Q151M and T69i. There are also equivalent issues to consider when analysing response to treatment conditional on patient characteristics and ART regimen. We were concerned that the analysis of a large number of potential risk (or predictive) factors with a small number of cases would lead to a high risk of false-positive results, and so we chose to carry out our analyses using a Bayesian framework that would penalise estimates of effect sizes without substantial evidence in the data; this approach also has the advantage that results regarding estimation of effect sizes can be interpreted in a directly probabilistic manner rather than purely dichotomised into present or absent.

Q151M

We found strong associations between D4T exposure and emergence of the Q151M mutation, a link previously identified by Nouhin et al. [15] who found the mutation in 14% (47/328) of patients failing a D4T-containing regimen with at least one resistance mutation present. Tang et al. found a prevalence for Q151M of 4.6% in a review of 1825 patients failing D4T-containing first-line ART [22] drawn largely from LMICs, considerably higher than the peak prevalence observed in the UK. The association with D4T was not identified by Scherrer et al. [14], but their cohort included a relatively small sample of 25 cases of the mutation. A secondary analysis of the EARNEST Trial found a much higher prevalence of Q151M amongst subtype-C patients failing first-line ART (11% vs negligible for other non-B subtypes) [23]. However, in their sample D4T use at failure was much higher (66%) in subtype-C patients than in others (7% when pooled), so this seems likely to have driven the observed difference.

D4T has been subject to a global phase-out over recent years, with a drop in total market share for NRTI use in adults from 29% in 2011 to just 0.2% in 2016 [24], and as such it can be expected that the emergence of this mutation will have undergone a corresponding decrease over this period. However, it is possible that the mutation may persist in a substantial number of patients whilst virological monitoring is limited.

The overall level of confirmed viral suppression (62/96:65%) was similar to that reported by Scherrer et al. (14/25:56%) [14]. We observed that rbPI use showed both a strong negative association with the emergence of the Q151M mutation and a strong association with viral suppression following detection of the mutation, suggesting that this may be a particularly effective treatment option for affected patients. The relative success of rbPI regimens despite broad NRTI resistance is consistent with the findings of secondary analyses of the SECOND-LINE [25] and EARNEST [26] trials of patients failing first-line NNRTI+NRTI regimens, in which those with NRTI resistance switched to rbPI+NRTI regimens showed better virological outcomes than those without resistance mutations. The fact that patients without resistance performed worse on second-line therapy in these studies could be the result of worse adherence within this group, but the results nonetheless indicate that rbPI regimens can be very successful despite viral resistance to the NRTI backbone.

We should note that owing to the historic nature of the cases described, no patients were switched to an integrase inhibitor regimen directly following detection of the mutation and so we have not provided any information on the relative efficacy of this drug class. Our models indicate that virological outcomes were substantially better for patients that had lower baseline VL at detection of the mutation, but it may now be possible to achieve better outcomes for patients with high VL using modern ART regimens.

We did not find evidence that presence of the Q151M mutation is associated with increased risk of mortality relative to comparable patients matched on ART initiation and resistance testing dates, but it is not possible to draw strong conclusions from the limited data available. Mortality outcomes will also be dependent on the availability of effective ART options, and rbPI regimens may not always be available in LMICs. Scherrer et al. [14] assessed mortality with matching to control patients with ≥ 3 TAMs, and in a multivariable model found a non-statistically significant but potentially strong association with the hazard of death (HR 7.5, 95% CI 0.9–64.6). In combination, these results are consistent with the Q151M mutation possibly being associated with the risk of death, but there is once again the caveat that the link could disappear with more modern ART regimens.

T69i

Recent data from LMICs has indicated that T69i remains a rare mutation, for example Tang et al. identified only two cases (0.1%) in a review of 1825 patients failing D4T-containing first-line ART [22] (this study also included a small minority of patients from the USA and Europe) and Villabona-Arenas et al. found four cases (0.3%) amongst 1599 patients failing first-line ART (ZDV/D4T+3TC+NVP/EFZ) from 10 West and Central African countries [19]. Scherrer et al. found an association between years spent receiving DDI and emergence of the T69i mutation [14]; we also found some evidence for this link, but we only found a definitive association for total years on ART with virological failure. However, it should be noted that Scherrer et al. carried out an analysis matched against patients with ≥ 3 TAMs, whereas we matched on the basis of ART-start date. The rationale for our choice was to allow investigation of factors associated with appearance of the mutation using comparable patients without requiring the controls to have also failed treatment. As has been reported previously, we found that TAM1 mutations were found in most patients with T69i [35].

The baseline VL prior to treatment switch (or initiation in ART-naïve patients) and continued D4T use were the strongest (negative) predictors of subsequent virological suppression, but the small sample size and large number of potentially important factors made it impossible to rule out important associations with other variables including drug choices and associated mutations. The overall level of confirmed viral suppression (33/45:73%) was very similar to that reported by Scherrer et al. (9/13:69%) [14]. As for the Q151M, we should note that improved outcomes may be possible using modern ART regimens. We did not find any evidence that the T69i was associated with increased mortality, consistent with the findings of Scherrer et al. [14], although we should again note that it is not possible to form strong conclusions given the limited data.

Conclusions

Our data confirm that modern ART and laboratory monitoring have greatly reduced the occurrence of multi-NRTI resistance due to T69i and Q151M in the UK, a change that is very likely to have also occurred in other developed countries. It remains to be seen whether similar progress can be achieved in LMICs. In addition this report demonstrates that ART regimen changes can be successful despite these mutations, although whether outcomes in patients with the poorest prognosis can be improved with more modern ART regimens also remains to be determined.

Abbreviations

3TC: lamivudine; ABC: abacavir; AIDS: acquired immune deficiency syndrome; ART: antiretroviral therapy; CRF: circulating recombinant form; CrI: credibility interval; D4T: stavudine; DDI: didanosine; FTC: emtricitabine; HIV: human immunodeficiency virus; HR: hazard ratio; LMICs: low- and middle-income countries; NNRTIs: non-nucleoside/nucleotide reverse transcriptase inhibitors; NRTIs: nucleoside/nucleotide reverse transcriptase inhibitors; OR: odds ratio; PI: protease inhibitor; rbPI: ritonavir-boosted PI; sHR: standardised HR; sOR: standardised OR; T69i: T69 insertion; TAMs: thymidine analogue mutations; TDF: tenofovir; ubPI: un-boosted PI; UK CHIC: UK Collaborative HIV Cohort; UK-HDRD: UK HIV Drug Resistance Database; VL: viral load; ZDV: zidovudine.

Authors' contributions

PC conceived the study and planned the analysis in conjunction with OTS and DTD. OTS carried out statistical analyses, with AT assisting in data preparation and processing. CS, AP, DA, AC, CO and FM were all involved in development of the datasets used and all contributed to interpretation of the results of statistical analyses in the context of existing scientific literature. OTS and PC wrote the first draft of the manuscript, with all other authors providing revisions. All authors read and approved the final manuscript.

Author details

[1] Centre for Clinical Research in Infection and Sexual Health, Institute for Global Health, University College London, London, UK. [2] Centre for Clinical Research, Epidemiology, Modelling and Evaluation, Institute for Global Health, University College London, Royal Free Campus, London, UK. [3] Chelsea and Westminster Hospital NHS Foundation Trust, London, UK. [4] Infection and Immunity laboratory, Charing Cross Hospital, London, UK. [5] Barts Health NHS Trust, London, UK. [6] Hull York Medical School, University of York, York, UK. [7] Faculty of Medicine, University of Queensland, Brisbane, Australia. [8] High Containment Microbiology, Public Health England, Salisbury, UK.

Acknowledgements

UK HIV Drug Resistance Database

Steering Committee:
David Asboe, Anton Pozniak (Chelsea & Westminster Hospital, London); Patricia Cane (Public Health England, Porton Down); David Chadwick (South Tees Hospitals NHS Trust, Middlesbrough); Duncan Churchill (Brighton and Sussex University Hospitals NHS Trust); Duncan Clark (Barts Health NHS Trust, London); Simon Collins (HIV i-Base, London); Valerie Delpech (National Infection Service, Public Health England); Samuel Douthwaite (Guy's and St. Thomas' NHS Foundation Trust, London); David Dunn, Esther Fearnhill, Kholoud Porter, Anna Tostevin, Oliver Stirrup (Institute for Global Health, UCL); Christophe Fraser (University of Oxford); Anna Maria Geretti (Institute of Infection and Global Health, University of Liverpool); Rory Gunson (Gartnavel General Hospital, Glasgow); Antony Hale (Leeds Teaching Hospitals NHS Trust); Stéphane Hué (London School of Hygiene and Tropical Medicine); Steve Kaye (Imperial College, London); Linda Lazarus (Expert Advisory Group on AIDS Secretariat, Public Health England); Andrew Leigh-Brown (University of Edinburgh); Tamyo Mbisa (National Infection Service, Public Health England); Nicola Mackie (Imperial NHS Trust, London); Samuel Moses (King's College Hospital, London); Chloe Orkin (Barts Health NHS Trust, London); Eleni Nastouli, Deenan Pillay, Andrew Phillips, Caroline Sabin (University College London, London); Erasmus Smit (Public Health England, Birmingham Heartlands Hospital); Kate Templeton (Royal Infirmary of Edinburgh); Peter Tilston (Manchester Royal Infirmary); Ian Williams (Mortimer Market Centre, London); Hongyi Zhang (Addenbrooke's Hospital, Cambridge).

Coordinating Centre:
Institute for Global Health, UCL (David Dunn, Keith Fairbrother, Esther Fearnhill, Kholoud Porter, Anna Tostevin, Oliver Stirrup).

Centres contributing data:
Clinical Microbiology and Public Health Laboratory, Addenbrooke's Hospital, Cambridge (Jane Greatorex); Guy's and St Thomas' NHS Foundation Trust, London (Siobhan O'Shea, Jane Mullen); PHE – Public Health Laboratory, Birmingham Heartlands Hospital, Birmingham (Erasmus Smit); Antiviral Unit, National Infection Service, Public Health England, London (Tamyo Mbisa); Imperial College Health NHS Trust, London (Alison Cox); King's College Hospital, London (Richard Tandy); Medical Microbiology Laboratory, Leeds Teaching Hospitals NHS Trust (Tracy Fawcett); Specialist Virology Centre, Liverpool (Mark Hopkins); Department of Clinical Virology, Manchester Royal Infirmary, Manchester (Peter Tilston); Department of Virology, Royal Free Hospital, London (Clare Booth, Ana Garcia-Diaz); Edinburgh Specialist Virology Centre, Royal Infirmary of Edinburgh (Lynne Renwick); Department of Infection & Tropical Medicine, Royal Victoria Infirmary, Newcastle (Matthias L Schmid, Brendan Payne); South Tees Hospitals NHS Trust, Middlesbrough (David Chadwick); Department of Virology, Barts Health NHS Trust, London (Duncan Clark, Jonathan Hubb); Molecular Diagnostic Unit, Imperial College, London (Steve Kaye); University College London Hospitals (Stuart Kirk); West of Scotland Specialist Virology Laboratory, Gartnavel, Glasgow (Rory Gunson, Amanda Bradley-Stewart).

UK Collaborative HIV Cohort

Steering Committee:
Jonathan Ainsworth, Sris Allan, Jane Anderson, Abdel Babiker, David Chadwick, Duncan Churchill, Valerie Delpech, David Dunn, Brian Gazzard, Richard Gilson, Mark Gompels, Phillip Hay, Teresa Hill, Margaret Johnson, Sophie Jose, Stephen Kegg, Clifford Leen, Fabiola Martin, Dushyant Mital, Mark Nelson, Chloe Orkin, Adrian Palfreeman, Andrew Phillips, Deenan Pillay, Frank Post, Jillian Pritchard, Caroline Sabin, Achim Schwenk, Anjum Tariq, Roy Trevelion, Andy Ustianowski, John Walsh.

Central Co-ordination:
University College London (Teresa Hill, Sophie Jose, Andrew Phillips, Caroline Sabin, Alicia Thornton, Susie Huntington); Medical Research Council Clinical Trials Unit at UCL, London (David Dunn, Adam Glabay, Shaadi Shidfar).

Participating Centres:
Barts Health NHS Trust, London (Chloe Orkin, Janet Lynch, James Hand, Carl de Souza); Brighton and Sussex University Hospitals NHS Trust (Duncan Churchill, Nicky Perry, Stuart Tilbury, Elaney Youssef, Duncan Churchill); Chelsea and Westminster Hospital NHS Foundation Trust, London (Brian Gazzard, Mark Nelson, Tracey Mabika, David Asboe, Sundhiya Mandalia); Homerton University Hospital NHS Trust, London (Jane Anderson, Sajid Munshi); King's College Hospital NHS Foundation Trust, London (Frank Post, Ade Adefisan, Chris Taylor, Zachary Gleisner, Fowzia Ibrahim, Lucy Campbell); Middlesbrough, South Tees Hospitals NHS Foundation Trust, (David Chadwick, Kirsty Baillie); Mortimer Market Centre, Central and North West London NHS Foundation Trust/University College London (Richard Gilson, Nataliya Brima, Ian Williams); North Middlesex University Hospital NHS Trust, London (Jonathan Ainsworth, Achim Schwenk, Sheila Miller, Chris Wood); Royal Free NHS Foundation Trust/University College London (Margaret Johnson, Mike Youle, Fiona Lampe, Colette Smith, Rob Tsintas, Clinton Chaloner, Samantha Hutchinson, Caroline Sabin, Andrew Phillips, Teresa Hill, Sophie Jose, Susie Huntington, Alicia Thornton); Imperial College Healthcare NHS Trust, London (John Walsh, Nicky Mackie, Alan Winston, Jonathan Weber, Farhan Ramzan, Mark Carder); The Lothian University Hospitals NHS Trust, Edinburgh (Clifford Leen, Alan Wilson, Sheila Morris); North Bristol NHS Trust (Mark Gompels, Sue Allan); Leicester, University Hospitals of Leicester NHS Trust (Adrian Palfreeman, Adam Lewszuk); Woolwich, Lewisham and Greenwich NHS Trust (Stephen Kegg, Akin Faleye, Victoria Ogunbiyi, Sue Mitchell), St. George's Healthcare NHS Trust (Phillip Hay, Christian Kemble); York Teaching Hospital NHS Foundation Trust (Fabiola Martin, Sarah Russell-Sharpe, Janet Gravely); Coventry, University Hospitals Coventry and Warwickshire NHS Trust (Sris Allan, Andrew Harte); Wolverhampton, The Royal Wolverhampton Hospitals NHS Trust (Anjum Tariq, Hazel Spencer, Ron Jones); Chertsey, Ashford and St. Peter's Hospitals NHS Foundation Trust (Jillian Pritchard, Shirley Cumming, Claire Atkinson); Milton Keynes Hospital NHS Foundation Trust (Dushyant Mital, Veronica Edgell, Julie Allen); The Pennine Acute Hospitals NHS Trust (Andy Ustianowski, Cynthia Murphy, Ilise Gunder); Public Health England, London (Valerie Delpech); i-Base (Roy Trevelion).

Competing interests
The authors declare that they have no competing interests.

Funding
This work was supported by the UK Medical Research Council (Award Number 164587). The funder supports maintenance and analysis of the UK-HDRD, but was not directly involved in the planning or write-up of this analysis.

References
1. UK HIV Drug Resistance Database. HIV drug resistance in the UK. 2017. http://www.hivrdb.org.uk/hiv-drug-resistance-uk. Accessed 13 Sept 2017.
2. Rocheleau G, Brumme CJ, Shoveller J, Lima V, Harrigan P. Longitudinal trends of HIV drug resistance in a large Canadian cohort, 1996–2016. Clin Microbiol Infect. 2018;24:185–91.
3. De Luca A, Dunn D, Zazzi M, Camacho R, Torti C, Fanti I, et al. Declining prevalence of HIV-1 drug resistance in antiretroviral treatment-exposed individuals in Western Europe. J Infect Dis. 2013;207:1216–20.
4. Scherrer AU, von Wyl V, Yang W-L, Kouyos RD, Böni J, Yerly S, et al. Emergence of acquired HIV-1 drug resistance almost stopped in Switzerland: a 15-year prospective cohort analysis. Clin Infect Dis. 2016;62:1310–7.
5. Ssemwanga D, Lihana RW, Ugoji C, Al Abimiku, Nkengasong J, Dakum P, et al. Update on HIV-1 acquired and transmitted drug resistance in Africa. AIDS Rev. 2015;17:3–20.
6. Stadeli KM, Richman DD. Rates of emergence of HIV drug resistance in resource-limited settings: a systematic review. Antivir Ther. 2013;18:115.
7. Phillips AN, Stover J, Cambiano V, Nakagawa F, Jordan MR, Pillay D, et al. Impact of HIV drug resistance on HIV/AIDS-associated mortality, new infections, and antiretroviral therapy program costs in Sub-Saharan Africa. J Infect Dis. 2017;215:1362–5.
8. Gupta RK, Hill A, Sawyer AW, Cozzi-Lepri A, von Wyl V, Yerly S, et al. Virological monitoring and resistance to first-line highly active antiretroviral therapy in adults infected with HIV-1 treated under WHO guidelines: a systematic review and meta-analysis. Lancet Infect Dis. 2009;9:409–17.
9. Rowley C, MacLeod I, Maruapula D, Lekoko B, Gaseitsiwe S, Mine M, et al. Sharp increase in rates of HIV transmitted drug resistance at antenatal clinics in Botswana demonstrates the need for routine surveillance. J Antimicrob Chemother. 2016;71:1361–6.
10. Roberts T, Cohn J, Bonner K, Hargreaves S. Scale-up of routine viral load testing in resource-poor settings: current and future implementation challenges. Clin Infect Dis. 2016;62:1043–8.
11. WHO. Global action plan on HIV drug resistance 2017–2021. Geneva: WHO; 2017.
12. Wensing AM, Calvez V, Günthard HF, Johnson VA, Paredes R, Pillay D, et al. 2017 update of the drug resistance mutations in HIV-1. Topics Antivir Med. 2017;24:132–41.
13. Stanford University Drug Resistance Database. NRTI Resistance Notes, version 8.4 (last updated 2017-06-16). 2017. https://hivdb.stanford.edu/dr-summary/resistance-notes/NRTI/. Accessed 14 Sept 2017.
14. Scherrer AU, von Wyl V, Joos B, Klimkait T, Bürgisser P, Yerly S, et al. Predictors for the emergence of the 2 multi-nucleoside/nucleotide resistance mutations 69 insertion and Q151M and their impact on clinical outcome in the Swiss HIV Cohort Study. J Infect Dis. 2011;203:791–7.
15. Nouhin J, Madec Y, Ngo-Giang-Huong N, Ferradini L, Nerrienet E. Increased risk of Q151M and K65R mutations in patients failing stavudine-containing first-line antiretroviral therapy in Cambodia. PLoS ONE. 2013;8:e73744.
16. Van Vaerenbergh K, Van Laethem K, Albert J, Boucher CA, Clotet B, Floridia M, et al. Prevalence and characteristics of multinucleoside-resistant human immunodeficiency virus type 1 among European patients receiving combinations of nucleoside analogues. Antimicrob Agents Chemother. 2000;44:2109–17.
17. Zaccarelli M, Perno CF, Forbici F, Soldani F, Bonfigli S, Gori C, et al. Q151M-mediated multinucleoside resistance: prevalence, risk factors, and response to salvage therapy. Clin Infect Dis. 2004;38:433–7.
18. Prasitsuebsai W, Teeraananchai S, Singtoroj T, Truong KH, Ananworanich J, Do VC, et al. Treatment outcomes and resistance patterns of children and adolescents on second-line antiretroviral therapy in Asia. JAIDS J Acquir Immune Defic Syndr. 2016;72:380–6.
19. Villabona-Arenas CJ, Vidal N, Guichet E, Serrano L, Delaporte E, Gascuel O, et al. In-depth analysis of HIV-1 drug resistance mutations in HIV-infected individuals failing first-line regimens in West and Central Africa. AIDS. 2016;30:2577–89.
20. Barennes H, Virak K, Rouet F, Buisson Y, Strobel M, Vibol U. Factors associated with the failure of first and second-line antiretroviral therapies therapy, a case control study in Cambodian HIV-1 infected children. BMC Res Notes. 2016;9:69.
21. Saravanan S, Kausalya B, Gomathi S, Sivamalar S, Pachamuthu B, Selvamuthu P, et al. Etravirine and rilpivirine drug resistance among HIV-1 subtype C infected children failing non-nucleoside reverse transcriptase inhibitor-based regimens in South India. AIDS Res Hum Retroviruses. 2017;33:567–74.
22. Tang MW, Rhee S-Y, Bertagnolio S, Ford N, Holmes S, Sigaloff KC, et al. Nucleoside reverse transcriptase inhibitor resistance mutations associated with first-line stavudine-containing antiretroviral therapy: programmatic implications for countries phasing out stavudine. J Infect Dis. 2013;207:S70–7.
23. Kityo C, Thompson J, Nankya I, Hoppe A, Ndashimye E, Warambwa C, et al. HIV drug resistance mutations in non-B subtypes after prolonged virological failure on NNRTI-based first-line regimens in Sub-Saharan Africa. JAIDS J Acquir Immune Defic Syndr. 2017;75:e45–54.
24. WHO. Combined global demand forecasts for antiretroviral medicines and HIV diagnostics in low- and middle-income countries from 2015 to 2020. Geneva: WHO; 2016.
25. Boyd MA, Moore CL, Molina J-M, Wood R, Madero JS, Wolff M, et al. Baseline HIV-1 resistance, virological outcomes, and emergent resistance in the SECOND-LINE trial: an exploratory analysis. Lancet HIV. 2015;2:e42–51.
26. Paton NI, Kityo C, Thompson J, Nankya I, Bagenda L, Hoppe A, et al. Nucleoside reverse-transcriptase inhibitor cross-resistance and outcomes from second-line antiretroviral therapy in the public health approach: an observational analysis within the randomised, open-label, EARNEST trial. Lancet HIV. 2017;4:e341–8.

27. The UK Collaborative HIV Cohort Steering Committee. The creation of a large UK-based multicentre cohort of HIV-infected individuals: The UK Collaborative HIV Cohort (UK CHIC) Study. HIV Med. 2004;5:115–24.
28. Carpenter B, Gelman A, Hoffman MD, Lee D, Goodrich B, Betancourt M, et al. Stan: a probabilistic programming language. J Stat Softw. 2017;76:32.
29. Stan Development Team. RStan: the R interface to Stan. 2016. http://mc-stan.org/. Accessed 14 Sept 2017.
30. Gelman A, Hill J, Yajima M. Why we (usually) don't have to worry about multiple comparisons. J Res Educ Effectiveness. 2012;5:189–211.
31. McKinnon EJ, James IR, John M, Mallal SA. Viral load detectability profiles for HIV infection. Stat Med. 2003;22:385–96.
32. Masquelier B, Race E, Tamalet C, Descamps D, Izopet J, Buffet-Janvresse C, et al. Genotypic and phenotypic resistance patterns of human immunodeficiency virus type 1 variants with insertions or deletions in the reverse transcriptase (RT): multicenter study of patients treated with RT inhibitors. Antimicrob Agents Chemother. 2001;45:1836–42.
33. Gupta RK, Jordan MR, Sultan BJ, Hill A, Davis DH, Gregson J, et al. Global trends in antiretroviral resistance in treatment-naive individuals with HIV after rollout of antiretroviral treatment in resource-limited settings: a global collaborative study and meta-regression analysis. Lancet. 2012;380:1250–8.
34. WHO. HIV drug resistance report 2017. Geneva: WHO; 2017.
35. Scherrer AU, von Wyl V, Götte M, Klimkait T, Cellerai C, Yerly S, et al. Polymorphic mutations associated with the emergence of the multinucleoside/tide resistance mutations 69 insertion and Q151M. JAIDS J Acquir Immune Defic Syndr. 2012;59:105–12.

19

Geographic patterns of poor HIV/AIDS care continuum in District of Columbia

Suparna Das[1*], Jenevieve Opoku[1], Michael Kharfen[2] and Adam Allston[1]

Abstract

Background: Concurrent with the UNAIDS 90-90-90 and NHAS plans, the District of Columbia (DC) launched its 90/90/90/50 plan (*Plan*) in 2015. The *Plan* proposes that by 2020, 90% of all DC residents will know their HIV status; 90% of residents living with HIV will be in sustained treatment; 90% of those in treatment will reach "Viral Suppression" and DC will achieve 50% reduction of new HIV cases. To achieve these goals targeted prevention strategies are imperative for areas where the relative risk (RR) of not being linked to care (NL), not retained in any care (NRC) and low viral suppression (NVSP) are highest in the District. These outcomes are denoted in this study as *poor outcomes of HIV care continuum*. This study applies the Bayesian model for RR for area specific random effects to identify the census tracts with poor HIV care continuum outcomes for DC.

Methods: This analysis was conducted using cases diagnosed from 2010 to 2015 and reported to the surveillance system from the District of Columbia Department of Health (DC DOH), HIV/AIDS, Hepatitis, STD and TB Administration. The jurisdictions of the District of Columbia is divided into 179 census tracts. It is challenging to plot sparse data in 'small' local administrative areas, characteristically which may have a single-count datum for each geographic area. Bayesian methods overcome this problem by assimilating prior information to the underlying RR, making the predicted RR estimates robust.

Results: The RR of NL is higher in 59 (33%) out of 179 census tracts in DC. The RR of NRC was high in 46 (26%) of the census tracts while 52 census tracts (29%) show a high risk of having NVSP among its residents. This study also identifies clear correlated heterogeneity or clustering is evident in the northern tracts of the district.

Conclusion: The study finds census tracts with higher RR of poor linkage to care outcomes in the District. These results will inform the *Plan* which aims to increase targeted testing leading to early initiation of antiretroviral therapy. The uniqueness of this study lies in its translational scope where surveillance data can be used to inform local public health programs and enhance the quality of health for the people with HIV.

Keywords: HIV care continuum, Bayesian relative risk, Disease mapping, District of Columbia, Area based prevention intervention strategies

Background

The HIV care continuum is an internationally-recognized framework, accepted in the United States as a series of stages from the time an individual receives a diagnosis of HIV through the successful treatment of their infection with HIV medications [1, 2]. The care continuum was introduced as the HIV treatment cascade in 2010 as a part of the United States National HIV/AIDS Strategy (NHAS). It proposes being in care not only leads to better health outcomes for people living with HIV, but it may also help reduce new transmissions within the community. Thus evaluating HIV care dynamics is a vital step to gauging the strengths of HIV programs and addressing the gaps in the care continuum [3]. Effective HIV treatment as prevention requires people be tested, know their HIV status, be linked and retained in care, and achieve

*Correspondence: suparna.das@dc.gov
[1] Strategic Information Division, HIV/AIDS, Hepatitis, STD and TB Administration (HAHSTA), District of Columbia Department of Health, Government of the District of Columbia, 899 North Capitol St., NE/Fourth Floor, Washington, DC 20002, USA

viral suppression through effective antiretroviral therapy (ART) [4, 5]. Treatment as prevention (TasP) is an HIV prevention intervention where treating an HIV-positive person with ART is used to diminish the potential of HIV transmission to the negative partner [6]. The core strategy of treatment as prevention in the context of the care continuum is to make ART available to the people. Early introduction of ART for people living with HIV (PLWH) is critical in ensuring better individual health outcomes and reducing HIV transmission [7, 8].

In 2016, concurrent with the UNAIDS 90-90-90 and NHAS plan, the District of Columbia (DC) launched its 90/90/90/50 plan (*Plan*). This *Plan* proposes that by 2020, 90% of all DC residents will know their HIV status; 90% of residents living with HIV will be in sustained treatment; 90% of those in treatment will reach "Viral Suppression"; and DC will achieve a 50% reduction in new HIV cases. One of the first significant steps to achieving these goals is to identify geographic areas with higher levels of relative risk (RR) of poor HIV care continuum outcomes. Areas of poor care continuum outcomes where the resident population is at greater risk of *not being linked to any care* (NL) or *not retained in any* care (NRC) or *have lower levels or no viral suppression* (NVSP).

Mapping health outcomes and detecting geographic disparities in care are valuable tools in public health, helping decision-makers to recognize areas which requires resources [9]. Local as well as federal agencies have used surveillance data to analyze the care continuum by demographic characteristics and HIV transmission risk [7, 10]. Studies have been conducted to understand spatial patterns along the HIV care continuum [11] and the feasibility of using the HIV care continuum to identify geographic areas at most risk for HIV and poor health outcomes [12].

There are different models and methods to develop maps of diseases including simple statistical illustration, informal methods, basic models, multilevel models etc. This study aims to identify areas of poor HIV care continuum outcomes in DC using Bayesian disease mapping methods. Disease mapping using Bayesian approach consists of prior information about variation in disease rates, in addition to observed events in each area. It also considers the spatial pattern of disease in which close geographic areas have more similar disease rates [13–16].

The results from this analysis will be used by DC Department of Health (DOH) to shape its HIV prevention and care programs as well as used to implement the targets mentioned in the 90/90/90/50 plan. Apart from the immediate impact of the study in shaping DC's care continuum, the study is also significant as it uses local surveillance data to identify areas of risks of being out of care continuum thus not relying on national estimates.

Methods and data

Disease mapping comprises of a set of statistical techniques, which assist in generating accurate maps based on estimations of incidence, prevalence, and mortality of disease [17]. Contemporary disease mapping, the cornerstone of spatial epidemiology, identifies geographical risk disparities and clustering within small areas. This is commonly called small-area disease or health mapping [18, 19]. The crucial question remains whether the patterns, variations, and clusters observed from the disease map are significant or simply variations due to small samples [19]. Spatial analysis and disease mapping of the HIV care continuum has been used to identify areas of poor outcomes as a tool for identifying target areas for prevention and intervention strategies [11, 20]. The principal limitation of using these traditional measures is the uneven distribution of the population among tracts [21]. This may lead to inflated rates yielding erroneous and inaccurate disease maps and risk identification. Another challenge in disease mapping is plotting sparse data in 'small' local administrative areas, which, characteristically, may have a single-count datum for each tract [18, 19]. These challenges are usually met by using standard mortality rate (SMR) for disease mapping. SMR is the ratio of between observed number of events in a study population and the expected number of events in the study population. Unfortunately, SMRs also suffers from several drawbacks [22]. The ratio estimators can yield large variations in approximation with comparatively minor changes in expected value [22, 23]. The SMR is essentially a saturated estimate of relative risk and hence is not parsimonious. SMR is a crude estimate and can provide unsteady estimations owing to its ratio formula, and does not consider the correlation among neighbors [24, 25].

Bayesian approach to disease mapping overcomes these drawbacks. Relative risk (RR) of disease in area i was shown as θ_i. Clayton and Kaldor [16] suggested a method (Besag, Mollie and York—BYM) that models the RR as a function of spatially structured and unstructured random effects [23]. The unstructured random effects are modeled on a Conditional AutoRegressive-prior or CAR-prior. These CAR models are frequently used both by statisticians and epidemiologists, and their application is enabled by existing software such as OpenBUGS [26]. The central feature of all these models is to deliver some shrinkage and spatial smoothing of the raw RR approximations that otherwise would be calculated individually for each area. Such shrinkage provides a further steady approximation of the pattern of underlying risk than that delivered by the raw estimates. The pattern of the raw risks, based on the size of the population at risk, leads to a noisy and fuzzy image of the true unobserved risks [27].

This paper uses a model for relative risks for area specific random effects which are deconstructed into a component that models the effects that vary in a structured manner in space (clustering or correlated heterogeneity) and a component that models the effects that vary in an unstructured way between areas (uncorrelated heterogeneity) [22]. The parameter of interest is θ_i, the RR that quantifies whether the area i has a higher ($\theta_i > 1$) or lower ($\theta_i < 1$) occurrence of cases than that expected from the background population.

The model was introduced by Clayton and Kaldor and extended by Besag, York, and Mollie, [16, 28] and its formulation is described as:

$$y_i = poisson(E_i\theta_i)$$

$$\log(\theta_i) = \alpha + u_i + v_i,$$

where α: trend component that is overall level of relative risk. u_i: [(spatial overdispersion) spatial correlated heterogeneity]: It is logical that the close areas have similar relative risks. To take this similarities into account, the random variable u_i which is uncorrelated with other (u_j) included in the model. For this component, spatial correlation structure is used where estimates relative risk in each area are dependent on adjacent areas. The conditional autoregressive model proposed by Besag et al. is:

$$\left[u_i|u_j,\ \mathrm{i} \neq \mathrm{j}, \tau_v^2\right] \sim N\left(\overline{\mathrm{u}}_i, \tau_v^2\right),$$

where $\overline{\mathrm{u}_i} = \frac{1}{\sum w_{ij}} \sum u_i w_{ij}, \tau_v^2 = \frac{1}{\sum_j w_{ij}}, w_{ij} = 1$ if i, j are adjacent (or 0 if they are not),v_i: [Non-Spatial over dispersion (spatial uncorrelated heterogeneity)]: By the formulation of the model for spatially correlated heterogeneities, the variance is dependent on the number of neighbors and independence couldn't be defined well. In order to justify this problem, another component (v_i) is introduced that is an uncorrelated over dispersion parameter. The prior distribution of this parameter is $v_i \sim N\left(0, \tau_v^2\right)$.

Parameters τ_v^2 and τ_u^2 control the variability of v and u [22] respectively. In a full Bayesian analysis, prior distributions must be specified for those parameters (Additional file 1: Figure S1). We considered gamma prior distribution for both τ_v^2 and τ_w^2, as suggested by Bernardinelli [29] (Additional file 1: Figure S1). The OpenBUGS Code used in the analysis was borrowed from Lawson [22]. Model fitting was done using two separate chains starting with different initial values. Convergence was checked by visual examination of time series plots of samples for each chain and by computing the Gelman and Rubin diagnostic [30]. The first 5000 samples were discarded as a burn-in; each chain run for a further 75,000 iterations for all the models [31]. Results were mapped using Maptitude software. To investigate how the models fit the data well, a deviance information criterion (DIC) was applied.

Data analyzed for the study were obtained from the Enhanced HIV/AIDS Reporting System (EHARS) of the District of Columbia Department of Health (DC DOH), HIV/AIDS, Hepatitis, STD and TB Administration (HAHSTA) for years 2010–2015. The variables were extracted using SAS code from persons and laboratory dataset of EHARS. For those cases NL (Not linked to care) outcome, the cases were based on the residence of diagnosis. NRC (Not retained in any care) outcome cases were based on the current address of the resident, cases with no laboratory information on being in any care after being linked were treated not retained in care outcome. For NVSP (Not Virally Suppressed) current addresses were geocoded; cases not suppressed or no viral load reported were treated as not virally suppressed. The geographic coordinates associated with each case of infection were assigned using Maptitude Geographic Information System (GIS) software. Between 2010 and 2015 there were 1125 eligible cases with an available address that could be geocoded. Post Office Box numbers, DC Detention centers, and homeless were not included in the analysis to avoid spatial bias. Overall, the District of Columbia comprises 179 census tracts, 8 wards and 49 neighborhoods (Fig. 1 boundary map of District of Columbia). The cartographic boundary map is based on the 2010 US census.

The following table (Table 1) have the socio-economic and demographic variables of people in the wards of DC. The data is obtained from Office of Planning, Government of District of Columbia. Ward six (84,290) has the highest number of people and Ward seven (73,290) has the lowest number of people. The district shows racial variation in distribution, with highest percent of black population is ward one (95.20%) while white population is highest in ward three (8.50%). Unemployment rates are highest in ward eight (12.70%) and lowest in ward three (2.60%). High school education does not show significant variation across the wards, with lowest in wards seven and eight (83.0%).

Table 2 defines the HIV care continuum measures followed and applied in the District of Columbia. The ultimate goal of HIV treatment is to achieve viral suppression, meaning the amount of HIV in the body is very low or undetectable. This is important for people with HIV to stay healthy, live longer and reduce their chances of passing HIV to others.

This study used Bayesian spatial statistics to find areas of poor outcomes along the HIV care continuum. This study used three measures of the care dynamics that were defined as poor outcomes of HIV care continuum: (1)

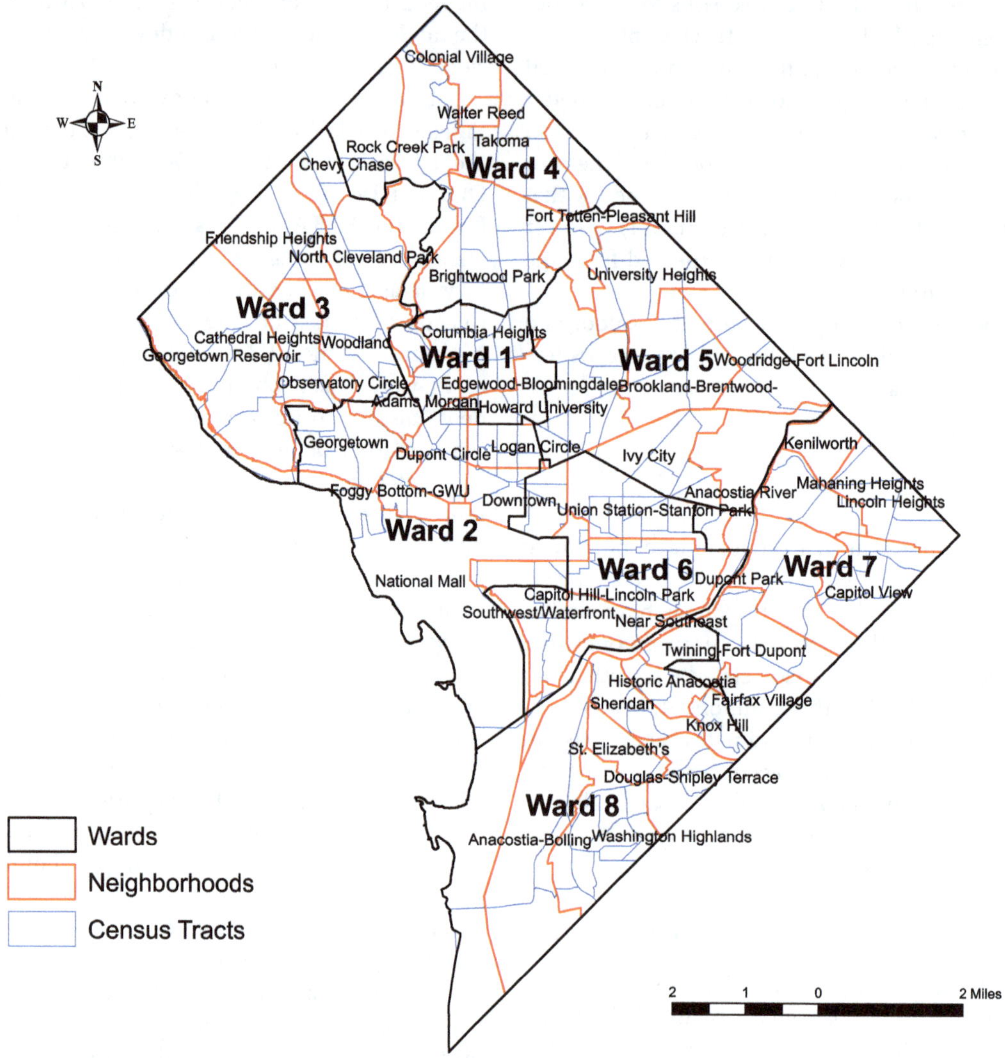

Fig. 1 The boundary map of District of Columbia, delineating Wards, Neighbourhoods and Census Tracts

Table 1 Social, economic and demographic characteristics of wards in District of Columbia

Variables	Ward 1	Ward 2	Ward 3	Ward 4	Ward 5	Ward 6	Ward 7	Ward 8
Total population[a]	82,859	77,645	83,152	83,066	82,049	84,290	73,290	81,133
Male[a]	49.90	50.5	44.7	48.60	47.20	47.90	46.30	43.80
Female[a]	50.10	49.50	55.30	51.40	52.80	52.10	53.70	56.20
White[a]	56.70	77.20	83.90	28.40	22.10	58.00	3.00	5.40
Black and African American[a]	31.50	9.80	8.50	57.90	71.90	36.80	95.20	93.60
Unemployment rate[a]	5.10	2.70	2.60	6.90	9.00	4.70	11	12.70
High school education[a]	87.7	94.90	97.60	87.10	86.30	92.60	83.0	83.0

[a] Office of planning, District of Columbia

not linked to care—diagnosed in District of Columbia, but do not have any evidence of a CD4 and/or viral load after initial lab in DC. For newly diagnosed, no evidence of a CD4 and/or viral load lab within 3 months of initial HIV diagnosis. (2) Not retained in care—comprises of those who have no lab reported within year of analysis or do not have two labs reported more than 90 days apart within the year of analysis. (3) Not achieving viral

Table 2 Care continuum outcome measures followed in DC

Measure	Definition	Levels
HIV cases living in DC	Number of cases diagnosed with HIV through 2015 and presumed living in DC at the end of 2016	
Linkage to care	Evidence of diagnosis date to first CD4 and/or viral load laboratory	Living in DC; any evidence of a CD4 and/or viral load after initial lab in DC Newly diagnosed: any evidence of a CD4 and/or viral load lab within 3 months initial HIV diagnosis
Retained in care	Stability of care in 2016	Two viral load and/or CD4 labs reported more than 90 days apart in the year Out of care: No lab reported in the year
Virally suppressed	Suppression any time after HIV disease diagnosis	Suppressed: reported viral load ≤ 200copies/ml Not suppressed: reported viral load ≥ 200 copies/ml No viral load reported

suppression—comprises those who have not achieved viral suppression and those with no viral load reported within the year analysis.

Results

The results compares three forms of disease mapping for HIV care continuum measures for the DC DOH, HAHSTA conducted an internal evaluation of the percentage of DC residents with undiagnosed HIV infection [32]. The analysis found 9–14% of the people in the District are unaware of their HIV diagnosis [33].

Not linked in care (NL)

Figure 2 (Not linked to care) shows disease mapping for people not linked to any care in the census tracts of the District. The simple rates, which is the percent of cases with no lab report by the total population. Two tracts in wards three and a single tract in ward 1 with more than 10% of NL, compared to the SMR map which has higher values across in all tracts except in ward eight. Tracts with SMR greater than 1.0 indicates not linked to HIV care compared to what was expected. The θ_i (RR) of NL is higher than 1 in 59 (33%) out of 179 census tracts in DC. θ_i map shows a smoother version of SMR in the Bayesian estimates showing parts of ward two, three, five and six with highest risk of not being linked to any care. The idea is that the smoothed estimate for each tract borrows strength from the data in the surrounding tracts making the results stable.

Figure 3 (NRC) shows disease mapping for people NRC in the census tracts of the District. The higher rates of NRC is evident in almost all the wards. For SMR most

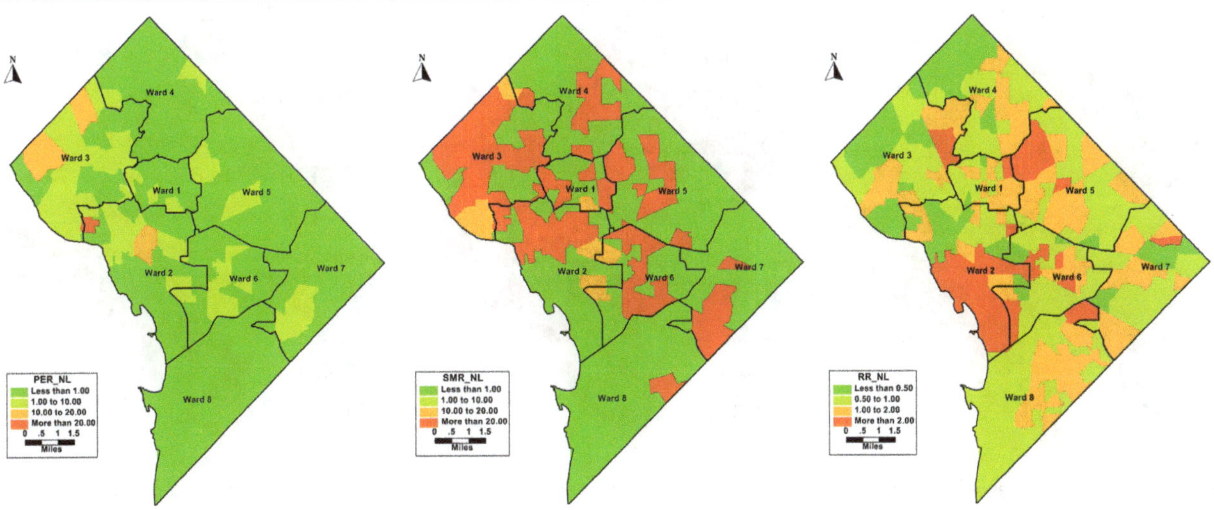

Fig. 2 Maps of simple rates (left), raw SMRs (middle) of *not linked to HIV care* compared to smoothed Relative Risks from Poisson log normal model (right) in District of Columbia (2010–2015)

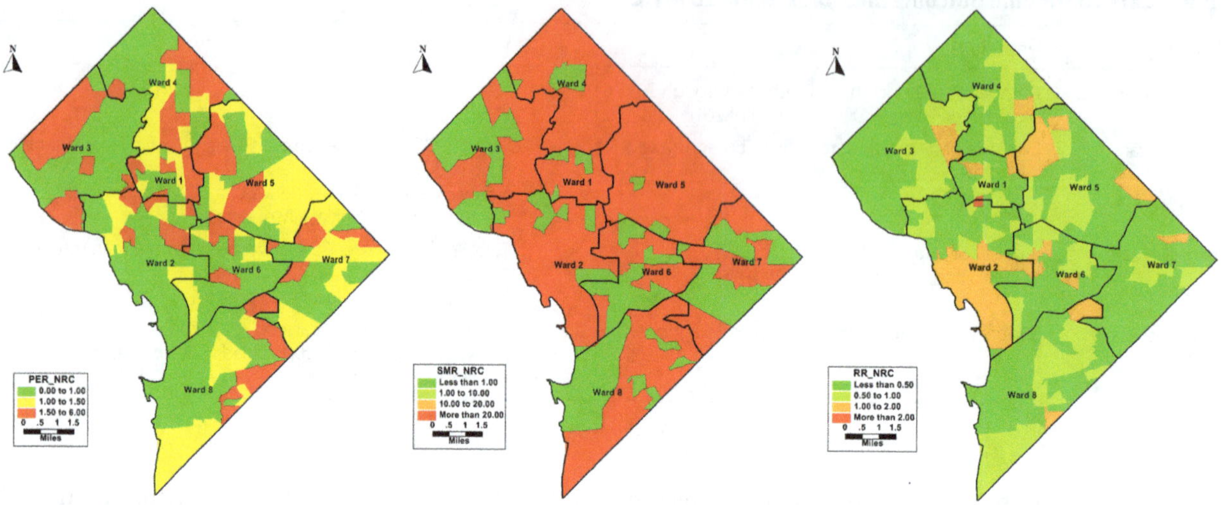

Fig. 3 Maps of simple rates (left), raw SMRs (left) of *not retained in any care* compared to smoothed Relative Risks from Poisson log normal model (right) in District of Columbia (2010–2015)

tracts have SMR more than 20. $\theta_i > 1$ for NRC is evident in 13 (7%) of the 179 census tracts. Compared to SMR disease map, θ_i maps shows smoothed results with RR more than in few tracts across DC.

Not virally suppressed (NVSP)

Figure 4 show simple rates mapping where the highest rates of NVSP are in the tracts of Wards two and six. SMR with greater than 1.00 are most prevalent in the tracts of Wards three, five, six and eight. θ_i (RR) of NVSP is more than 1 in 52 (29%) of the 179 census tracts in the DC by the end of the study period. Bayesian estimates of θ_i display a smoother map compared to SMR, tracts in wards three, five and eight have θ_i more than 1.

Table 3 shows α (intercept) which is the overall level of RR poor outcomes in DC of NL (− 0.02389), NRC (− 0.3182) and NVSP (− 0.4891). The table also shows the posterior mean and 95% credible intervals of the variance components for the model. The variability of the relative risk is attributed more to the uncorrelated

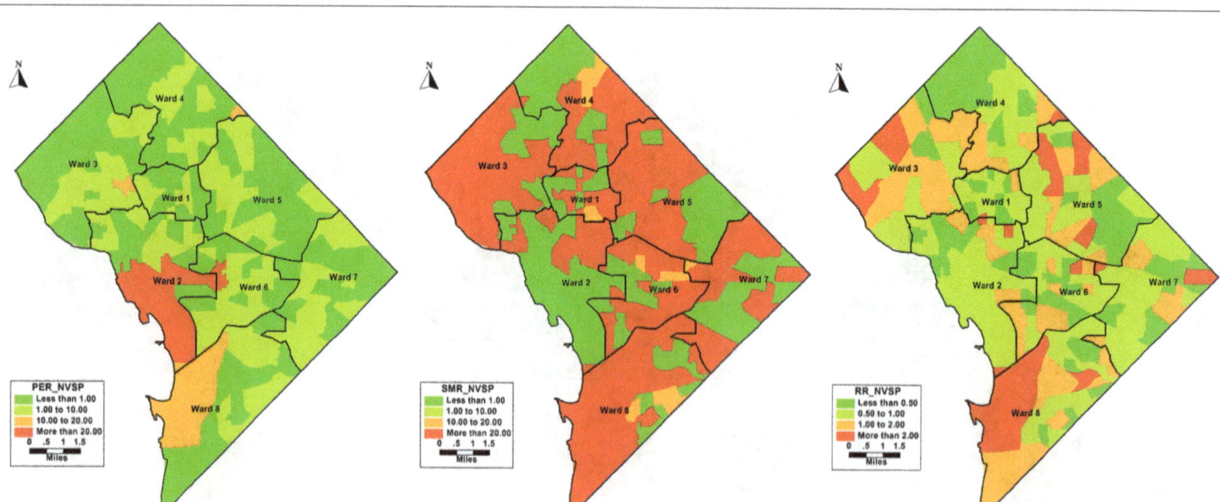

Fig. 4 Maps of simple rates (left), raw SMRs (left) of *not retained in any care* compared to smoothed Relative Risks from Poisson log normal model (right) in District of Columbia (2010–2015)

Table 3 Posterior statistics of the variance components and model

Not linked to care				Not retained to care				Not virally suppressed			
	Mean	STD dev	Credible interval		Mean	STD dev	Credible interval		Mean	STD dev	Credible interval
α	−0.2389	0.09904	−0.4424, −0.05504	α	−0.3182	0.09017	−0.5017, -0.1474	α	−0.4891	0.096	−0.6847, −0.3074
τ_u^2	34.21	247.8	0.3736, 276.1	τ_u^2	233.4	790.1	0.9515, 2544	τ_u^2	0.8418	1.429	0.2251, 3.847
τ_v^2	639.7	1231	1.369, 4364	τ_v^2	1.578	0.4645	0.9697, 2.708	τ_v^2	541.2	1192	0.9033, 4113
DIC			442.8	DIC			664.7	DIC			484.7
PD			21.78	PD			80.63	PD			−28.41

heterogeneity than to the spatial structure effects. The τ_u^2 for the NL is 34.21 vs. 233.4 for the NRC model, are substantial number indicating that the risk in any given tract in DC does not have any similarities to that of the neighboring tracts. Comparatively, the τ_u^2 for NVSP is smaller than the preceding values at 0.8418; thus the risk of NVSP in any given tract in DC may be similar to that in the neighboring areas. The DIC is low for all the models, but lowest for the NL.

For NVSP results in the spatial blocks with low values are evident in the north as well as in the south, but a pattern of spatial association is not as clear as in the previous two outcomes, which the low τ_u^2 results. The τ_u^2 is large for NL and NRC outcomes, indicating areas of correlated heterogeneity. Figure 5 maps areas of correlated heterogeneity over space in the district, which displays blocks of values for all the three models. The resulting correlated heterogeneity is the random effect that arises from a model where the spatial unit is correlated with neighboring spatial units. This denotes spatial autocorrelation of the outcomes among the census tracts.

Discussion

This study used surveillance data to identify geographic patterns of the areas of poor adherence to the HIV care continuum for people living with HIV in DC. The smoothed Bayesian estimate for each 'borrow strength' (precision) from the data in the surrounding areas which takes into account a spatial pattern of the outcome (i.e. Tobler's First Law of Geography, things that are nearby are more related than things that are far away). From the results it is evident that percentages (will be addressed as rates) used to identify the areas of lower care continuum outcome is specially unstable as much of the variation in the rates is attributable to the statistical noise due to the small number in low-population tracts [24]. Traditional standard mortality rates calculated simply as a ratio of observed and expected is another approach that is widely used by epidemiologists. There are shortcomings [34] in SMR which is calculated as the following: $SMR = \frac{Observerd}{Expected}$. The results produced through the SMR are not robust enough to be used for policy implementation particularly in DC which calls for small area

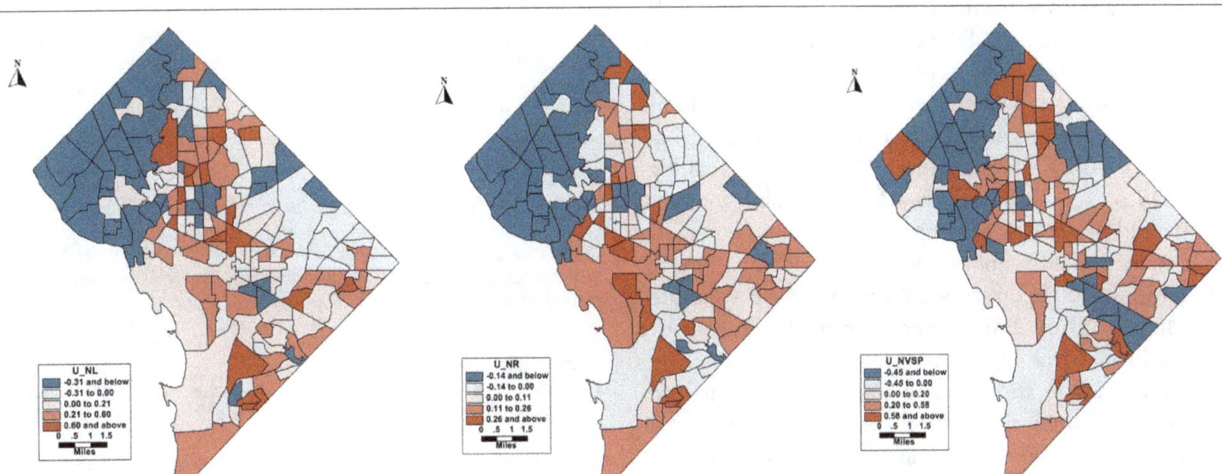

Fig. 5 Posterior expectation of u (correlated heterogeneity) for the Bayesian model

estimation. The results in accordance with Clayton and Kaldor's methods are smoothed for areas of poor HIV care continuum outcomes. The smoothed estimates points the tracts where people are at higher risk of being not linked to care, not retained in care and not virally suppressed. The statistical noise which rates and SMRs suffer from is smoothed in the bayesian results.

Tracts in wards two, three, five and six have show the highest risk for people being not linked to care (NL). The total number of tracts of NL with $\theta_i > 1$ was 59 (33%) of the 179 tracts. The results will help DOH shape its programs to the areas with higher risk. The lower linkage areas would be monitored and evaluated on the factors of the suboptimal performance to inform and design an enhanced comprehensive linkage service system. Upon diagnosis, it is critical for patients to be linked with medical treatment and anti-retroviral therapy in order for them to stay healthy. Timely linkage to care is a significant focus of DOH's Plan. This would involve area based expansion of access to treatment and related services which also includes AIDS Drug Assistance Program (ADAP) as well as other medical assitance programs.

Results show the tracts across DC where the risk of retention to care (NRC) are higher. The total number tracts where the risk of NRC is $\theta_i > 1$ is only 13 (7%). The lower retained areas would guide strategies in identifying and recapture people living with HIV who have been out of care. Though low in number yet DOH would target these areas to offer facilities in order to assist people to remain in care. It is important for the linked and diagnosed individuals to be retained in case as drug therapy can improve health outcomes and lowers transmission risk.

There are 52 tracts where the residents are at higher risk ($\theta_i > 1$) of not achieving viral suppression. DOH will use the results to inform its strategies for ending HIV epidemic in the district. DOH is currently working with providers to remove barriers to care and adhering in care. In 2015, Whitman-Walker Health launched the Mobile Outreach Retention and Engagement (MORE) initiative, supported by funding from DOH and the Washington AIDS partnership [33]. The MORE mobile medical team would provide evaluation, lab tests, and counseling services in patients' home and at pop-up locations in the community. The areas would help MORE to strategize where pop-up clinics could be most helpful. In the areas of lower viral suppression DOH would work with the pharmacies in the areas to improve access to prescriptions and track medication treatment adherence as well as promote telemedicine approaches for adherence support. These results would also be used to find areas to support the *Plan's* approach where DOH would partner with other DC government agencies to address the social support needs of the person living with HIV in the District.

DOH will also be able to evaluate the barriers to be linked to care in the census tracts where the risk of NL is high. Under the *Plan* DC is targeting to implement several programs that would help end the HIV epidemic in the district. Those programs include targeted expansion of access to treatment and related services.

Conclusion

The analysis identified the areas for District of Columbia's 90/90/90/50 plan which will be used to target testing activities and care activities of the DC DOH. The results also show clustering of the outcomes of HIV care continuum. The exact reason for clustering is not addressed in the study. Clustering may naturally be present in the are or may also stem from the presence of undetected ecological or "frailty effects" [22], which provides a scope for further exploration.

There are a few limitations to this study. The results are based on surveillance data reported by providers and laboratories to the HAHSTA. Therefore data for patients not reported to HAHSTA or those that moved out of the jurisdiction were not included in the analysis. Those addresses which could not be geocoded were not included in the analysis. Further it needs to be evaluated in social-determinants of health have any impact on HIV care continuum measures across space and time in DC.

Authors' contributions

SD conceived the idea of the analysis, did the data analysis as well wrote the majority of the text. JO was also a great support in developing the document and editing. The data extraction code was written and prepared by JO. AA assisted in scientific inputs and draft editing. MK was instrumental in draft editing. All authors read and approved the final manuscript.

Author details

[1] Strategic Information Division, HIV/AIDS, Hepatitis, STD and TB Administration (HAHSTA), District of Columbia Department of Health, Government of the District of Columbia, 899 North Capitol St., NE/Fourth Floor, Washington, DC 20002, USA. [2] HIV/AIDS, Hepatitis, STD & TB Administration (HAHSTA), District of Columbia Department of Health, Government of the District of Columbia, 899 N. Capitol St., NE, Washington, DC 20002, USA.

Acknowledgements

The Authors would like to thank everyone at Strategic Information Division, HAHSTA, DC DOH for their inputs particularly Kate Drezner for editing the paper.

Presented in part at the HIV Research for Prevention Conference in October, 2015 as a poster in Chicago, Illinois.

Competing interests

The authors declare that they have no competing interests.

Funding source

This work was not supported by any grants.

References

1. Centers for Disease Control and Prevention. Understanding the HIV Care Continuum. 2014;1–5.
2. Mugavero MJ, Amico KR, Horn T, Thompson MA. The state of engagement in HIV care in the United States: from cascade to continuum to control. Clin Infect Dis. 2013;57:1164–71.
3. District of Columbia Department of Health HIV/AIDS, Hepatitis, STD and TA (HAHSTA). Retained HIV Care and Ryan White Care Dynamics Data through December 2015. 2015.
4. Gardner EM, McLees MP, Steiner JF, Del Rio C, Burman WJ. The spectrum of engagement in HIV care and its relevance to test-and-treat strategies for prevention of HIV infection. Clin Infect Dis. 2011;52:793–800.
5. Hall HI, Tang T, Westfall AO, Mugavero MJ. HIV care visits and time to viral suppression, 19 US jurisdictions, and implications for treatment, prevention and the National HIV/AIDS Strategy. PLoS ONE. 2013;8:1–7.
6. Van de Laar MJ, Pharris A. Treatment as prevention: will it work? Euro surveillance. 2011;16:1–3.
7. Hall HI, Frazier EL, Rhodes P, Holtgrave DR, Furlow-Parmley C, Tang T, et al. Differences in human immunodeficiency virus care and treatment among subpopulations in the United States. JAMA Intern Med. 2013;173:1337–44.
8. Attia S, Egger M, Muller M, Zwahlen M, Low N. Sexual transmission of HIV according to viral load and antiretroviral therapy: systematic review and meta-analysis. AIDS. 2009;23:1397–404.
9. Rebeiro PF, Gange SJ, Horberg MA, Abraham AG, Napravnik S, Samji H, et al. Geographic variations in retention in care among HIV-infected adults in the United States. PLoS ONE. 2016;11:4–9.
10. Nosyk B, Montaner JSG, Colley G, Lima VD, Chan K, Heath K, et al. The cascade of HIV care in British Columbia, Canada, 1996–2011: a population-based retrospective cohort study. Lancet Infect Dis. 2014;14:40–9.
11. Eberhart MG, Yehia BR, Hillier A, Voytek CD, Blank MB, Frank I, et al. Behind the cascade: analyzing spatial patterns along the HIV care continuum. J Acquir Immune Defic Syndr (1999). 2013;64 Suppl 1:S42–51. http://www.ncbi.nlm.nih.gov/pubmed/24126447.
12. Castel AD, Kuo I, Mikre M, Young T, Haddix M, Das S, et al. Feasibility of using HIV care-continuum outcomes to identify geographic areas for targeted HIV testing. J Acquir Immune Defic Syndr. 2017;74:96–103.
13. Carlin BP, Louis TA. Bayes and empirical bayes methods for data analysis. 2nd ed. London: Chapman and Hall; 2000.
14. Manton KG, Woodbury MA, Stallard E. A variance components approach to categorical data models with heterogeneous cell populations: analysis of spatial gradients in lung cancer mortality rates in North Carolina counties. Biometrics. 1981;37:259–69.
15. Tsutakawa RK. Mixed model for analyzing geographic variability in mortality rates. J Am Stat Assoc. 1988;83:37–42.
16. Clayton D, Kaldor J. Empirical bayes estimates of age-standardized relative risks for use in disease mapping. Biometrics. 1987;43:671–81. http://www.jstor.org/stable/2532003.
17. Mahaki B, Mehrabi Y, Kavousi A, Mohammadian Y, Kargar M. Applying and comparing empirical and full Bayesian models in study of evaluating relative risk of suicide among counties of Ilam province. J Educ Health Promot. 2015;4:50 **(eCollection 2015)**.
18. Robertson C, Nelson TA, MacNab YC, Lawson AB. Review of methods for space-time disease surveillance. Spat Spatiotemporal Epidemiol. 2010;1:105–16. https://doi.org/10.1016/j.sste.2009.12.001.
19. MacNab YC. On identification in Bayesian disease mapping and ecological-spatial regression models. Stat Methods Med Res. 2014;23:134–55. http://www.ncbi.nlm.nih.gov/pubmed/22573502.
20. Goswami ND, Hecker EJ, Vickery C, Ahearn MA, Cox GM, Holland DP, et al. Geographic information system-based screening for TB, HIV, and syphilis (GIS-THIS): a cross-sectional study. PLoS ONE. 2012;7:1–8.
21. Sturtevant L. The new district of columbia: what population growth and demographic change mean for the city. J Urban Aff. 2014;36:276–99.
22. Lawson A. Bayesian disease mapping: hierarchical modeling in spatial epidemiology. Boca Raton: Chapman and Hall: Taylor and Francis; 2013.
23. Aregay M, Lawson AB, Faes C, Kirby R. Bayesian multiscale modeling for aggregated disease mapping data. Proceedings of the Third ACM SIGSPATIAL International Workshop on the Use of GIS in Public Health—HealthGIS'14. 2014;45–8. http://www.scopus.com/inward/record.url?eid=2-s2.0-84926369237&partnerID=tZOtx3y1.
24. Gelman A, Price PN. All maps of parameter estimates are misleading. Stat Med. 1999;18:3221–34.
25. Gelman A. Multilevel (hierarchical) modeling: what it can and cannot do. Technometrics. 2006;48:432–5.
26. Spiegelhalter DJ, Best NG, Carlin BP, van der Linde A. Bayesian measures of model complexity anf Fit. J R Stat Soc. 2002;64:583–639.
27. Richardson S, Thomson A, Best N, Elliott P. Interpreting posterior relative risk estimates in disease-mapping studies. Environ Health Perspect. 2004;112:1016–25.
28. Besag J, York J, Mollié A. Bayesian image restoration, with two applications in spatial statistics. Ann Inst Stat Math. 1991;43:1–20. https://doi.org/10.1007/BF00116466.
29. Bernardinelli L, Clayton D, Pascutto C, Montomoli C, Ghislandi M, Songini M. Bayesian analysis of space—time variation in disease risk. Stat Med. 1995;14:2433–43. https://doi.org/10.1002/sim.4780142112.
30. Gelman A, Rubin DB. Inference from iterative simulation using multiple sequences. Stat Sci. 1995;7:354–63.
31. Lawson AB, Browne WJ, CLVR. Disease Mapping with WinBUGS and MLwiN. Hoboken: Wiley; 2004.
32. Unaids. 90-90-90. An ambitious treatment target to help end the AIDS epidemic. 2014;40. http://www.unaids.org/sites/default/files/media_asset/90-90-90_en.pdf.
33. HAHSTA DC DEPT OF HEALTH, DC Appleseed WA partnership. 90-90-90-50 Plan. 2016.
34. Lawson AB, Biggeri A, Boehning D, Lesaffre E, Viel JF, Clark A, et al. Disease mapping models: an empirical evaluation. Disease mapping collaborative group. Stat Med. 2000;19:2217–41.

20

Prevalence of lower limb deep venous thrombosis among adult HIV positive patients attending an outpatient clinic at Mulago Hospital

Sosthene Tsongo Vululi[1*], Samuel Bugeza[2], Muyinda Zeridah[3], Henry Ddungu[4], Akello Betty Openy[5], Mubiru Frank[6] and Rosalind Parkes-Ratanshi[7]

Abstract

Background: Deep venous thrombosis (DVT) and its major complication pulmonary embolism (PE) are collectively known as venous thromboembolism. In Uganda, the prevalence of DVT among HIV patients has not been previously published. The aim of the study was to determine the prevalence and sonographic features of lower limb deep venous thrombosis among HIV positive patients on anti-retroviral treatment (ART).

Methods: This was a cross sectional study in which HIV positive patients on ART were recruited from an out-patient HIV clinic at Mulago National Referral Hospital. Patients were randomly selected and enrolled until a sample size of 384 was reached. Study participants underwent compression and Doppler ultrasound studies of both lower limb deep veins using Medison Sonoacer7 ultrasound machine.

Resuts: We found a prevalence of DVT of 9.1% (35 of 384 participants) among HIV patients on ART. The prevalence of latent (asymptomatic) DVT was 2.3%. Among 35 patients with DVT, 42.8% had chronic DVT; 31.1% had acute DVT and the rest had latent DVT. Among the risk factors, the odds of occurrence of DVT among patients with prolonged immobility were 4.81 times as high as in those with no prolonged immobility ($p = 0.023$; OR = 4.81; 95% CI 1.25–18.62). Treatment with second line anti-retroviral therapy (ART) including protease inhibitors (PIs) was associated with higher odds of DVT occurrence compared with first line ART ($p = 0.020$; OR = 2.38; 95% CI 1.14–4.97). The odds of DVT occurrence in patients with a lower CD4 count (< 200 cells/μl) were 5.36 times as high as in patients with CD4 counts above 500 cells/μl ($p = 0.008$). About 48.6% patients with DVT had a low risk according to Well's score.

Conclusion: DVT was shown in nearly 10% of HIV patients attending an out-patient clinic in an urban setting in Uganda. Risk factors included protease inhibitors in their ART regimen, prolonged immobility, and low CD4 count (< 200 cells/μl). Clinicians should have a low threshold for performing lower limb Doppler ultrasound scan examination on infected HIV patients on ART who are symptomatic for DVT. Therefore, clinicians should consider anti-coagulant prophylaxis and lower deep venous ultrasound screening of patients who are on second line ART regimen with low CD4 cell counts and/or with prolonged immobility or hormonal contraception.

Keywords: Lower limb veins anatomy, Well's score, Doppler ultrasound, DVT echo pattern

*Correspondence: sosthenetsongo@gmail.com
[1] Makerere University College of Health Sciences (MakCHS), Kampala, Uganda
Full list of author information is available at the end of the article

Background

Deep venous thrombosis is one of the most prevalent medical conditions [1]. The risk of DVT in the general population of South Africa is 0.10% a year [2]. HIV infection has been recognised as a hypercoagulable condition since the late 1980s and the current and other studies indicate that the prevalence in HIV positive patients is significantly increased [3, 4] with a two to tenfold increased risk in HIV infected patients compared to the general population. A large number of worldwide studies reported the frequency of DVT in HIV-infected patients ranging from 0.19 to 8% [5]. There is some evidence to suggest that anti-retroviral therapy (ART) may increase the risk of DVT [6]. There is limited work on DVT in sub-Saharan Africa, especially Uganda. A study done by Mangeni et al. in 2003 at Mulago Hospital showed that out of 86 patients clinically suspected to have lower limb DVT, 38 (44.2%) were found to have DVT after sonography [7]. Doppler ultrasound of lower limb deep veins presents an echo-pattern of the thrombus usually found in DVT. The thrombus may be anechoic, hypoechoic, heterogeneous or hyper-echoic depending on the age of the clot. To our knowledge, there has been no study conducted in Eastern Africa to determine the prevalence of DVT in HIV positive patients. The aim of this study was to determine the prevalence of DVT in HIV outpatients on ART in Uganda and to appreciate the association between clinical presentation and sonographic features of DVT.

Materials/methods

This study was conducted from May 2014 to January 2015. This was a cross sectional study in which adult HIV positive outpatients on ART were recruited from the Infectious Diseases Institute and HIV clinic at Mulago Hospital. Participants were attending for routine follow-up of their HIV. Participants unable to understand the procedure and unable to consent for ultrasound scan examination were excluded. Using systematic sampling [8], patients who met the inclusion criteria were enrolled until the sample size of 384 was reached. Informed consent was signed by each participant before ultrasound scan examination. Study participants underwent Doppler ultrasound studies of both lower limb deep veins using an ultrasound machine (Medison Sonoacer7).

The patients were categorized depending on the ultrasound findings: latent DVT when there was lack of venous compressibility or reduction of blood flow on ultrasound; acute DVT was diagnosed in the presence of hypoechoic thrombus with limited venous compressibility; chronic DVT when there was hyper echoic or heterogeneous thrombus and limitation of venous compressibility. Proximal DVT was diagnosed in the presence of a thrombus in common femoral vein up to popliteal vein whereas distal DVT was seen below the popliteal fossa. A Wells score was calculated for each patient based on the presence of clinical symptoms. At the time of the study, WHO and Ugandan guidelines recommended first line ART to be backbone of nucleoside reverse transcriptase inhibitors (lamivudine/zidovudine or lamivudine/tenofovir) with either nevirapine or efavirenz non-nucleoside reverse transcriptase inhibitors. Second line regimens for those who had failed first line was either of these backbones with a protease inhibitor; either ritonavir boosted lopinavir or ritonavir boosted atazanavir. A structured non-disguised questionnaire was used and acquired data were entered using EPI—DATA 3.02 and exported to be analysed using a statistical software program STATA 13.

The study was approved by the IDI Scientific Review Committee (SRC) and the School of Medicine Research and Ethics Committee (SOMREC).

Results

Three hundred eighty-four patients were enrolled. 286 participants were aged between 18 and 50 years (74.5%) and the remainder were above 50 years (25.5%). The most common occupation in 38.5% of participants was business (see Table 1).

Out of 384 study participants, 229 (59.6%) were on first line ART regimen and 155 (40.4%) participants were on second line.

The prevalence of lower limb DVT was 9.1% (35/384) (Table 2). Among 35 participants found with DVT, 26 (74.3%) were symptomatic and 9 (25.7%) participants asymptomatic for DVT. The prevalence of latent DVT among HIV patients on ART was 2.3%. Among

Table 1 Study participants by gender, age-group categories and occupation

Demographics	Number (n)	Percentage (%)
Gender		
Male	126	32.8
Female	258	67.2
Age (years)		
18–29	40	10.4
30–39	110	28.7
40–49	136	35.4
≥ 50	98	25.5
Occupation		
Business	148	38.5
Driver	18	4.7
Farmer	43	11.2
House wife	28	7.3
Work in office	30	7.8
Others	117	30.5

Table 2 Prevalence of DVT in the study population

DVT	Type of DVT			
	n (%)	n (%)		
Present	35 (9.1)	Symptomatic for DVT	Acute	11 (31.4)
			Chronic	15 (42.9)
		Asymptomatic for DVT	Latent	9 (25.7)
Absent	349 (90.9)			

35 patients with DVT, 31.1% had acute DVT, 42.8% had chronic DVT, and the rest had latent DVT (Figs. 1, 2). Among the patients with DVT, 30 (80.7%) had proximal DVT and 5 had distal DVT. Bilateral deep venous thrombosis was noted in 3/35 (0.08%) participants.

Among participants who had DVT, 4 (11.4%) reported the use of hormonal contraception. Patients with hormonal contraception use had a high probability of DVT ($p = 0.024$).

On the Wells scoring out of 35 patients with DVT, 17 (48.6%) patients had a low probability of DVT, 8 (22.9%) patients had moderate probability of DVT and 10 patients had high probability of DVT. Study findings showed that among 35 patients with DVT, 23 (65.7%) patients had leg swelling ($p < 0.0001$).

In the bivariate analysis, study findings showed that prolonged immobility, platelets count, latest CD4 count, and ART line regimen had an association with deep venous thrombosis (see Table 3).

In the multivariate analysis (Table 4), the odds of occurrence of DVT among patients with prolonged immobility are 4.81 times as high as in those with no prolonged immobility. Being on second line ART regimen, is associated with higher odds of DVT occurrence compared with being on ART first line (OR = 2.38; 95% CI 1.14–4.97). Patients with a lower CD4 count (cd4 < 200 cells/μL) had 5.36 times the odds of DVT occurrence than those with higher CD4 count (cd4 > 500 cells/μL).

Discussion

We found the prevalence of DVT in ambulatory HIV positive patients on ART to be 9.1% at the National Referral Hospital, Kampala, Uganda. This prevalence is higher

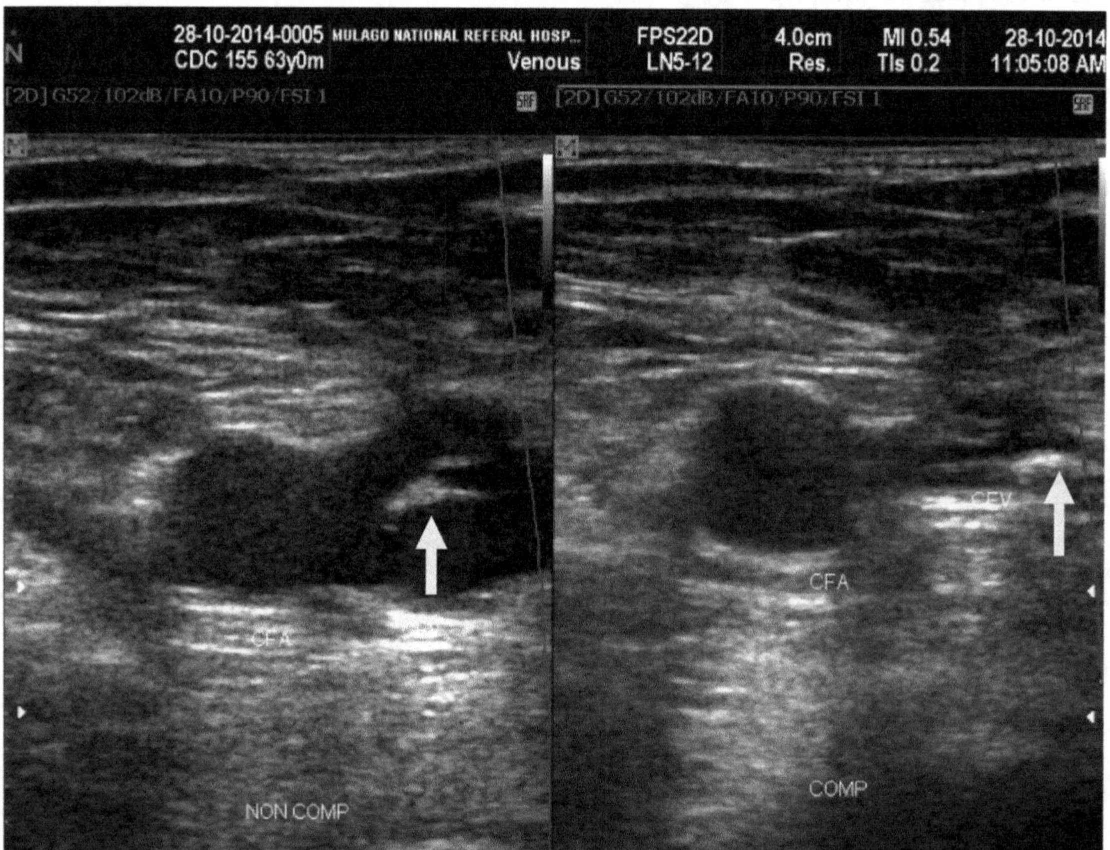

Fig. 1 Chronic DVT. Transverse sonogram of 63 years old male HIV positive patient on HAART shows echogenic thrombus (white arrow) in the right common femoral vein (CFV) causing partial compressibility of the vein

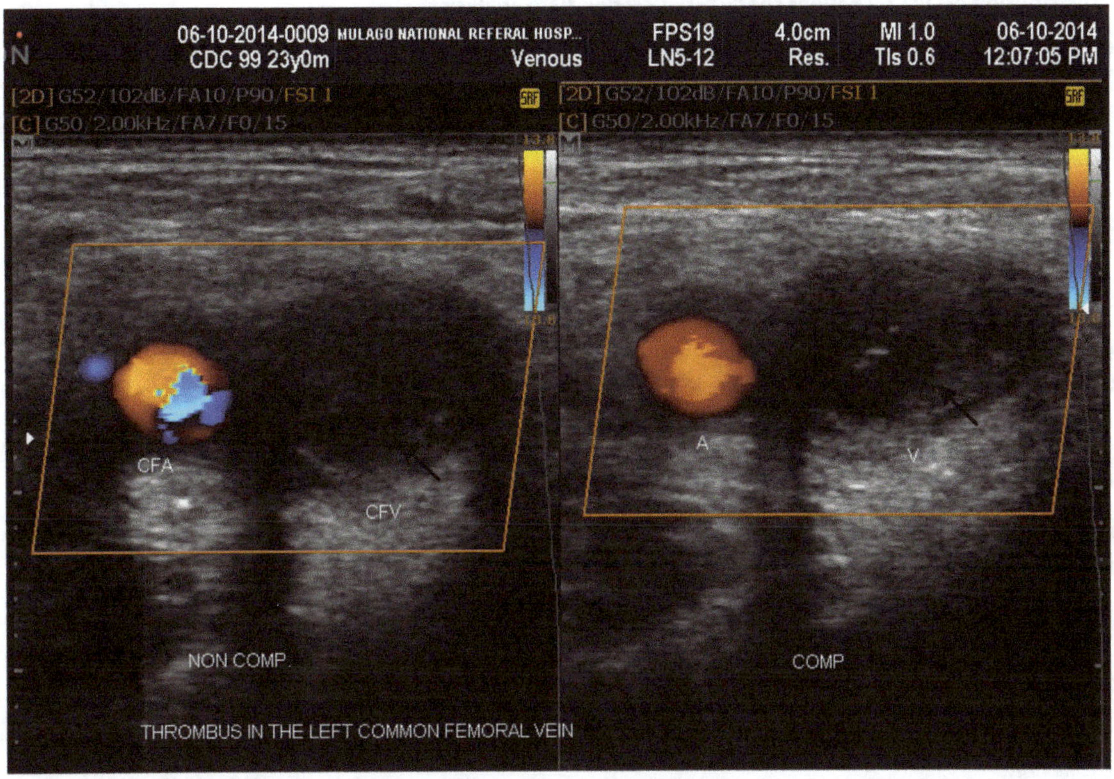

Fig. 2 Acute DVT. Transverse sonogram of a 23 years old man on second line HAART who presented with acute DVT of CFV. Ultrasound scan shows lack of compressibility of the left CFV, presence of heterogeneous thrombus (black arrow) in the lumen and absence of spontaneous Doppler signal

than previously reported in several studies among HIV-infected patients in Western and African countries ranging from 0.19 to 8% per year [6, 9–11] The prevalence of DVT in HIV-infected patients is within limits from previous studies although a little higher than in the general population in Uganda [12] (1/1000 person-years of observation). This is especially striking as these patients were attending for routine follow up for their HIV and were not admitted as in-patients or attending hospital because they were unwell. To our knowledge, this is the first study to determine the prevalence of DVT among HIV sero-positive out patients on ART in Eastern Africa.

In this study, 15 of 35 patients found with DVT had hyperechoic thrombus (42%). The other sonographic characteristic of DVT noted in this study were the same characteristics reported in other studies [13, 14].

Majority of participants found with DVT had clinical symptoms of this pathology (Table 2) and only few patients had latent DVT (2.3%). Almost half of HIV patients with DVT (48.6%) had a lower Wells score for DVT (Table 3). This suggests that DVT in this population is difficult to predict clinically therefore Well's score need to be altered to account for HIV infection although other studies have shown that patients with high score are likely to develop DVT [5]. This study demonstrates that infected HIV patients on ART may be asymptomatic for DVT according Wells score findings however they may develop an asymptomatic DVT. Based on the results of Wells score in this study, a compression ultrasound screening in HIV positive patients on ART may be helpful for early diagnosis.

There was a significant association between PIs containing second line ART and deep venous thrombosis in patients ($p = 0.02$) which is in keeping with several other studies. HIV-infected patients on second line ART regimen (PIs) have higher risk for blood clot formation than those on first line treatment [5, 8, 15, 16]. Studies supporting this association reported high rate of DVT among HIV-infected patients after the introduction of protease inhibitors in ART regimen [4].

This study shows significant association between hormonal contraception use and DVT ($p = 0.024$) as per well known evidence for increased risk of VTE associated with combined hormonal contraceptive use generally [22].

Eleven (2.9%) of 384 participants had history of immobility in the last 3 months. Among 35 participants with DVT, 4 (11.4%) had history of immobility ($p = 0.005$).

Table 3 Distribution of DVT by patient characteristics: bivariate analysis

Characteristic	Total population n (%) n = 384	DVT present n = 35 (9.1%)	DVT absent 349 (89.1%)	Chi square	p value
Gender				0.88	0.35
Male	126 (32.8%)	9 (25.7%)	117 (33.5%)		
Female	258 (67.2%)	26 (74.3%)	232 (66.5%)		
Age (years)				0.32	0.574
< 50	286 (74.5)	26 (74.3)	260 (74.5)	0.001	0.98
50 years and above	98 (25.5)	9 (25.7)	89 (25.5)		
Duration on ART (mean of years)	4.5 (2.5–8.5)	5.5 (2.5–8.5)	4.5 (2.5–8.5)		0.80
ART line status				6.17	*0.01*
First line	229 (59.6%)	14 (40.0%	215 (61.6%)		
Second line	155 (40.4%)	21 (60%)	134 (38.4%)		
Latest CD4 cell counts				6.73	*0.04*
Less than 200	23 (6.0%)	5 (14.3%)	18 (5.2%)		
200–500	194 (50.5%)	20 (57.1%)	174 (49.9%)		
Above 500	167 (43.5)	10 (28.6%)	157 (45.0%)		
Occupation				2.78	0.73
Business	148 (38.5%)	11 (31.4%)	137 (39.3%)		
Driver	18 (4.7%)	2 (5.7%)	16 (4.6%)		
Farmer	43 (11.2%)	5 (14.3%)	38 (10.9%)		
House wife	28 (7.3%)	3 (8.7%)	25 (7.2)		
Work in office	30 (7.8%)	1 (2.9%)	29 (8.3%)		
Others	117 (30.5%	13 (37.1%)	104 (29.8%)		
Prolonged immobility				10.21	*0.005*
Yes	11 (2.9%)	4 (11.4%)	7 (2.0%)		
No	373 (97.1%)	31 (88.6%)	342 (98.0%)		
Platelets count	235 (185–301)	206 (178–287)	236 (186–303)		0.10
BMI (median (IQR)	23.5 (21.5–26.9)	24.6 (21.9–28.1)	23.4 (21.5–26.8)		0.37

This is also in line with other studies suggesting that chronic immobility (> 30 days) is a high risk for deep venous thrombosis [17–19]. These study findings were similar to the case–control study in 2008 conducted by Leibson and colleagues in 2008 [20, 21]. HIV patients are susceptible to develop opportunistic infections responsible of hospitalization, and this will put them at increased risk for DVT [15, 21–23].

Our study showed that among 23 participants (6%) with low CD4 cell counts (< 200 cells/mm^3), 5 participants (14.3%) had DVT. Therefore, correlation between low CD4 and DVT was significant even after correcting for immobility which may be associated with higher rates of opportunistic infections in people with low CD4 counts. Several studies reported the same findings [5–24]. The association between low CD4 count and DVT may be related to progressive immunosuppression and increasing hypercoagulable state [25]. Having a low CD4 count can be associated with having an uncontrolled high HIV viral load. HIV with a high viral load is associated with hypercoagulable state. Unfortunately, viral load was not done in all patients recruited in this study therefore it was not possible to analyse any association between DVT and viral load.

Whilst newer lower molecular weight anti-coagulation is expensive for low resource settings, traditional anti-coagulation with warfarin is cheap, although logistically difficult. Research into the cost–benefit of use of newer anti-coagulation or point of care monitoring of warfarin in patients at highest risk of DVT in our setting should be considered. The blood tests such as D-dimer, tissue factor (TF) and analysis of other coagulation biomarkers should also be considered in relation to blood clot formation in this population with hypercoagulable state.

Conclusion and recommendations

The prevalence of DVT among ambulatory HIV positive patients on ART is 9.1%. Majority of participants with DVT were symptomatic. Prolonged immobility, low CD4 count (< 200 cells/μl) and ART second line (PIs) were associated with risk of DVT. It is advisable to perform lower limb Doppler ultrasound scan examination on infected HIV patients on ART who are symptomatic for DVT. However, half of patients with a DVT had a

Table 4 Multivariate analysis: study findings

Characteristic	Crude odds ratio (95% CI)	p-value	Adjusted odds ratio (95% CI)	p-value
Gender				
Male	1.00		1.00	
Female	1.46 (0.66–3.21)	0.350	1.94 (0.84–4.47)	0.119
Age (years)				
< 50 years	1.00			
50 years and above	1.37 (0.45–4.15)	0.98		
Duration on ART (years)	1.02 (0.934–1.11)	0.679		
ART line status				
First line	1.00		1.00	
Second line	2.40 (1.18–4.89)	0.015	2.38 (1.14–4.97)	*0.020*
Latest CD4 count (cells/μl)				
Above 500	1.00		1.00	
200–500	1.80 (0.82–3.97)	0.143	1.82 (0.80–4.14)	0.153
Less than 200	4.36 (1.34–14.18)	0.014	5.31 (1.54–18.35)	*0.008*
Occupation				
Business	1.00			
Driver	1.56 (0.32–7.69)	0.586	–	–
Farmer	1.64 (0.54–5.00)	0.386	–	–
House wife	1.50 (0.39–5.74)	0.558	–	–
Work in office	0.43 (0.01–3.46)	0.430	–	–
Others	1.56 (0.68–3.61)	0.303	–	–
History of immobility				
No	1.00		1.00	
Yes	6.30 (1.75–22.72)	0.005	4.81 (1.25–18.62)	*0.023*
Platelets count	0.99 (0.96–1.00)	0.103	0.99 (0.97–1.02)	0.110
Body mass index	1.02 (0.94–1.09)	0.687	–	–

low Wells score suggesting that they did not have typical clinical features of DVT. Therefore, clinicians should consider prophylactic anti-coagulation or routine Doppler ultrasound scan monitoring in HIV patients with low CD4 counts and PIs who are immobile knowing that they may develop an asymptomatic DVT. Patients using oral contraception on PIs and with low CD4 count should be counselled on signs and symptoms of DVT that they should report to their doctor and should be monitored closely for DVT.

Abbreviations
ART: antiretroviral therapy; DVT: deep venous thrombosis; HAART: highly active antiretroviral therapy; HIV: human immunodeficiency virus; IDI: infectious disease institute; PE: pulmonary embolism; PIs: protease inhibitors; VTE: venous thromboembolism.

Authors' contributions
All listed authors have contributed all the time in the design of the study and collection, analysis, and interpretation of data and in writing this manuscript. All authors read and approved the final manuscript.

Author details
[1] Makerere University College of Health Sciences (MakCHS), Kampala, Uganda. [2] Radiology Department of Mulago Hospital, Lecturer at MakCHS, Kampala, Uganda. [3] Mulago Hospital, Kampala, Uganda. [4] Uganda Cancer Institute, Kampala, Uganda. [5] MakCHS, Kampala, Uganda. [6] Stastician-IDI-Kampala, Kampala, Uganda. [7] Prevention Care Treatment, Infectious Diseases Institute (IDI), Kampala, Uganda.

Acknowledgements
I really appreciate AusHEAL, Sonic Healthcare Limited and Dr. Murray Thorn in Australia for advices and financial support through HEAL Africa Hospital in Goma D. R. Congo. My thanks go to IDI and Mulago Hospital in Uganda for assistance in data collection and analysis. I'm very grateful to Dr. Rosalind Parkes-Ratanshi for assistance in preparation of this manuscript.

Competing interests
The authors declare that they have no competing interests.

Funding
Funding from AusHEAL, Sonic Healthcare Limited and Dr. Murray Thorn in Australia through HEAL Africa Hospital Goma/North Kivu/D. R. Congo. Mulago Hospital through radiology department provided the ultrasound machine and room for examination. IDI/Mulago Hospital provided a room for examination. IDI/Mulago Hospital helped also in analysis by allowing the assistance of the statistician Frank Mubiru.

References
1. Malani PN. Harrison's principles of internal medicine. JAMA. 2012;308(17):1813–4.

2. Louw S, Jacobson BF, Büller H. Human immunodeficiency virus infection and acute deep vein thromboses. Clin Appl Thromb Hemost. 2008;14(3):352–5.
3. Eyal A, Veller M. HIV and venous thrombotic events: vascular surgery: review. S Afr J Surg. 2009;47(2):54–6.
4. Aquila AM. Deep venous thrombosis. J Cardiovasc Nurs. 2001;15(4):25–44.
5. Veller M, Pillai J. Lower-limb venous thrombosis. Contin Med Educ. 2009;27(7):306–11.
6. Crum-Cianflone NF, Weekes J, Bavaro M. Review: thromboses among HIV-infected patients during the highly active antiretroviral therapy era. AIDS Patient Care STDs. 2008;22(10):771–8.
7. Mangeni F, Kawooya M, Kiguli-Malwadde E, Ssali F. Sonography and risk factors for lower limb deep venous thrombosis at Mulago hospital, Uganda. East Afr Med J. 2006;83(8):443–9.
8. Gordis Leon. Epidemiology. 3rd ed. Philadelphia: Elsevier; 2004.
9. Geerts W, Cook D, Selby R, Etchells E. Venous thromboembolism and its prevention in critical care. J Crit Care. 2002;17(2):95–104.
10. Bibas M, Biava G, Antinori A. HIV-associated venous thromboembolism. Mediterr J Hematol Infect Dis. 2011;3(1):e2011030.
11. Saif M. Thromboembolism associated with HIV infection: a case report and review of the literature. AIDS Reader. 2000;10(8):492–6.
12. Friedman AC. Diagnostic ultrasound, vols. 1 and 2. Am J Roentgenol. 2006;187(1):W139.
13. Chaer RA, et al. Multimodal therapy for acute and chronic venous thrombotic and occlusive disease. Vasc Endovasc Surg. 2005;39(5):375–80.
14. Khaladkar SM, Thakkar DK, et al. Deep vein thrombosis of the lower limbs: a retrospective analysis of doppler ultrasound findings. Med J Dr DY Patil Univ. 2014;7(5):612.
15. De Cock KM, Jaffe HW, Curran JW. The evolving epidemiology of HIV/AIDS. Aids. 2012;26(10):1205–13.
16. Shen Y, Frenkel EP. Thrombosis and a hypercoagulable state in HIV-infected patients. Clin Appl Thromb Hemost. 2004;10(3):277–80.
17. Aldington S, Pritchard A, Perrin K, James K, Wijesinghe M, Beasley R. Prolonged seated immobility at work is a common risk factor for venous thromboembolism leading to hospital admission. Intern Med J. 2008;38(2):133–5.
18. Cushman M. Epidemiology and risk factors for venous thrombosis. Semin Hematol. 2007;44(2):62–9.
19. Rocha AT, et al. Risk of venous thromboembolism and efficacy of thromboprophylaxis in hospitalized obese medical patients and in obese patients undergoing bariatric surgery. Obes Surg. 2006;16(12):1645–55.
20. Leibson CL, Petterson TM, Bailey KR, Melton LJ, Heit JA. Risk factors for venous thromboembolism in nursing home residents. In: Mayo clinic proceedings vol. 83, no. 2. New York: Elsevier; 2008. p. 151–7.
21. Zarowitz BJ, et al. Thrombotic risk and immobility in residents of long-term care facilities. J Am Med Direct Assoc. 2010;11(3):211–21.
22. Klein SK, Slim EJ, De Kruif MD, Keller TT, Ten Cate H, van Gorp EC, et al. Is chronic HIV infection associated with venous thrombotic disease? A systematic review. Neth J Med. 2005;63(4):129–36.
23. Sullivan PS, Dworkin MS, Jones JL, Hooper WC. Epidemiology of thrombosis in HIV-infected individuals. Aids. 2000;14(3):321–4.
24. Lifson AR, et al. Development of diagnostic criteria for serious non-AIDS events in HIV clinical trials. HIV Clin Trials. 2010;11(4):205–19.
25. Levine AM, et al. Progressive prothrombotic state in women with advancing HIV disease. JAIDS J Acquir Immune Defic Syndr. 2006;42(5):572–7.

21

Social-support needs among adolescents living with HIV in transition from pediatric to adult care in Cambodia

Graham Toth[1], Gitau Mburu[2], Sovannary Tuot[3], Vohith Khol[4], Chanrith Ngin[3], Pheak Chhoun[3] and Siyan Yi[3,5*]

Abstract

Background: Understanding the circumstances of adolescents living with HIV is critical in designing adolescent-friendly services that will facilitate successful transition from pediatric to adult care. This study describes access, utilization and ongoing social support needs among adolescents living with HIV aged 15–17 in transition from pediatric to adult HIV care in Cambodia.

Methods: A cross-sectional study was conducted among 328 adolescents, randomly selected from 11 antiretroviral therapy (ART) clinics across the country. Descriptive analyses were conducted to summarize their characteristics, access to social support and ongoing support needs among male and female adolescents.

Results: Mean age of the study participants was 15.8 (SD=0.8) years. Just over half (55.2%) were male. Most had at least one deceased parent (mother 50.9%; father 60.5%), and majority were living with biological parents (40.8%) or relatives (49.3%). A third came from families with an ID poor card, and 21.0% were working for pay. Almost half (46.6%) reported that their family had received social support for their health care, including food support (76.5%), school allowance (62.1%), transport allowance to ART clinics (53.6%), psychosocial counseling (35.3%), vocational training (22.9%) or home visits (11.1%). Several ongoing social support needs were identified, including ongoing inability to cover health expenses unless they are supported by health insurance or health equity fund (55.0%). In addition, adolescents reported having been asked to come back earlier than their scheduled appointment (13.7%), having had to purchase their own drugs (2.7%), experiencing HIV stigma (32.0%), having been denied housing or food due to HIV (8.2%) or failing to attend school within the past month partly because of HIV (16.8%). Two-thirds did not have access to peer support groups.

Conclusions: Social protection mechanisms are reaching some adolescents in need, while other remain without social support due to discontinuities in health and social care. Multi-sectoral interventions, supporting school attendance, adolescent-friendly clinic scheduling, reductions in child employment, mitigation of HIV-related stigma and strengthening of peer-to-peer support are required to improve coverage of social protection interventions for adolescents in transition.

Keywords: HIV, Adolescents, Transition, Social support, Social protection, Cambodia

*Correspondence: siyan@doctor.com
[3] KHANA Center for Population Health Research, No. 33, Street 71, Phnom Penh, Cambodia
Full list of author information is available at the end of the article

Background

Adolescents, defined as people aged 10–19 years, undergo rapid psychological, sexual and physical maturity [1]. Adolescents experience marked changes in sexuality [2], mental capacity [3], self-efficacy and independence [4]. At the same time, adolescents are one of the most affected populations by HIV. Globally, over two million adolescents are living with HIV [5]. Given the dynamic changes during adolescence, studies exploring outcomes of HIV care tend to distinguish adolescents living with HIV from both pediatric and adult populations.

Evidence from these studies shows that adolescents' access and outcomes of care are generally sub-optimal. Compared to adults, adolescents have poorer rates of HIV testing, disclosure [6], treatment adherence [7], long-term immunologic recovery [8] and viral suppression [9, 10]. In addition, adolescents often face denial of care by their legal guardians and parents [11], are inexperienced in negotiation for safer sex during sexual debut [12, 13] and may be unable to obtain services due to restrictive parental consent laws [14]. Exploration of causes and potential solutions to these poor outcomes have generally focused on biomedical and health system solution [15].

However, the issues of social support for adolescents living with HIV are increasingly occupying a center stage. Due to the increasing survival of children living with HIV into adolescence [16], some of whom were orphans or had lost their primary caregivers [17, 18], there is rising recognition that they require social support to adjust socially and psychologically to living with HIV [19, 20].

The influence of social support on adolescent's self-efficacy [4], uptake of new services, acceptance of their diagnosis and treatment adherence [21, 22] have been documented in recent studies. Additionally, peer support groups have been shown to have a positive impact on disclosure, mental health [23] and uptake of HIV services [24] among adolescents. Furthermore, structural social protection interventions—such as cash transfers, food security, school fees and feeding programs—have been shown to have a positive impact on adolescents' adherence to antiretroviral therapy (ART) and general wellbeing [25].

These findings suggest that social support and protection are essential in achieving positive health outcomes among adolescents living with HIV. However, adolescents are not a homogenous group, but instead, they have evolving social needs in tandem with their physical and psychological maturity [26]. Studies suggest that older adolescents are particularly at risk of poorer HIV outcomes during their transition from pediatric to adult HIV care [27]. During this period, adolescents living with HIV are at high risk of poor adherence to ART [28], disengagement from HIV care [29], immunological deterioration [30] and death [5, 31].

However, there is a paucity of research exploring social support during adolescents' transition from pediatric to adult HIV care. Most of the existing studies tend to focus on clinical and biomedical (e.g., virological, retention and mortality) outcomes during and after transition to adult care [28, 29, 32, 33], with little focus on the social support interventions or needs specific to this group. As a result, social support for adolescents living with HIV remain undocumented and unaddressed [30]. This paper describes utilization and ongoing social support needs among adolescents living with HIV aged 15–17 in transition from pediatric to adult care in Cambodia and discusses the implications of the findings on a successful transition from pediatric to adult HIV care.

Methods

Study design and settings

This cross-sectional study was conducted in August 2016 among 328 adolescents living with HIV, randomly selected from 11 ART clinics throughout Cambodia. The details of the study have been reported elsewhere [34]. Briefly, we applied a two-stage sampling design to identify 598 eligible participants from the 18 major ART clinics countrywide. Twenty-one clinics with less than 10 adolescents living with HIV each were excluded to minimize cost. The sample size was set at 320, calculated to estimate a high level of preparedness of 60% with a confidence interval (CI) of 95% and design effect of 1.4 using a probability proportional to size method [35]. Eligible subjects were selected using a random number table.

Participant recruitment

Selected adolescents were screened via telephone and informed of research objectives as well as place, date and time of the interview. Adolescents would be asked to participate if they were between 15 and 17 years of age, receiving treatment and care services, able to communicate in Khmer, allowed by a parent or guardian to participate, their parent or caregiver was willing to provide a written consent, able to present themselves on the day of the interview and physically and mentally stable to provide verbal assent to participate. Upon confirming eligibility, a written consent from their parent or guardian was obtained. Recruitment continued until the required sample size for each clinic was achieved.

Questionnaire development

Questionnaire development was guided by existing literature [36, 37]. Information on socio-demographic characteristics, perceived health status, school attendance, disclosure, stigma experience, psychosocial support and medication supply and ART adherence were collected through self-reported interviews. Clinical and immunological data, including HIV status, ART history and laboratory values for CD4 and viral loads were obtained from medical records.

Data collection and training

Data were collected by two teams of interviewers and moderators who were trained on study protocol, questionnaire administration, confidentiality and issues related to research with human participants [38]. Pretesting was conducted among 20 adolescents living with HIV and 10 parents and guardians, and questionnaire adjustments were made.

Data analyses

Data were classified and scaled continuously or categorically as appropriate and recorded into a computerized database using EpiData version 3 (Odense, Denmark). Double data entry was implemented to minimize errors. Descriptive analyses were performed to determine frequency distribution for categorical variables and mean with standard deviation (SD) for continuous variables. Chi square, Fisher's exact or t-test tests for significance were used to compare characteristics of male and female adolescents. p-values of less than 0.05 were considered statistically significant.

Ethical considerations

The study was approved by the National Ethics Committee for Health Research, Ministry of Health in Cambodia (Ref: 297NECHR). Assent from participants and a written informed consent from a parent or guardian was obtained. Data were collected in private locations, and confidentiality protected by removing all personal identifiers from questionnaires. Participants were provided with a token of $2.5–$5 for transportation.

Results

Characteristics and of the study sample

Of the 328 adolescents, 51.3% had completed secondary (7–9 years) school, less than half (42.7%) were living with one or both parents, and 55.2% were male. Parents (40.8%) or relatives (33.6%) were the most frequently reported caregivers. More than half of respondents had at least one deceased parent (mother 50.9%; father 60.5%). Maternal and paternal educational levels were both 20% for high school (10–12 years) or university education (Table 1).

Access and adherence to ART

On average, ART refills were dispensed every two months. Forty-five participants (13.7%) reported having to return earlier than their scheduled appointment due to inadequate supply of medicines (22.2%) or the need for an additional check-up (46.7%). A small number (2.7%) had been asked to purchase their own drugs. Notably, sharing of ART was not reported (Table 2).

Stigma and discrimination

Thirty-two percent reported negative attitudes or being mistreated (10.7%) because of their HIV status; 8.2% had been denied housing or food (Table 3).

School attendance, employment and social support

Within the past month, 22.9% experienced disruptions with attendance at school, and 16.8% reported that they were no longer enrolled. Being too ill (34.1%), lack of fees (14%) or poor academic performance (18.6%) were the most frequently reported reasons for being absent. Only a fraction (0.6%) of the 69 adolescents currently working for pay sought employment outside of their hometown. Almost half (46.6%) reported that their family had received social support for their health care, including food support (76.5%), school allowance (62.1%), transport allowance to ART clinic (53.6%), emotional counseling (35.3%), vocational training (22.9%) and home visit (11.1%). Thirty percent belonged to a peer support group (Table 4).

Assessment of preparedness for transition

The majority (72.0%) of respondents were able to recognize when they were getting sick, and 80.5% knew when they needed to call a health care provider. However, less than half (46.0%) reported being the one responsible for scheduling follow-up visits, and 13.4% indicated that they felt comfortable asking health questions during appointments. An approximately equal number of males and females reported some degree of difficulty with ART adherence. The average visual adherence scale score between the two groups was 95.4% (SD = 9.6%) (Table 5).

Significantly, females were less likely to retain copies of their health records and doctor contacts (32.7% vs. 57.4%, $p < 0.001$), less likely to report having a method for organizing HIV-related appointments (47.9% vs. 72.8%, $p < 0.001$) and more likely to report that they would discontinue ART when feeling ill (7.1% vs. 15.1%, $p = 0.02$) (Table 5).

Experiences of preparation for transition

About one-third (29.6%) had received counseling on the transition to adult services. However, only 2.7% of them had completed a transfer form, and 19.7% had visited an adult ART clinic to prepare for the transition. About one-forth (24.7%) reported that a case manager had been identified to support them during the transition. The

Table 1 Socio-demographic characteristics of male and female adolescents living with HIV

Socio-demographic characteristics	Total (*n* = 328), *n* (%)	Male (*n* = 169), *n* (%)	Female (*n* = 159), *n* (%)	*P*-value*
Mean age (in years)	15.9 ± 0.8	15.8 ± 0.8	16.0 ± 0.8	0.06
Type of ART regimen				0.91
First line	183 (82.4)	140 (82.8)	131 (82.4)	
Second line	36 (16.2)	29 (17.2)	27 (17.6)	
Duration on ART (in months)	101 ± 40	99.8 (40.7)	94.0 (39.6)	0.20
Initial CD4 count (cells/mm^3)	632 ± 110	777 ± 1460	632 ± 460	0.35
Latest CD4 count (cells/mm^3)	672 ± 284	683 ± 314	660 ± 250	0.44
First viral load count (copies)	34,375 ± 13,958	37,868 ± 13,205	30,662 ± 14,748	0.64
Latest viral load count (copies)	9268 ± 6407	4103 ± 1573	14,759 ± 9041	0.13
Visual adherence scale (%)	95.4 ± 9.6	95.3 ± 9.6	95.4 ± 9.7	0.91
Travel time to ART clinic (min)	48.2 ± 43.4	46.1 ± 41.2	55.5 ± 45.5	0.36
Cost to travel to clinic (USD)	3.4 ± 3.9	3.5 ± 3.9	3.3 ± 4.0	0.61
Level of formal education[a]				0.76
Primary school or lower	92 (28.0)	50 (20.7)	42 (26.4)	
Secondary school	168 (51.3)	86 (50.9)	82 (51.6)	
High school or higher	68 (20.7)	33 (19.5)	35 (22.0)	
Ability to cover health expenses				0.11
No	181 (55.2)	86 (50.9)	95 (59.7)	
Yes	147 (44.8)	83 (49.3)	64 (40.3)	
Family has an ID poor card				0.04
No	190 (57.9)	88 (52.1)	102 (64.2)	
Yes	112 (34.2)	63 (37.3)	49 (30.8)	
Don't know	26 (7.9)	18 (10.7)	8 (5.0)	
Access to the health equity fund				<0.001
No	185 (56.4)	109 (64.5)	76 (47.8)	
Yes	126 (38.4)	45 (35.7)	81 (50.9)	
Don't know	17 (5.2)	15 (8.9)	2 (1.3)	
Covered by health insurance				0.02
No	289 (88.1)	148 (87.6)	141 (88.7)	
Yes	148 (87.6)	0 (0.0)	6 (3.8)	
Don't know	33 (10.1)	21 (12.4)	12 (7.5)	
Currently living with				0.33
Parents	140 (42.7)	73 (43.2)	67 (42.1)	
Grandparents	49 (14.9)	29 (12.7)	20 (12.6)	
Relatives	106 (32.3)	54 (32.0)	52 (32.7)	
In an orphanage	27 (8.2)	12 (7.1)	15 (9.4)	
Other	6 (1.8)	1 (0.6)	5 (3.1)	
Type of accommodation				0.94
Flat/apartment	19 (8.9)	10 (8.7)	9 (8.4)	
Hut	12 (5.4)	7 (6.1)	5 (4.7)	
Mid-size country house	173 (73.7)	88 (78.7)	85 (79.4)	
Mansion/large country house	12 (5.4)	6 (5.2)	6 (5.6)	
Other	6 (2.7)	4 (3.5)	2 (1.9)	
Family possessions				
Running water	123 (55.4)	61 (53.0)	62 (57.9)	0.46
Electricity	195 (87.8)	102 (88.7)	93 (86.9)	0.69
Television	167 (75.2)	88 (76.5)	79 (73.8)	0.64
Radio	77 (34.7)	45 (39.1)	32 (29.9)	0.15
Fridge	30 (13.5)	13 (11.3)	17 (15.9)	0.32
Private latrine	182 (82.0)	96 (83.5)	86 (80.4)	0.55

Table 1 continued

Socio-demographic characteristics	Total ($n=328$), n (%)	Male ($n=169$), n (%)	Female ($n=159$), n (%)	P-value*
Mother is still alive				0.18
No	167 (50.9)	80 (47.3)	87 (54.7)	
Yes	161 (49.1)	89 (52.7)	72 (45.3)	
Mother's education level[a]				0.12
No education	20 (12.7)	7 (8.1)	13 (18.1)	
Primary school	53 (33.5)	27 (31.4)	26 (36.1)	
Secondary school	24 (15.2)	14 (16.3)	10 (13.9)	
High school or higher	24 (15.2)	12 (14.0)	12 (16.7)	
Don't know	37 (23.4)	26 (30.2)	11 (15.3)	
Father is still alive				0.82
No	198 (60.4)	101 (59.8)	97 (61.0)	
Yes	130 (39.6)	68 (40.2)	62 (39.0)	
Father's education level[a]				0.04
No education	9 (5.6)	4 (6.2)	3 (4.3)	
Primary school	33 (26.2)	12 (18.8)	21 (33.9)	
Secondary school	18 (14.3)	8 (12.5)	10 (16.1)	
High school or higher	28 (24.3)	9 (14.1)	14 (22.6)	
Don't know	45 (35.7)	31 (48.4)	14 (22.6)	
Main daily caregiver				0.57
Parent	187 (57.0)	102 (60.4)	85 (53.5)	
Grand parent	5 (1.5)	2 (1.2)	3 (1.9)	
Sibling	24 (7.3)	9 (5.3)	15 (9.4)	
Relatives	100 (30.5)	50 (29.6)	50 (31.4)	
Orphanage/NGO staff	12 (3.7)	6 (3.6)	6 (3.8)	
Main caregiver's education level[a]				<0.001
Primary school or lower	14 (7.2)	2 (2.1)	12 (12.1)	
Secondary school	40 (20.5)	8 (8.3)	32 (32.3)	
High school	11 (5.6)	6 (6.2)	5 (5.1)	
University or higher	29 (14.9)	16 (16.7)	13 (13.1)	
Don't know	101 (51.8)	64 (66.7)	37 (37.4)	

ART antiretroviral therapy, *HIV* human immunodeficiency virus, *NGO* non-governmental organization, *USD* United States Dollar

* Chi square or Fisher's exact test was used as appropriate for categorical variables, Student's t-test was used for continuous variables

[a] Primary = less than or equal to 6 years, secondary = 7–9 years, high school = 10–12 years

majority of them felt supported during the preparation process for transition with 14.5% feeling very supported, and 59.5% felt somewhat supported. Sixty-six percent preferred to receive pediatric HIV-related care. Issues related to health, sexuality or daily life were most frequently discussed with family (47.9%), health providers (20.4%) and friends (13.4%). However, health care providers (79%) were reported as the most trusted source of information for HIV care and treatment (Table 6).

Males were significantly more likely to discuss health problems with medical providers (26.6% vs. 13.8%, $p=0.01$), and they were also more likely to trust friends or family members the most for their treatment (14.8% vs. 6.9%, $p=0.02$). Preparation strategies among males were more likely to include a visit to an adult clinic (34.9% vs. 21.4%, $p=0.007$) despite having a lower likelihood of being assigned a case manager (33.7% vs. 49.7%, $p=0.003$) or of including counselors or peer-educators in their transition plans (1.8% vs. 6.9%, $p=0.02$). Overall, male participants reported feeling more prepared for the transition to adult services (96.5% vs. 80.5%, $p<0.001$), despite being more likely to report feeling inadequately supported (77.6% vs. 92.4%, $p=0.006$) (Table 6).

Discussion

Our cross-sectional study describes the dynamic social circumstances unique to Cambodian adolescents living with HIV as they transition to adult clinics. We found that social protection mechanism are reaching some adolescents living with HIV in need. Almost half reported

Table 2 Access and adherence to ART among male and female adolescents living with HIV

Access and adherence to ART	Total ($n=328$) n (%)	Male ($n=169$) n (%)	Female ($n=159$) n (%)	p-value*
Mean number of days the drug supply is usually given	58.4±53.9	61.4±73.7	55.1±14.9	0.3
Ever shared your drugs to other persons				–
No	328 (100)	169 (100)	159 (100)	
Yes	0 (0.0)	0 (0.0)	0 (0.0)	
Having been asked to come back earlier than appointment				0.56
No	283 (86.3)	144 (85.2)	139 (87.4)	
Yes	45 (13.7)	25 (14.8)	20 (12.6)	
Reasons for coming back earlier than appointment				0.35
Lack of medicines	10 (22.2)	5 (20.0)	5 (25.0)	
Additional check up	21 (46.7)	10 (40.0)	11 (55.0)	
Other	14 (31.1)	10 (40.0)	4 (20.0)	
Having been asked to buy any other medicines				0.81
No	319 (97.3)	164 (97.0)	155 (97.5)	
Yes	9 (2.7)	5 (3.0)	4 (2.5)	

Table 3 Experiences of stigma and discrimination among male and female adolescents living with HIV

Experiences of stigma and discrimination	Total ($n=328$) n (%)	Male ($n=169$) n (%)	Female ($n=159$) n (%)	p-value*
Someone has mistreated you because of your HIV-infected status				0.28
No	293 (89.3)	154 (91.1)	139 (87.4)	
Yes	35 (10.7)	15 (8.9)	20 (12.6)	
Having experienced negative attitudes because of your HIV-infected status				0.09
No	223 (68.0)	122 (72.2)	101 (63.5)	
Yes	105 (32.0)	47 (27.8)	58 (36.5)	
Having been refused to share housing/other materials because of your HIV-infected status				0.66
No	301 (91.8)	154 (91.1)	147 (92.5)	
Yes	27 (8.2)	15 (8.9)	12 (7.5)	

that their family had received at least one element of social support for their health care, ranging from food support, school allowance, transport allowance to ART clinics, psychosocial counseling, vocational training, or home visits. Of these, food support and school allowance had the highest coverage.

At the same time, significant social support needs were identified, including ongoing inability ability to cover health expenses (55.0%), stigma and discrimination and lack of access to peer support groups. Some of these needs intersected with health system factors such as lack of HIV treatment, failure to received counselling on transition, low rate of familiarization with adult clinics and allocation of a transition case manager.

The numbers of participants accessing the social supports indicate that current interventions have the capacity-building potential to reach adolescents living with HIV from poorer communities. This is important given that socioeconomic and social health protection status are significant determinants of a successful move to adult-oriented medical care [30, 39]. Evidence from other setting suggests that both adolescents living with HIV and their health care providers consider poor socioeconomic conditions to be a significant barrier to the transition process [30].

We uncovered remarkable differences in how male and female adolescents living with HIV communicate their health needs and manage their care and treatment. Our data shows that female adolescents have difficulty managing their own care, including discussing their medical concerns with their health care providers, which may explain the more frequent reports of ART non-adherence among female adolescents when feeling sick. Future studies may elucidate how gender and gender responsibilities

Table 4 School attendance and employment history among male and female adolescents living with HIV

School attendance and employment history	Total (*n* = 328), *n* (%)	Male (*n* = 169), *n* (%)	Female (*n* = 159), *n* (%)	*p*-value*
School attendance in the past month				0.79
Never	55 (16.8)	29 (17.2)	26 (16.4)	
With disruptions	75 (22.9)	36 (21.3)	39 (24.5)	
Full time	198 (60.4)	104 (61.5)	94 (59.1)	
Age when stopped going to school	14.7 ± 1.5	14.7 ± 1.2	14.6 ± 1.8	0.48
Reasons for not attending school				0.25
No money to go to school	18 (14.0)	6 (9.4)	12 (18.5)	
Too sick to go to school	44 (34.1)	20 (31.2)	24 (36.9)	
Not successful at school	24 (18.6)	15 (23.4)	9 (13.8)	
Other	43 (33.3)	23 (35.9)	20 (30.9)	
Currently working for pay				0.34
No	259 (79.0)	137 (81.1)	122 (76.7)	
Yes	69 (21.0)	32 (18.9)	37 (23.3)	
Mean age when started working	14.8 ± 1.9	15.0 ± 1.2	14.7 ± 2.3	0.54
Ever travelled outside of hometown for work				0.23
No	326 (94.4)	169 (100)	157 (98.7)	
Yes	2 (0.6)	0 (0.0)	2 (1.3)	
Family received social support for your health				0.85
No	175 (53.4)	91 (53.8)	84 (52.8)	
Yes	153 (46.6)	78 (46.2)	75 (47.2)	
Types of support received by family				
Transportation allowance	82 (53.6)	43 (55.1)	39 (52.0)	0.7
Food support	117 (76.5)	57 (73.1)	60 (80.0)	31
School allowance	95 (62.1)	46 (59.0)	49 (65.3)	0.42
Emotional counseling	54 (35.3)	24 (30.8)	30 (40.0)	0.23
Vocational training	35 (22.9)	14 (17.9)	21 (28.0)	0.14
Home visit	17 (11.1)	10 (12.8)	7 (9.3)	0.49
Family received financial support for your health				0.95
No	214 (65.2)	110 (65.1)	104 (65.4)	
Yes	114 (34.8)	59 (34.9)	55 (34.6)	
Belonged to a patient group				0.63
No	231 (70.4)	121 (71.6)	110 (69.2)	
Yes	97 (27.9)	48 (28.4)	49 (30.8)	

ART antiretroviral therapy, *HIV* human immunodeficiency virus

* Chi square or Fisher's exact test was used as appropriate for categorical variables, Student's t-test was used for continuous variables

influence the doctor-patient relationship in this setting and could form the basis for effective gender-sensitive interventions [24].

Addressing social factors

The proportion (22%) of adolescents working for pay is concerning and may explain the lower school attendance rate in our study population. Education exerts a positive influence on adolescents living with HIV [24] and is a considerable protective factor against poor mental outcomes, risky sexual behavior and substance abuse [40, 41]. Our findings offer additional rationale to improve school retention by confronting discrimination in schools and normalizing HIV. HIV-related stigma is a primary determinant in adolescent health and is also a decisive motivator in the transition process [42]. In addition, expansion of peer support to the two-thirds of adolescents who did not belong to such groups is needed, as participation in peer support is associated with improved medical adherence [24, 43]. Given that access to available social protection support was suboptimal, our results argue for adolescent-focused interventions at multiple layers of the sociological context [24] to ensure that every needy adolescent has access to available wrap around services to support successful adolescent transition. In addition, future analyses are needed to explore

Table 5 Assessment of preparedness for transition from pediatric to adult care among male and female adolescents living with HIV

Assessment of preparedness for transition	Total (*n* = 328), *n* (%)	Male (*n* = 169), *n* (%)	Female (*n* = 159), *n* (%)	*p*-value*
Can you recognize when you are getting sick?				0.28
No	92 (28.0)	43 (25.4)	49 (30.8)	
Yes	236 (72.0)	126 (74.6)	110 (69.2)	
Do you know when you need to call the doctor?				1.00
No	64 (19.5)	33 (19.5)	31 (19.5)	
Yes	264 (80.5)	136 (80.5)	128 (80.5)	
Are you responsible for making your own appointments?				0.40
No	177 (54.0)	95 (56.2)	82 (51.6)	
Yes	151 (46.0)	74 (43.8)	77 (48.4)	
Are you responsible for refilling your own medications?				0.79
No	151 (46.0)	79 (46.7)	72 (45.3)	
Yes	177 (54.0)	90 (53.3)	87 (54.7)	
Do you feel comfortable asking questions at your appointments?				0.04
No	284 (86.6)	140 (82.8)	144 (90.6)	
Yes	44 (13.4)	29 (17.2)	15 (9.4)	
Do you have a copy of your health records and doctor contacts?				< 0.001
No	179 (54.6)	72 (42.6)	107 (67.3)	
Yes	149 (45.4)	97 (57.4)	52 (32.7)	
Do you have a method of keeping track of your healthcare appointments?				< 0.001
No	126 (38.4)	46 (27.2)	80 (50.3)	
Yes	202 (61.6)	123 (72.8)	79 (49.7)	
Do you find it difficult to remember to take your medicine?				0.21
No	250 (76.2)	124 (73.4)	126 (79.2)	
Yes	78 (26.8)	45 (26.6)	33 (20.8)	
When you feel better, do you stop taking your medicine?				0.14
No	326 (99.4)	169 (100)	157 (98.7)	
Yes	2 (0.6)	0 (0.0)	2 (1.3)	
If you feel worse when you take the medicine, do you stop taking it?				0.02
No	292 (89.0)	157 (92.9)	135 (84.9)	
Yes	36 (11.0)	12 (7.1)	24 (15.1)	
Thinking back over the past 4 days, have you missed any of your medicine?				0.81
No	282 (86.0)	147 (87.0)	135 (84.9)	
Not sure	41 (12.5)	20 (11.8)	21 (13.2)	
Yes	5 (1.5)	2 (1.2)	3 (1.9)	
Visual adherence scale (%)	95.4 ± 9.6	95.3 ± 9.6	95.4 ± 9.7	0.91

HIV human immunodeficiency virus

Values are number (%) for categorical variables and mean (± SD) for continuous variables

* Chi square or Fisher's exact test was used for categorical outcome variables and Student's t-test was used for continuous outcome variables

the socioeconomic factors driving these students out of school and into the workforce.

Addressing health system factors

An inadequate drug supply was common which may affect ART adherence and partially contribute to the high rate of school absences. Improved medication adherence is associated with a daily routine [39], which is reliant upon a consistent supply of medication. Moreover, the transition from pediatric to adult care has the potential for being a significant psychological burden [44] on adolescents living with HIV, which requires adequate supply and adolescent-friendly services, devoid of stigma. In the current context, strengthening supply of ARV will be essential. At the same time, there is a need to strengthen the provision of counselling on transition and enhance adolescent familiarization with adult clinics as part of the transition. Furthermore, despite policies requiring

Table 6 Experience of transition from pediatric and adult care among male and female adolescents living with HIV

Experience of transition from pediatric and adult care	Total ($n = 328$), n (%)	Male ($n = 169$), n (%)	Female ($n = 159$), n (%)	p-value*
Facility you prefer to receive care and treatment				0.46
Pediatric pre ART/ART services	217 (66.2)	115 (68.8)	102 (64.2)	
Adult pre ART/ART service	111 (33.8)	54 (32.0)	57 (35.8)	
Preferred to discuss questions related to health, sexuality, or daily life with				0.01
Health providers	67 (20.4)	45 (26.6)	22 (13.8)	
Counselors/peer educators	19 (5.8)	6 (3.6)	13 (8.2)	
Friends	44 (13.4)	17 (10.1)	27 (17.0)	
Family	157 (47.9)	81 (47.9)	76 (47.8)	
Other	41 (12.5)	20 (11.8)	21 (13.2)	
Person who you trust the most for your treatment				0.02
Health providers	259 (79.0)	132 (78.1)	127 (79.9)	
Counselors/peer educators	14 (4.3)	3 (1.8)	11 (6.9)	
Friends/family	36 (11.0)	25 (14.8)	11 (6.9)	
Other	19 (5.8)	9 (5.8)	10 (6.3)	
Sources of information about health				< 0.001
Pre ART/ART clinic	199 (60.7)	118 (69.8)	81 (50.9)	
NGOs	21 (6.4)	10 (5.9)	11 (6.9)	
Family	80 (24.7)	25 (14.8)	55 (34.6)	
Other	28 (8.5)	16 (9.5)	12 (7.5)	
Current HIV care provider				0.06
Health provider for adults	105 (32.0)	46 (27.2)	59 (37.1)	
Health provider for children	223 (68.8)	123 (72.8)	100 (62.9)	
Received counseling on transition to adult services				0.49
No	190 (57.9)	101 (59.8)	89 (56.0)	
Yes	138 (42.1)	68 (40.2)	70 (44.0)	
Person who provided the counseling				0.34
Health providers	56 (40.9)	31 (45.6)	25 (36.2)	
Counselors/peer educators	64 (46.7)	31 (45.6)	33 (47.8)	
Other	17 (12.4)	6 (8.8)	11 (15.9)	
Ever completed a transfer form				0.58
No	292 (89.0)	152 (89.9)	140 (88.1)	
Yes	36 (11.0)	17 (10.1)	19 (11.9)	
Ever visited an adult clinic to prepare for transition				0.007
No	235 (71.6)	110 (65.1)	125 (78.6)	
Yes	93 (28.4)	59 (34.9)	34 (21.4)	
Person who took you to visit the adult clinic to prepare for transition				0.07
Health providers	8 (8.7)	4 (6.8)	4 (12.1)	
Counselors/peer educators	8 (8.7)	2 (3.4)	6 (18.2)	
Friends/family	58 (63.0)	41 (69.5)	17 (51.5)	
Other	18 (19.6)	12 (20.3)	6 (18.2)	
The visit was helpful for you to cope with the transition				0.83
No	5 (5.6)	3 (5.2)	2 (6.3)	
Yes	85 (94.4)	55 (94.8)	30 (93.8)	
A 'Case Manager' has been identified to support you during the transition				0.003
No	192 (58.5)	112 (66.3)	80 (50.3)	
Yes	136 (41.5)	57 (33.7)	79 (49.7)	
Preparedness to manage your treatment going forward				< 0.001
Very prepared	42 (12.8)	27 (16.0)	15 (9.4)	
Somewhat prepared	249 (75.9)	136 (80.5)	113 (71.1)	

Table 6 continued

Experience of transition from pediatric and adult care	Total ($n = 328$), n (%)	Male ($n = 169$), n (%)	Female ($n = 159$), n (%)	p-value*
Somewhat unprepared	21 (6.4)	4 (2.4)	17 (10.7)	
Very unprepared	16 (4.9)	2 (1.2)	14 (8.8)	
Feeling supported during your transition from pediatric care to adult care				0.006
Very supported	45 (25.4)	17 (20.0)	28 (30.4)	
Somewhat supported	106 (59.9)	49 (57.6)	57 (62.0)	
Somewhat unsupported	13 (7.3)	7 (8.2)	6 (6.5)	
Very unsupported	13 (7.3)	12 (14.1)	1 (1.1)	
Satisfaction you with your transition experience in general				0.34
Very satisfied	53 (16.2)	29 (17.2)	24 (15.1)	
Somewhat satisfied	107 (32.6)	51 (30.2)	56 (35.2)	
Somewhat dissatisfied	34 (10.4)	14 (8.3)	20 (12.6)	
Very dissatisfied	134 (40.7)	75 (44.4)	59 (37.1)	

ART antiretroviral therapy, *HIV* human immunodeficiency virus

Values are number (%) for categorical variables and mean (± SD) for continuous variables

* Chi square or Fisher's exact test was used for categorical outcome variables and Student's t-test was used for continuous outcome variables

allocation of a transition case manager, only a quarter of adolescents in this study had been allocated one. This will also need to be enhanced in order to support successful transition of adolescents to adult HIV care. Transition managers provide and link adolescents to available social support and protection.

Limitations

Our study offers a picture of the HIV epidemic among Cambodian adolescents and the sociocultural phenomena they experience while transitioning from pediatric to adult HIV care. However, and despite our sampling methodology, the generalizability of our results to the entire population of adolescents living with HIV in Cambodia may be limited. Potential for bias due to social desirability or recall biases were minimized by validating responses against medical records whenever possible, but may not have been eliminated.

Conclusions

The considerable advancements made in reducing new infections from mother-to-child transmission indicates that a focused worldwide effort, robust political commitment and leadership at the national level can produce substantial results. The same type of concentrated focus must now be shifted to adolescents. Our study reports that social protection mechanisms are reaching a number of adolescents living with HIV in need, but others remain without support. Multi-sectoral interventions, boosting school attendance, mitigating HIV-related stigma, and expanding coverage of social protection mechanisms are necessary to improving the health and quality of life of all adolescents living with HIV in Cambodia.

Authors' contributions

SY, ST and VK conceived the study. PC and ST were responsible for data collection and data entry. SY, CN, GM and GT analyzed data interpreted the results and wrote the manuscript. All authors read and approved the final manuscript.

Author details

[1] Fielding School of Public Health, University of California Los Angeles, Los Angeles, USA. [2] Division of Health Research, Lancaster University, Lancaster, UK. [3] KHANA Center for Population Health Research, No. 33, Street 71, Phnom Penh, Cambodia. [4] National Center for HIV/AIDS, Dermatology and STD, Phnom Penh, Cambodia. [5] Center for Global Health Research, Touro University California, Vallejo, USA.

Acknowledgements

The authors thank the National Center for HIV/AIDS, Dermatology and STD and KHANA's programs teams, research assistants and all participants and family for their contribution to this study. Authors thank Morten Skovdal for comments on an earlier draft. The authors' views expressed in this manuscript do not necessarily reflect the views of UNICEF Cambodia or the authors' affiliated institutions.

Competing interests

The authors declare that they have no competing interests.

Funding

Data used for this analysis were collected as part of a larger study funded by UNICEF Cambodia.

References

1. Patton GC, Viner RM, le Linh C, Ameratunga S, Fatusi AO, Ferguson BJ, et al. Mapping a global agenda for adolescent health. J Adolesc Health. 2010;47(5):427–32.
2. Friedman HL. Changing patterns of adolescent sexual behavior: consequences for health and development. J Adolesc Health. 1992;13(5):345–50.
3. Viner RM, Ozer EM, Denny S, Marmot M, Resnick M, Fatusi A, et al. Adolescence and the social determinants of health. Lancet. 2012;379(9826):1641–52.
4. Mburu G, Hodgson I, Teltschik A, Ram M, Haamujompa C, Bajpai D, et al. Rights-based services for adolescents living with HIV: adolescent self-

efficacy and implications for health systems in Zambia. Reprod Health Matters. 2013;21(41):176–85.
5. Idele P, Gillespie A, Porth T, Suzuki C, Mahy M, Kasedde S, et al. Epidemiology of HIV and AIDS among adolescents: current status, inequities, and data gaps. J Acquir Immune Defic Syndr. 2014;66(Suppl 2):S144–53.
6. Mburu G, Hodgson I, Kalibala S, Haamujompa C, Cataldo F, Lowenthal ED, et al. Adolescent HIV disclosure in Zambia: barriers, facilitators and outcomes. J Int AIDS Soc. 2014;17:18866.
7. Kim SH, Gerver SM, Fidler S, Ward H. Adherence to antiretroviral therapy in adolescents living with HIV: systematic review and meta-analysis. AIDS. 2014;28(13):1945–56.
8. Nachega JB, Hislop M, Nguyen H, Dowdy DW, Chaisson RE, Regensberg L, et al. Antiretroviral therapy adherence, virologic and immunologic outcomes in adolescents compared with adults in southern Africa. J Acquir Immune Defic Syndr. 2009;51(1):65–71.
9. Cruz ML, Cardoso CA, Darmont MQ, Souza E, Andrade SD, D'Al Fabbro MM, et al. Viral suppression and adherence among HIV-infected children and adolescents on antiretroviral therapy: results of a multicenter study. J Pediatr. 2014;90(6):563–71.
10. Zanoni BC, Mayer KH. The adolescent and young adult HIV cascade of care in the United States: exaggerated health disparities. AIDS Patient Care STDS. 2014;28(3):128–35.
11. Busza J, Strode A, Dauya E, Ferrand RA. Falling through the gaps: how should HIV programmes respond to families that persistently deny treatment to children? J Int AIDS Soc. 2016;19(1):20789.
12. Fernet M, Wong K, Richard ME, Otis J, Levy JJ, Lapointe N, et al. Romantic relationships and sexual activities of the first generation of youth living with HIV since birth. AIDS Care. 2011;23(4):393–400.
13. Fair C, Albright J. "Don't tell him you have HIV unless he's 'the one'": romantic relationships among adolescents and young adults with perinatal HIV infection. AIDS Patient Care STDS. 2012;26(12):746–54.
14. Binagwaho A, Fuller A, Kerry V, Dougherty S, Agbonyitor M, Wagner C, et al. Adolescents and the right to health: eliminating age-related barriers to HIV/AIDS services in Rwanda. AIDS Care. 2012;24(7):936–42.
15. Judd A, Sohn AH, Collins IJ. Interventions to improve treatment, retention and survival outcomes for adolescents with perinatal HIV-1 transitioning to adult care: moving on up. Curr Opin HIV AIDS. 2016;11(5):477–86.
16. Ben-Farhat J, Schramm B, Nicolay N, Wanjala S, Szumilin E, Balkan S, et al. Mortality and clinical outcomes in children treated with antiretroviral therapy in four African vertical programs during the first decade of paediatric HIV care, 2001–2010. Trop Med Int Health. 2017;22(3):340–50.
17. Bryant M, Beard J. Orphans and vulnerable children affected by human immunodeficiency virus in sub-Saharan Africa. Trop Med Int Health. 2017;22(3):340–50.
18. Andrews G, Skinner D, Zuma K. Epidemiology of health and vulnerability among children orphaned and made vulnerable by HIV/AIDS in sub-Saharan Africa. AIDS Care. 2006;18(3):269–76.
19. Brown LK, Lourie KJ, Pao M. Children and adolescents living with HIV and AIDS: a review. J Child Psychol Psychiatry. 2000;41(1):81–96.
20. Schenk KD, Michaelis A, Sapiano TN, Brown L, Weiss E. Improving the lives of vulnerable children: implications of Horizons research among orphans and other children affected by AIDS. Public Health Rep. 2010;125(2):325–36.
21. Midtbo V, Shirima V, Skovdal M, Daniel M. How disclosure and antiretroviral therapy help HIV-infected adolescents in sub-Saharan Africa cope with stigma. Afr J AIDS Res. 2012;11(3):261–71.
22. Hodgson I, Ross J, Haamujompa C, Gitau-Mburu D. Living as an adolescent with HIV in Zambia—lived experiences, sexual health and reproductive needs. AIDS Care. 2012;24(10):1204–10.
23. Menon A, Glazebrook C, Campain N, Ngoma M. Mental health and disclosure of HIV status in Zambian adolescents with HIV infection: implications for peer-support programs. J Acquir Immune Defic Syndr. 2007;46(3):349–54.
24. Mburu G, Ram M, Oxenham D, Haamujompa C, Iorpenda K, Ferguson L. Responding to adolescents living with HIV in Zambia: a social-ecological approach. Child Youth Serv Rev. 2014;45:9–17.
25. Cluver LD, Toska E, Orkin FM, Meinck F, Hodes R, Yakubovich AR, et al. Achieving equity in HIV-treatment outcomes: can social protection improve adolescent ART-adherence in South Africa? AIDS Care. 2016;28(Suppl 2):73–82.
26. Lowenthal ED, Bakeera-Kitaka S, Marukutira T, Chapman J, Goldrath K, Ferrand RA. Perinatally acquired HIV infection in adolescents from sub-Saharan Africa: a review of emerging challenges. Lancet Infect Dis. 2014;14(7):627–39.
27. Lee S, Hazra R. Achieving 90-90-90 in paediatric HIV: adolescence as the touchstone for transition success. J Int AIDS Soc. 2015;18(Suppl 6):20257.
28. Kakkar F, Van der Linden D, Valois S, Maurice F, Onnorouille M, Lapointe N, et al. Health outcomes and the transition experience of HIV-infected adolescents after transfer to adult care in Quebec, Canada. BMC Pediatr. 2016;16:109.
29. Ryscavage P, Macharia T, Patel D, Palmeiro R, Tepper V. Linkage to and retention in care following healthcare transition from pediatric to adult HIV care. AIDS Care. 2016;28(5):561–5.
30. Wiener LS, Kohrt BA, Battles HB, Pao M. The HIV experience: youth identified barriers for transitioning from pediatric to adult care. J Pediatr Psychol. 2011;36(2):141–54.
31. Bygrave H, Mtangirwa J, Ncube K, Ford N, Kranzer K, Munyaradzi D. Antiretroviral therapy outcomes among adolescents and youth in rural Zimbabwe. PLoS ONE. 2012;7(12):e52856.
32. Westling K, Naver L, Vesterbacka J, Belfrage E. Transition of HIV-infected youths from paediatric to adult care, a Swedish single-centre experience. Infect Dis. 2016;48(6):449–52.
33. Righetti A, Prinapori R, Nulvesu L, Fornoni L, Viscoli C, Di Biagio A. Transitioning HIV-infected children and adolescents into adult care: an Italian real-life experience. J Assoc Nurses AIDS Care. 2015;26(5):652–9.
34. Yi S, Ngin C, Pal K, Khol V, Tuot S, Sau S, et al. Transition into adult care: factors associated with level of preparedness among adolescents living with HIV in Cambodia. AIDS Res Ther. 2017;14:33.
35. Skinner J. Probability proportional to size (PPS) sampling. London: Wiley; 2006.
36. Sharma N, Willen E, Garcia A, Sharma TS. Attitudes toward transitioning in youth with perinatally acquired HIV and their family caregivers. J Assoc Nurses AIDS Care. 2014;25(2):168–75.
37. Bakeera-Kitaka S, Nabukeera-Barungi N, Nostlinger C, Addy K, Colebunders R. Sexual risk reduction needs of adolescents living with HIV in a clinical care setting. AIDS Care. 2008;20(4):426–33.
38. World Medical Association (WMA). Declaration of Helsinki: ethical principles for medical research involving human subjects (2008 Revision). Seoul: World Medical Association; 2008.
39. Dowshen N, D'Angelo L. Health care transition for youth living with HIV/AIDS. Pediatrics. 2011;128(4):762–71.
40. Magnani RJ, Karim AM, Weiss LA, Bond KC, Lemba M, Morgan GT. Reproductive health risk and protective factors among youth in Lusaka, Zambia. J Adolesc Health. 2002;30(1):76–86.
41. Shackleton N, Jamal F, Viner RM, Dickson K, Patton G, Bonell C. School-based interventions going beyond health education to promote adolescent health: systematic review of reviews. J Adolesc Health. 2016;58(4):382–96.
42. Seng SDT, Welle E, Mok S, Soch K, Tep S, et al. Stigma and discrimination as factors affecting the transition from paediatric to adult HIV care services by children living with HIV aged 12–17 in Cambodia: a qualitative exploratory study. In: International AIDS conference Abstract TUPE-286. Melbourne, Australia; 2014.
43. Mupambireyi Z, Bernays S, Bwakura-Dangarembizi M, Cowan FM. "I don't feel shy because I will be among others who are just like me…": the role of support groups for children perinatally infected with HIV in Zimbabwe. Child Youth Serv Rev. 2014;45:106–13.
44. Miles K, Edwards S, Clapson M. Transition from paediatric to adult services: experiences of HIV-positive adolescents. AIDS Care. 2004;16(3):305–14.

Validation of a questionnaire to monitor symptoms in HIV-infected patients during hepatitis C treatment

Edward R. Cachay[1,2*], Craig Ballard[3], Bradford Colwell[3], Francesca Torriani[1,2], Charles Hicks[1,2] and Wm. Christopher Mathews[1]

Abstract

Background: Clinicians are incorporating patient-reported outcomes in the management of HIV-infected persons co-infected with hepatitis C virus (HCV), but there are no validated inventories to monitor symptoms of patients during HCV therapy.

Design: Five-year retrospective cohort analysis of persons living with HIV (PLWH) treated for HCV.

Methods: The HCV symptom-inventory (HCV-SI) was administered before, during, and after HCV treatment. Discriminant validity was assessed, separately, in mixed model linear regression of HCV-SI T-scores on treatment regimens (pegylated-interferon and ribavirin; pegylated-interferon, ribavirin, and telaprevir; and interferon-free antivirals); and side effect-related premature treatment discontinuation (SE-DC).

Results: From the 103 patients who completed the HCV-SI, 7% were female, 26% non-white, 32% cirrhotics and 91% had undetectable HIV viral loads. Most had genotype 1 (83%) and were HCV treatment-naïve (78%). We treated 19% of patients with pegylated-interferon and ribavirin, 22% with pegylated-interferon, ribavirin, and telaprevir and 59% received interferon-free antivirals. Overall, 77% achieved a sustained virologic response, and 6% discontinued HCV treatment due to side effects. In the treatment discrimination model, compared to the no treatment period, HCV-SI scores were significantly ($p < 0.01$) lower for interferon-free antivirals and higher for interferon-containing regimens. In the SE-DC model, the total HCV-SI, somatic and neuropsychiatric scores significantly predicted those patients who prematurely discontinued HCV treatment ($P < 0.05$).

Conclusions: The HCV-SI effectively differentiated among treatment regimens known to vary by side effect profiles and between patients with and without treatment discontinuation due to side effects. The HCV-SI may have value as a patient-reported outcome instrument predicting the risk of HCV treatment discontinuation.

Keywords: HIV, HCV treatment, Symptoms, Monitoring

Background

Direct-acting antivirals (DAA) provide safe and curative treatment for hepatitis C virus (HCV) in patients who start and complete therapy successfully [1].

Clinicians treating HCV are increasingly incorporating patient-reported outcomes in clinical trials and routine care settings to better understand the interaction of complex patient-related factors [2]. Although clinical trials have used instruments that mainly focus on disease-specific health quality of life such as The Chronic Liver Disease Questionnaire-Hepatitis C Virus [3], there are no standard quantitative monitoring tools that can systematically track different symptom domains of patients while on HCV therapy. Assessing symptoms of persons living with HIV (PLWH) while undergoing HCV-related health management is important as many PLWH may still present with non-specific psychosomatic symptoms

*Correspondence: ecachay@ucsd.edu
[1] Department of Medicine-Owen Clinic, University of California at San Diego, 200 W. Arbor Drive, San Diego, CA 92103-8681, USA
Full list of author information is available at the end of the article

before providers recognize potentially causative issues. These potential issues include relapse of substance/alcohol with resultant worsening depression, low perceived self-esteem, and/or poor adherence to HCV or antiretroviral medications [4]. PLWH have a high prevalence of medical comorbidities and ongoing barriers to care such as substance/alcohol use, unstable housing, and neuropsychiatric disease [5]. These factors can unfavorably impact patient medication tolerance, perception and willingness to complete HCV therapy, even when treating their HCV with shorter, better-tolerated, interferon (IFN)-free DAA [6, 7].

We previously validated a 41-item HCV symptom inventory (HCV-SI) as a predictor of HCV treatment initiation using pegylated interferon and ribavirin in PLWH. The inventory consists of a clinically meaningful, three-factor structure that includes neuropsychiatric, somatic, and sleep symptoms. The three-factor subscales demonstrated excellent internal consistency, reliability, and predictive validity [8].

The composition of HCV treatment regimens can serve as a validation criterion for an HCV symptom inventory, based on findings from clinical trials that symptom burden reflects the components of the HCV regimen. Therefore, we conducted the present study to compare the potential of a multidimensional HCV-SI score: (1) to discriminate between IFN-containing and IFN-free treatment regimens; and (2) to identify patients with premature treatment discontinuation and/or loss to follow-up due to worsening symptoms or side effects.

Methods

The Owen Hepatitis Co-Infection Clinic was founded in April 2008 as a multidisciplinary HCV primary care-based program at the University of California San Diego (UCSD) Medical Center. Since its inception, it has used inclusive protocols aimed at increasing HCV treatment uptake among PLWH, including those with ongoing drug use, alcohol consumption, neuropsychiatric disease, and unstable housing while fulfilling our minimum eligibility criteria [9]. In short, the pre-treatment assessment for HCV treatment eligibility among patients with ongoing barriers to care required only: (1) consistent undetectable HIV viral load, (2) stable concurrent medical comorbidities, (3) favorable assessment by the team's psychiatrist when there is a history of a psychiatric condition that may interfere with treatment, (4) encouraging registration with a needle exchange program for those with ongoing injection drug use, and (5) alcohol sobriety or controlled drinking for at least one month before HCV treatment initiation [9]. To further investigate the psychometric properties of the HCV-SI, we assembled a retrospective longitudinal cohort of adult PLWH treated for HCV between December 2011 and May 2016.

The HCV-SI is incorporated in the substance, alcohol and depression screening as part of our standard of care every time a patient attends the Owen HCV Hepatitis Co-Infection Clinic. The testing is conducted before, during, and after HCV treatment. The first page of the evaluation contains a standard validated depression inventory (PHQ-9/CES-D), the second page includes the NIDA-ASSIST for illegal substance use and AUDIT-C for alcohol abuse assessment, and the third page contains the HCV-SI questions (Additional file 1: Table S1). We use the online survey platform SurveyGizmo for the HCV-SI. Regarding the HCV-SI, each symptom item includes a 5-category, Likert-scaled symptom severity response, ranging from 0 (symptom absent) to 4 (symptom very severe). The total HCV-SI score could range from 0 to 164. As previously reported [4], the 41-item HCV-SI yielded a three-factor structure explaining 60% of the variance for the inventory. Factor 1 (neuropsychiatric symptoms) had 17 items, factor 2 (somatic symptoms) had eleven items, and factor 3 (sleep symptoms) had two items, explaining 28, 22 and 11% of the variance, respectively. Internal consistency reliability estimates of the three subscales were 0.93, 0.89 and 0.79 for neuropsychiatric, somatic and sleep symptoms, respectively. The possible ranges of observable raw scores for the HCV-SI and its subscales were: 0–164 (HCV-SI total), 0–44 (somatic), 0–8 (sleep), and 0–68 (neuropsychiatric). We present raw sum scores, T-scores, and POMP-scores (percent of maximum possible) [10].

Per our HCV clinic protocol, following HCV therapy initiation patients are assessed monthly for the duration of the treatment. After treatment completion, patients returned after 1, 2 and 6 months during the INF-based era and, in the IFN-free DAA era, they returned after 1 and 3 months for SVR ascertainment. The HCV-SI is self-administered by patients prior to their clinic visit, taking approximately 5 min to complete. The last time that HCV-SI was administered in any given patient was during the clinical visit for SVR ascertainment. Patients who completed the HCV-SI during at least two phases of HCV treatment (before, during, or after treatment) were included in the analysis. Demographic data, substance use, psychiatric history, and comorbidity data were obtained from medical records.

Total HCV-SI scores were examined in longitudinal scatter plots with linear and lowess smoothing to select the distribution that best fits study data. Discriminant validity was assessed separately for criteria treatment regimen composition and premature treatment discontinuation, in a mixed model linear regression that accounts for repeated measures of the HCV-SI T-scores.

Raw summated total HCV-SI and subscale scores were transformed to T-scores (with mean 50 and standard deviation 10) to facilitate comparison of regression model coefficients across models varying by SI total or subscale dependent variables [11]. Our analyses focused on four dependent variables (T-scores for the total HCV-SI and the somatic, sleep, and neuropsychiatric subscales) and two independent discrimination variables (regimen composition and premature treatment discontinuation). To examine all selected variables, we fit by maximum likelihood separate mixed model random intercept linear regressions with robust standard errors using xtmixed (StataCorp. 2016. Stata Statistical Software: Release 14.2. College Station, TX).

Examination of discriminant validity of the HCV-SI was conducted using mixed model regression to compare HCV-SI scores while patients were receiving HCV treatment in the three-different groups, as follows: patients treated with pegylated interferon/ribavirin; those treated with pegylated interferon/ribavirin/telaprevir; and those treated with IFN-free DAA regimens. We estimated the treatment regimen effects using the non-treatment periods as the comparison reference category. For the premature treatment discontinuation criterion, we dichotomized patients into two groups according to whether they completed (reference category) or prematurely discontinued treatment due to side effects or loss to follow-up. We reported the intraclass correlation coefficient (ICC) for each model as a measure of the proportion of total variance in the dependent variable accounted for by clustering within subjects [12].

We conducted Harrell's c-statistics, equivalent to the receiver operating characteristics (ROC) area, to evaluate the ability of the HCV-SI and its subscales to discriminate between the levels of the two discriminating criteria. The Harrell's c-statistic was estimated for binary specifications of the criteria while taking into account within-subject clustering for (1) treatment regimen composition (combining both interferon-containing regimens in comparison with the combined no treatment and interferon-free DAA arms [reference category]) and (2) premature treatment continuation. The c-statistic was estimated using the Stata function somersd, which decomposes the ROC area into between and within cluster components [13]. Finally, we compared the discrimination (Harrell's c) of the total HCV Symptom Inventory T-score for the two discriminating outcomes to the comparable discrimination of PROMIS depression T-scores ascertained at the same clinic visits. Because both PHQ-9 and CES-D depression instruments were utilized during the study, we employed linking tables to transform both PHQ-9 and CES-D depression scores to PROMIS depression T-scores that were used in the analysis [14].

Results

During the study period, we treated 156 PLWH for HCV. Two patients (1.3%) were not eligible to complete the HCV-SI due language barriers. Of the remaining 154, 51 were excluded [five (3.2%) declined to participate, and 46 (29.5%) had fewer than two-time phases completed HCV-SI)] leaving 103 to comprise the study population. There were no differences in demographic characteristics or prevalence of barriers to care (drug or alcohol use, active psychiatric disease or unstable housing), HIV risk factors, CD4 cell count, HIV viral suppression, HCV genotype distribution, cirrhosis diagnosis, prior liver decompensation or prior HCV treatment history outcomes between those patients included versus those excluded from the study (Additional file 2: Table S2). Among the 46 patients who completed the HCV-SI in only one-time phase and were excluded from the main analysis, 25 had documented reasons for lack of completion such as a new competing medical priority (12), failure to return for follow-up and required outreach efforts to ascertain their HCV treatment outcome (5), relocated soon after starting HCV therapy (4), and incarceration (4). Likely patient fatigue was the main reason in 45.6% of patients who completed only one time-phase the HCV-SI (21 of 46). Table 1 shows the demographic, clinical, and HIV characteristics of the study population which were mostly male (93%), white (74%), and had a history of intravenous drug use (IDU—70%). Most patients had HCV genotype 1 infections and were naïve to HCV treatment. Overall, 32% of included patients had cirrhosis. Intolerance to previous HCV treatment was rare (6%). At the time of first HCV-SI measurement, 91% of patients had a suppressed HIV viral load.

By HCV treatment group, 19% (n = 19) of study patients were treated with pegylated interferon/ribavirin, 22% (n = 23) with pegylated-interferon/ribavirin/telaprevir, and 59% (n = 61) with IFN-free DAA. The IFN-free DAA regimens included sofosbuvir/ledipasvir (n = 39), sofosbuvir/simeprevir (n = 11), sofosbuvir/ribavirin (n = 8), sofosbuvir/daclatasvir (n = 1) and two patients received ombitasvir/paritaprevir/ritonavir plus dasabuvir and ribavirin. There were no differences between treatment groups in gender, race/ethnicity, HIV risk factor, the proportion of patients with suppressed HIV viremia and prior HCV treatment history outcomes (Table 1). Overall, 77% of patients achieved an HCV sustained viral response (SVR). Patients treated with IFN-free DAA achieved the highest SVR (88%) despite the high proportion of patients with cirrhosis in this group. Patients treated with pegylated interferon/ribavirin and

Table 1 Demographic, HCV and HUV related characteristics of study patients

Factor	Total cohort (n = 103)	Peg-IFN + RBV (n = 19)	Peg-IFN + RBV + TPV (n = 23)	IFN-free DAA (n = 61)	P value*
Age in years, mean (SD)	49.7 (9.3)	43.6 (12.1)	45.3 (7.8)	53.2 (7.0)	< 0.001
Sex					
Female	7 (6.8%)	2 (11%)	3 (13%)	2 (3%)	0.17
Male	96 (93.2%)	17 (89%)	20 (87%)	59 (97%)	
Race					
Non-white	27 (26.2%)	5 (26%)	6 (26%)	16 (26%)	1.00
White	76 (73.8%)	14 (74%)	17 (74%)	45 (74%)	
Ethnicity					
Not hispanic	85 (82.5%)	14 (74%)	17 (74%)	54 (89%)	0.14
Hispanic	18 (17.5%)	5 (26%)	6 (26%)	7 (11%)	
HIV risk factor					
MSM	24 (23.3%)	4 (21%)	3 (13%)	17 (28%)	0.55
Heterosexual	1 (1.0%)	0 (0%)	0 (0%)	1 (2%)	
Hemophilia	6 (5.8%)	0 (0%)	3 (13%)	3 (5%)	
MSM + IDU	45 (43.7%)	11 (58%)	11 (48%)	23 (38%)	
Heterosexual IDU	27 (26.2%)	4 (21%)	6 (26%)	17 (28%)	
CD4 + in cells/mm^3, median (IQR)	476.0 (341, 693)	607.0 (419, 719)	584.0 (426, 772)	417 (306, 598)	0.045
HIV viral load in copies/mL					
≤ 50	94 (91.3%)	17 (89%)	20 (87%)	59 (97%)	1.00
> 50	9 (8.7%)	5 (26%)	6 (26%)	16 (26%)	
HCV viral load in millions IU/L, median (IQR)	2.0 (0.4, 5.8)	3.8 (0.3, 9.7)	3.6 (1.2, 17)	1.3 (0.4, 3.5)	0.017
HCV genotype					
1/1A/1B	86 (83.5%)	13 (68%)	23 (100%)	50 (83%)	0.014
2	4 (3.8%)	1 (5%)	0 (0%)	3 (5%)	
3	11 (10.7%)	5 (26%)	0 (0%)	6 (10%)	
4	2 (1.9%)	0 (0%)	0 (0%)	2 (3%)	
HCV treatment history					
Naïve	80 (77.7%)	19 (100%)	16 (70%)	45 (74%)	0.19
IFN-intolerant	6 (5.8%)	0 (0%)	1 (4%)	5 (8%)	
Relapser	10 (9.7%)	0 (0%)	5 (22%)	5 (8%)	
Null responder	6 (5.8%)	0 (0%)	1 (4%)	5 (8%)	
Cure but reinfected	1 (1.0%)	0 (0%)	0 (0%)	1 (2%)	
Cirrhosis status					
Non-cirrhotic	70 (68.0%)	17 (89%)	17 (74%)	36 (59%)	0.032
Cirrhotic	33 (32.0%)	2 (11%)	6 (26%)	25 (41%)	
Prior decompensation or CPS > B					
Compensated cirrhosis	20 (19.4%)	2 (11%)	4 (17%)	14 (23%)	0.13
Prior decompensated cirrhosis	13 (12.6%)	0 (0%)	2 (9%)	11 (18%)	
Non-cirrhotic	70 (68.0%)	17 (89%)	17 (74%)	36 (59%)	
SVR on treatment 1					
Yes	78 (76.5%)	12 (63%)	13 (57%)	53 (88%)	1.00
No, null response	7 (6.9%)	2 (11%)	5 (22%)	0 (0%)	
No, relapse	4 (3.9%)	3 (16%)	0 (0%)	1 (2%)	
No, sides effects/adverse events	9 (8.8%)	2 (11%)	5 (22%)	2 (3%)	
No, died during treatment	4 (3.9%)	0 (0%)	0 (0%)	4 (7%)	
Discontinuation due to severe adverse events (1st regimen)					
No	93 (91.2%)	17 (89%)	18 (78%)	58 (97%)	0.021
Yes	9 (8.8%)	2 (11%)	5 (22%)	2 (3%)	

Table 1 continued

Factor	Total cohort (n = 103)	Peg-IFN + RBV (n = 19)	Peg-IFN + RBV + TPV (n = 23)	IFN-free DAA (n = 61)	P value*
No. HCV-SI observations, median (IQR)	7.0 (4.0, 12.0)	8.0 (6.0, 15.0)	15.0 (11.0, 20.0	5.0 (4.0, 7.0)	< 0.001
Barriers to care					
Ongoing drugs/alcohol use	30 (29%)	8 (42%)	7 (30%)	15 (25%)	0.34
Active psychiatric disease	28 (27%)	8 (42%)	6 (26%)	14 (23%)	0.26
Unstable housing	5 (5%)	1 (5%)	3 (13%)	1 (2%)	0.10

Peg-IFN Pegylated interferon, *IFN* Interferon, *RBV* Ribavirin, *DAA* Direct acting antiviral, *MSM* Men who have sex with men, *IDU* Intravenous drug use, *HCV* Hepatitis C virus, *SVR* Sustained viral response, *CPS* Child–Pugh score, *SD* Standard deviation, *IQR* Interquartile range, *HCV-SI* Hepatitis C symptom inventory

* P value for comparison of the 3 groups: Peg-IFN + RBV vs. Peg-IFN + RBV + TPV vs. IFN-Free DAA

pegylated interferon/ribavirin/telaprevir achieved an HCV SVR in 63 and 57%, respectively.

Table 2 presents the HCV-SI total and subscale score distributions of 868 responses from 103 patients. The median number of times that the HCV-SI was completed by each patient while on HCV therapy was 7 (range 4–12). Patients receiving IFN-containing regimens developed worsening neuropsychiatric and somatic symptoms (with stable sleep symptoms) compared to those who did not receive HCV treatment. In contrast, those treated with IFN-free DAA had significantly fewer reported symptoms than those who did not receive HCV treatment (Table 2). The estimated coefficient beta (b) of the models presented in Table 3 may be interpreted using the following example for the total HCV-SI T-score as the dependent variable. For patients not on HCV therapy (reference group), the average total symptom score was 49.42. For patients treated with IFN-free DAA, the average total symptom score was 47.24 (49.42–2.18), while the corresponding scores for patients treated with pegylated interferon/ribavirin/telaprevir, and pegylated interferon/ribavirin were 53.48 (49.42 + 4.06) and 52.31 (49.42 + 2.89), respectively. Figure 1a, depicts the findings of the treatment discrimination model, compared to no treatment period, where the predicted total HCV-SI marginal scores (fixed portion) of patients treated with IFN-free DAA are significantly lower than those treated with IFN-containing regimens ($p < 0.001$).

Eleven patients (11%) discontinued HCV therapy due to treatment-related side effects (9) or being lost to

Table 2 Distribution of HCV-SI total and subscale scores (raw, T-scores, and percent of maximum possible scores)

Scale	Mean (SD)
Number of patients	**103**
Number of responses	**868**
HCV-SI all symptoms [raw]	26.9 (24.0)
T-score, all symptoms	50.0 (10.0)
HCV-SI total, POMP	16.4 (14.6)
Neuropsychiatric symptoms [raw]	10.1 (9.8)
T-Score, neuropsychiatric	50.0 (10.0)
Neuropsychiatric, POMP	14.9 (14.4)
Somatic symptoms [raw]	7.2 (7.9)
T-score, somatic	50.0 (10.0)
Somatic, POMP	16.5 (18.0)
Sleep symptoms [raw]	2.3 (2.4)
T-Score, sleep	50.0 (10.0)
Sleep, POMP	29.3 (30.1)

SD standard deviation, *HCV-SI* hepatitis c symptom inventory, POPM percent of maximum possible scores

Table 3 Mixed model regression: symptom (subscales) T-scores on treatment category

Treatment group (Reference: no treatment)	T-score, all symptoms B (95% CI)	T-score, somatic B (95% CI)	T-score, sleep B (95% CI)	T-score, neuropsychiatric B (95% CI)
Peg-IFN + RBV	2.89 (1.03, 4.75)**	2.36 (0.33, 4.38)*	1.85 (−0.21, 3.91)	2.43 (0.48, 4.39)*
Peg-IFN + RBV + TPV	4.06 (2.23, 5.89)***	4.22 (2.54, 5.89)***	0.59 (−1.68, 2.85)	2.88 (0.94, 4.82)**
IFN-free DAA	−2.18 (−3.78, − 0.58)**	−1.763 (−3.22, − 0.31)*	−0.99 (−2.53, − 0.55)	−2.23 (−3.95, − 0.52)*
Constant	49.42 (47.69, 51.15)***	49.29 (47.64, 50.95)***	49.93 (48.35, 51.52)***	49.95 (48.16, 51.75)***
No. of patients	103	103	103	103
ICC	0.62	0.63	0.60	0.59

B Beta coefficient, *CI* Confidence intervals, *Peg-IFN* Pegylated interferon, *RBV* Ribavirin, *TPV* telaprevir, *ICC* intraclass correlation coefficient

t statistic p values: * $p < 0.05$; ** $p < 0.01$; *** $p < 0.001$

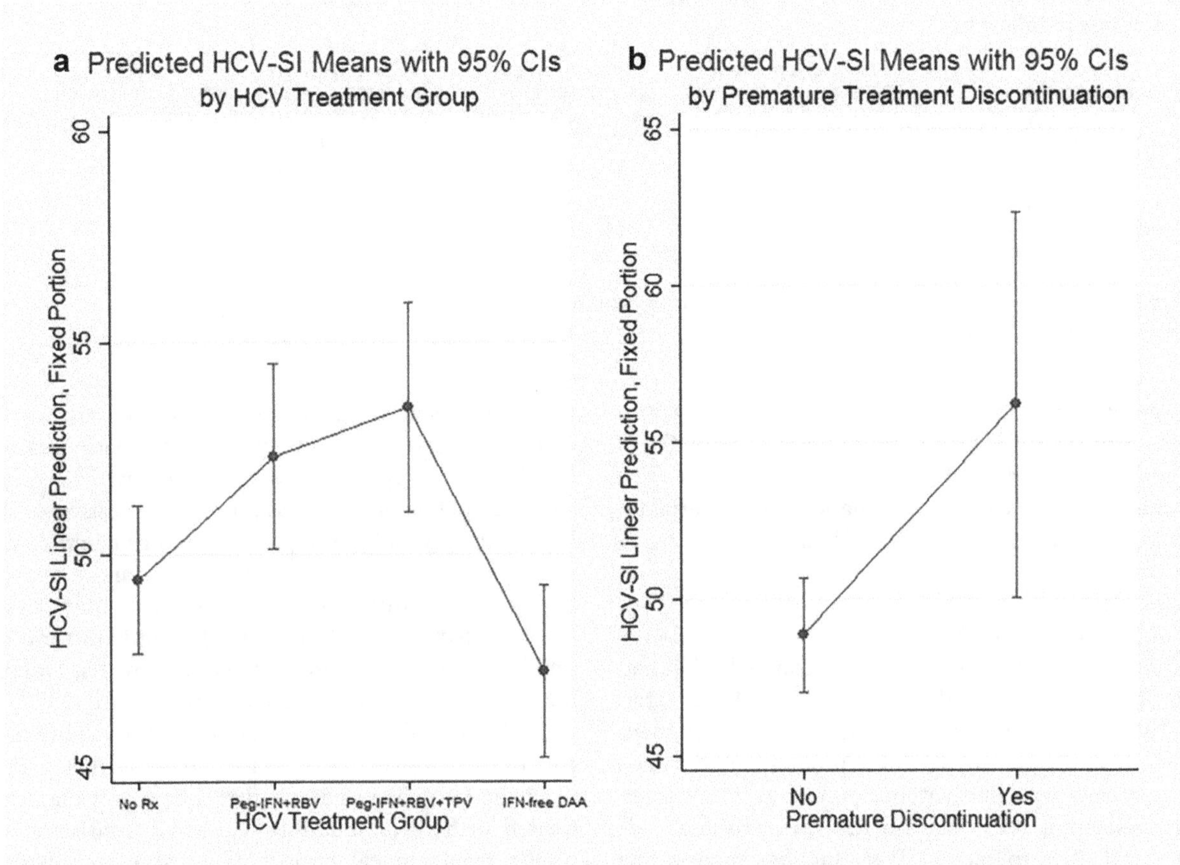

Fig. 1 **a** Shows plots with 95% confidence interval of the average T-scores of the symptoms of each treatment group while undergoing HCV therapy. **b** Illustrates plots with 95% confidence intervals of the symptom scores when patients were dichotomized based on their hepatitis C treatment premature discontinuation status due to adverse events or lost to follow-up

follow-up (2). A higher proportion of patients treated with IFN-containing regimens prematurely discontinued therapy due to side effects than those treated with IFN-free DAA (12.8% vs. 3.1%, P = 0.02). The two patients lost to follow-up received IFN-DAA treatment with sofosbuvir/ledipasvir. Two patients discontinued their IFN-free DAA due to worsening insomnia, gastrointestinal side effects, and severe fatigue. One of the latter two patients had a history of decompensated cirrhosis and received sofosbuvir/ledipasvir. The other patient had minimal liver fibrosis and received ombitasvir/paritaprevir/ritonavir plus dasabuvir and ribavirin. The mean and standard deviation of the total HCV-SI T-scores of the 11 patients discontinuing treatment were 55.66 and 11.96, respectively. In the HCV premature treatment discontinuation model, the predicted total HCV-SI marginal scores (fixed portion) during treatment were higher ($p < 0.05$) among those discontinuing early due to side effects than among those who completed treatment (Fig. 1b). Table 4 presents the mixed model results for the regression of HCV-SI T-scores on premature treatment discontinuation, demonstrating that the total HCV-SI significantly predicted those patients who prematurely discontinued HCV treatment. We observed similar effects for the somatic and neuropsychiatric subscales but not for the sleep scores.

Additional file 3: Table S3 presents ROC areas adjusted for within-subject clustering by the source of variation (between- and within- subject) and by discriminating criteria for total HCV-SI and its subscales, as discussed in Methods. Discrimination was poorest for the sleep subscale and tended unsurprisingly to be higher for within-subject discrimination than between subject discrimination. For the binary regimen composition criterion, ROC area confidence intervals excluded the null value of 0.5 for the total HCV-SI and the somatic and neuropsychiatric subscales on both between and within-subject estimates. For the premature treatment discontinuation criterion, ROC area confidence intervals excluded 0.5 for all within-subject estimates but only for

Table 4 Mixed model regression: symptom (subscales) T-scores on premature HCV treatment discontinuation due to side effects or loss to follow-up

Factor (Reference: all others)	T-score, all symptoms B (95% CI)	T-score, somatic B (95% CI)	T-score, sleep B (95% CI)	T-score, neuropsyp. B (95% CI)
Non-completer, AE/side effects	7.33 (1.05, 13.61)*	7.46 (0.70, 14.22)*	3.72 (−0.67, 8.10)	6.28 (1.31, 11.24)*
Constant	48.85 (47.03, 50.68)***	48.90 (47.12, 50.68)***	49.53 (47.85, 51.20)***	49.06 (47.24, 50.87)***
No. of patients	103	103	103	103
ICC	0.6	0.59	0.57	0.58

B Beta coefficient, *CI* Confidence intervals, *AE* Adverse events, *ICC* intraclass correlation coefficient

t statistic p-values: * $p < 0.05$; *** $p < 0.001$

the neuropsychiatric subscale for between-subject estimates. Comparing the discrimination of the total HCV SI to that of the PROMIS depression score, the total HCV SI was somewhat more discriminating for both criteria, for both within and between subject estimates.

Discussion

This study used the HCV-SI to evaluate the evolution of symptoms of PLWH before, during and after HCV treatment, and across three different HCV treatment eras. The HCV-SI discriminated among treatment regimens known to vary by their side effect profiles, and between those patients with and without premature HCV treatment discontinuation due to treatment-related side effects or loss to follow-up. These findings suggest that the HCV-SI can be used to monitor PLWH symptoms while undergoing HCV therapy.

If treating HCV with IFN-free DAA is shorter, better tolerated and more effective than the previous IFN-based therapies, why are quantitative instruments to monitor symptoms during HCV treatment with DAA of value? Improved access to contemporary HCV treatment regimens in patients with ongoing barriers to care and medical comorbidities is likely [15]. Ongoing structured screening of patient symptoms during treatment could provide counseling opportunities for symptom management and dosing recommendations (e.g. correcting the inappropriate use of antacids with sofosbuvir/ledipasvir) [16]. Use of a standardized assessment tool (such as the HCV-SI) facilitates a consistent approach for less experienced providers (such as nurse practitioners, physician assistants, and clinical pharmacists) to recognize patients at risk of treatment discontinuation [17, 18]. Hence, the HCV-SI allows standardization of patients' self-reported safety issues. Additionally, initial licensing studies suggested that discontinuation of DAA treatment among PLWH due to side effects or lost to follow-up was exceedingly rare [19]. However, data from actual clinical care in our clinic showed that during the first 2-years of DAA use, 5% of PLWH discontinued HCV therapy due to side effects or loss to follow-up [20]. Moreover, unlike with IFN-based treatments, patients discontinuing IFN-free DAA therapy are at risk of developing HCV resistance and potential transmission of HCV resistance [21]. Finally, incorporating symptom monitoring and concurrent drug and alcohol screening during and after HCV therapy can identify behaviors that put patients at risk for HCV reinfection [22]. The value of quantitative inventories such as the one presented here to direct appropriate behavior change will be valuable in this regard [23].

The HCV-SI demonstrated discriminant validity based on HCV treatment composition, showing that patients receiving DAA had significantly lower scores than those treated with IFN-containing regimens. Consistent with results from clinical trials [24], most of our patients treated with IFN-Free DAA tolerated their regimens well, despite having a high proportion of patients with cirrhosis and even prior liver decompensation. In fact, among HCV-infected PLWH, those treated with IFN-free DAA had lower symptom scores than did untreated patients, particularly notable given that 10% of the patients treated with IFN-free DAA also received ribavirin.

Importantly, the HCV-SI effectively predicted patients who prematurely discontinued HCV therapy either due to side effects or loss to follow-up. Patients who discontinued HCV therapy due to side effects had significantly higher symptom scores than those who finished HCV therapy successfully.

This study had several limitations. First, the limited number of patients who prematurely discontinued IFN-free DAA therapy limits the ability to fully explore the value of the instrument since changes were primarily reported as averages across patient groups. Secondly, while the mixed effect models demonstrated statistical significance, the ROC areas, especially for between-subject estimates, were only moderate. Third, the sample size is relatively small, and the results may not be generalizable to other populations with different sociodemographic and clinical characteristics. Finally, although we found no major differences between those completing HCV-SI and those not completing it, it is possible that unmeasured differences existed between the included and excluded treated patients. Nevertheless, the results of this study highlight the value of incorporating quantitative tools such as the HCV-SI to measure and track subjective manifestations of PLWH to help identify those patients at risk of treatment discontinuation.

Conclusions

The HCV-SI showed discriminant validity across different HCV regimen compositions and identified patients at risk of HCV treatment discontinuation due to adverse events. Medical providers treating HCV among PLWH could consider the HCV-SI as a patient-reported outcome.

Authors' contributions

EC and Wm CM conceived study. EC, CB, BC and FT provided clinical care and participated in data collection and data entry. EC and Wm CM wrote the manuscript. WM CM conducted main statistical analyses. CB provided critical inputs for writing the manuscript. All authors read and approved the final manuscript.

Author details

[1] Department of Medicine-Owen Clinic, University of California at San Diego, 200 W. Arbor Drive, San Diego, CA 92103-8681, USA. [2] Division of Infectious Diseases, University of California at San Diego, 9500 Gilman Drive #0711, La Jolla, CA 92093-0711, USA. [3] Skaggs School of Pharmacy and Pharmaceutical Sciences, UC San Diego, 9500 Gilman Drive, La Jolla, CA 92093-0021, USA.

Acknowledgements

We would like to thank The Owen Clinic Medical Assistants for supervising that the inventories were timely completed. We wish to thank Ms. Huifang Qin for providing logistic support and data management.

Competing interests

The authors declare that they have no competing interests.

Funding

This work was supported in part by the Clinical Investigation Core of the University of California San Diego Center for AIDS Research [AI036214], the CFAR Network of Integrated Clinical Systems (CNICS) [R24 AI067039-01A1], and the Pacific AIDS Education and Training Center (PAETC). The funders had no role in study design, data collection, and analysis, decision to publish, or preparation of the manuscript.

References

1. Kim A. Hepatitis C Virus. Ann Intern Med. 2016;165:ITC33–48.
2. Younossi ZM, Stepanova M, Sulkowski M, Naggie S, Henry L, Hunt S. Sofosbuvir and ledipasvir improve patient-reported outcomes in patients co-infected with hepatitis C and human immunodeficiency virus. J Viral Hepat. 2016;23:857–65.
3. Younossi ZM, Guyatt G, Kiwi M, Boparai N, King D. Development of a disease specific questionnaire to measure health-related quality of life in patients with chronic liver disease. Gut. 1999;45:295–300.
4. Hall CS, Charlebois ED, Hahn JA, Moss AR, Bangsberg DR. Hepatitis C virus infection in San Francisco's HIV-infected urban poor. J Gen Intern Med. 2004;19:357–65.
5. Cachay ER, Hill L, Wyles D, Colwell B, et al. The hepatitis C cascade of care among HIV-infected patients: a call to address ongoing barriers to care. PLoS ONE. 2014;9:e102883.
6. Cachay ER, Soriano V. Is HIV still a special population for the treatment of hepatitis C? AIDS. 2016;30:2001–3.
7. Soriano V, Labarga P, de Mendoza C, et al. New hepatitis C therapies for special patient populations. Expert Opin Pharmacother. 2016;17:217–29.
8. Cachay ER, Wyles DL, Goicoechea M. Reliability and predictive validity of a hepatitis-related symptom inventory in HIV-infected individuals referred for hepatitis C treatment. AIDS Res Ther. 2011;8:29.
9. Cachay ER, Hill L, Ballard C, et al. Increasing Hepatitis C treatment uptake among HIV-infected patients using an HIV primary care model. AIDS Res Ther. 2013;10:9.
10. Cohen P, Cohen J, Aiken LS, West SG. The problem of units and the circumstance for POMP. Multivar Behav Res. 1999;34:315–46.
11. Rust J, Golombok S. Modern psychometrics: the science of psychological assessment. 3rd ed. New York: Routledge; 2009. p. 84.
12. Rabe-Hesketh S, Skrondal A. Multilevel and longitudinal modeling using stata, volume I: continuous responses. 3rd ed. College Station: Stata Press; 2008. p. 80–2.
13. Newsom Roger. Confidence intervals for rank statistics: somers' D and extensions. Stata J. 2006;6:309–34.
14. Choi SW, Schalet B, Cook KF, Cella D. Establishing a common metric for depressive symptoms: linking the BDI-II, CES-D, and PHQ-9 to PROMIS depression. Psychol Assess. 2014;26:513–27.
15. Alavi M, Raffa JD, Deans GD, et al. Continued low uptake of treatment for hepatitis C virus infection in a large community-based cohort of inner city residents. Liver Int. 2014;34:1198–206.
16. Marcellin F, Roux P, Protopopescu C, Duracinsky M, Spire B, Carrieri MP. Patient-reported outcomes with direct-acting antivirals for the treatment of chronic hepatitis C: current knowledge and outstanding issues. Expert Rev Gastroenterol Hepatol. 2017;11:259–68.
17. Gross C, Akoth E, Price A, Kattakuzhy S, Silk R, Rosenthal E. HIV/HCV co-infection: overcoming barriers to Treatment. J Assoc Nurses AIDS Care. 2016;27:524–9.
18. Mohammad RA, Bulloch MN, Chan J, et al. Provision of clinical pharmacist services for individuals with chronic hepatitis C viral infection: joint opinion of the gi/liver/nutrition and infectious diseases practice and research networks of the American College of Clinical Pharmacy. Pharmacotherapy. 2014;34:1341–54.
19. Naggie S, Cooper C, Saag M, et al. Ledipasvir and sofosbuvir for HCV in patients coinfected with HIV-1. N Engl J Med. 2015;373:705–13.
20. Cachay E, Ballard C, Colwell B and Torriani F. Real-world effectiveness of direct-acting antivirals for hepatitis C among HIV-infected patients with genotype 1. 5th International Conference on Viral Hepatitis (ICVH 2016). San Francisco, CA. March 14–15 [Oral Abstract 036].
21. Benitez-Gutierrez L, Barreiro P, Labarga P, et al. Prevention and management of treatment failure to new oral hepatitis C drugs. Exp Opin Pharmacother. 2016;17:1215–23.
22. Falade-Nwulia O, Sulkowski M. The HCV care continuum does not end with cure: a call to arms for the prevention of reinfection. J Hepatol. 2017;66:267–9.
23. Innes HA, McDonald SA, Dillon JF, et al. Toward a more complete understanding of the association between a hepatitis C sustained viral response and cause-specific outcomes. Hepatology. 2015;62:355–64.
24. Younossi ZM, Stepanova M, Sulkowski M, et al. Ribavirin-free regimen with sofosbuvir and velpatasvir is associated with high efficacy and improvement of patient-reported outcomes in patients with genotypes 2 and three chronic hepatitis c: results from astral-2 and -3 clinical trials. Clin Infect Dis. 2016;63:1042–8.

Permissions

All chapters in this book were first published in AIDS R&T, by BioMed Central; hereby published with permission under the Creative Commons Attribution License or equivalent. Every chapter published in this book has been scrutinized by our experts. Their significance has been extensively debated. The topics covered herein carry significant findings which will fuel the growth of the discipline. They may even be implemented as practical applications or may be referred to as a beginning point for another development.

The contributors of this book come from diverse backgrounds, making this book a truly international effort. This book will bring forth new frontiers with its revolutionizing research information and detailed analysis of the nascent developments around the world.

We would like to thank all the contributing authors for lending their expertise to make the book truly unique. They have played a crucial role in the development of this book. Without their invaluable contributions this book wouldn't have been possible. They have made vital efforts to compile up to date information on the varied aspects of this subject to make this book a valuable addition to the collection of many professionals and students.

This book was conceptualized with the vision of imparting up-to-date information and advanced data in this field. To ensure the same, a matchless editorial board was set up. Every individual on the board went through rigorous rounds of assessment to prove their worth. After which they invested a large part of their time researching and compiling the most relevant data for our readers.

The editorial board has been involved in producing this book since its inception. They have spent rigorous hours researching and exploring the diverse topics which have resulted in the successful publishing of this book. They have passed on their knowledge of decades through this book. To expedite this challenging task, the publisher supported the team at every step. A small team of assistant editors was also appointed to further simplify the editing procedure and attain best results for the readers.

Apart from the editorial board, the designing team has also invested a significant amount of their time in understanding the subject and creating the most relevant covers. They scrutinized every image to scout for the most suitable representation of the subject and create an appropriate cover for the book.

The publishing team has been an ardent support to the editorial, designing and production team. Their endless efforts to recruit the best for this project, has resulted in the accomplishment of this book. They are a veteran in the field of academics and their pool of knowledge is as vast as their experience in printing. Their expertise and guidance has proved useful at every step. Their uncompromising quality standards have made this book an exceptional effort. Their encouragement from time to time has been an inspiration for everyone.

The publisher and the editorial board hope that this book will prove to be a valuable piece of knowledge for researchers, students, practitioners and scholars across the globe.

List of Contributors

Kolab Chhim, Sovannary Tuot, Ratana Sopha, Pheak Chhoun and Siyan Yi
KHANA Center for Population Health Research, No. 33, Street 71, Phnom Penh, Cambodia

Gitau Mburu
Division of Health Research, Lancaster University, Lancaster, UK

Vohith Khol
National Center for HIV/AIDS, Dermatology and STD, Phnom Penh, Cambodia

Siyan Yi
Saw Swee Hock School of Public Health, National University of Singapore and National University Health System, Singapore, Singapore
Center for Global Health Research, Touro University California, Vallejo, CA, USA

Sasisopin Kiertiburanakul
Department of Medicine, Faculty of Medicine Ramathibodi Hospital, Mahidol University, 270 Rama VI Road, Bangkok 10400, Thailand

David Boettiger
The Kirby Institute, University of New South Wales, Sydney, Australia

Oon Tek Ng
Tan Tock Seng Hospital, Singapore, Singapore

Nguyen Van Kinh
National Hospital of Tropical Diseases, Hanoi, Vietnam

Pacharee Kantipong
Chiangrai Prachanukroh Hospital, Chiang Rai, Thailand

Fujie Zhang
Beijing Ditan Hospital, Capital Medical University, Beijing, China

Jun Yong Choi
Division of Infectious Diseases, Department of Internal Medicine, Yonsei University College of Medicine, Seoul, South Korea

Evy Yunihastuti
Faculty of Medicine Universitas Indonesia, Dr. Cipto Mangunkusumo General Hospital, Jakarta, Indonesia

Sanjay Pujari
Institute of Infectious Diseases, Pune, India

Jeremy L. Ross
TREAT Asia, amfAR, The Foundation for AIDS Research, Bangkok, Thailand

Ne Myo Aung, Josh Hanson, Mar Mar Kyi and Htin Aung Saw
Department of Medicine, University of Medicine Yangon, Myanmar. Menzies School of Health Research, Darwin, Australia

Josh Hanson, David A. Cooper and Mark A. Boyd
The Kirby Institute, Sydney, Australia

Tint Tint Kyi
Department of Medical Care, Ministry of Health, Nay Pyi Taw, Myanmar

Zaw Win Htet
Insein General Hospital, Yangon, Myanmar

Mark A. Boyd
University of Adelaide, Adelaide, Australia

Hellen N. Siril and Sylvia F. Kaaya
Department of Psychiatry and Mental Health, Muhimbili University of Health and Allied Sciences, Dar es Salaam, Tanzania

Hellen N. Siril
Management and Development for Health (MDH), Plot number 802, Mwai Kibaki Road, 255 Dar es Salaam, Tanzania

Mary Kay Smith Fawzi
Department of Global Health and Social Medicine, Harvard Medical School, Boston, MA, USA

Expeditho Mtisi, Magreat Somba, Anna Minja and Anna Kaale
African Academy for Public Health (AAPH), Dar es Salaam, Tanzania

Japheth Kilewo
Department of Epidemiology, Muhimbili University of Health and Allied Sciences, Dar es Salaam, Tanzania

Ferdinand Mugusi
Department of Internal Medicine, Muhimbili University of Health and Allied Sciences, Dares Salaam, Tanzania

Jim Todd
National Institute for Medical Research (NIMR), Mwanza, Tanzania
Department of Epidemiology and Biostatistics, Kilimanjaro Christian Medical University College, Moshi, Tanzania
Population Health Department, London School of Hygiene and Tropical Medicine, London, UK

Jose Catalan
CNWL NHS Foundation Trust, South Kensington and Chelsea Mental Health Centre, London, UK

Veronica Tuffrey and Damien Ridge
Faculty of Science and Technology, University of Westminster, London, UK

Dana Rosenfeld
School of Social Science and Public Policy, Keele University, London, UK

Giovanni Guaraldi, Stefano Zona, Marianna Menozzi, Federica Carli, Chiara Stentarelli, Giovanni Dolci, Antonella Santoro and Cristina Mussini
Department of Medical and Surgical Sciences for Adults and Children, Clinic of Infectious Diseases, University of Modena and Reggio Emilia, Emilia-Romagna, Modena, Italy

Thomas D. Brothers
Faculty of Medicine, Dalhousie University, Halifax, NS, Canada

Julian Falutz
McGill University Health Center, Montreal, QC, Canada

Ana Rita Domingues Da Silva
Infectious Disease Department, Hospital Beatriz Ângelo, Regiao de Lisboa, Loures, Portugal

Elisa Rossi
Health Care Department, Cineca-Interuniversity Consortium, Casalecchio di Reno, Emilia-Romagna, Bologna, Italy

Alexander Kwarteng and Samuel Terkper Ahuno
Department of Biochemistry and Biotechnology, Kwame Nkrumah University of Science and Technology (KNUST), PMB, Kumasi, Ghana

Alexander Kwarteng
Kumasi Centre for Collaborative Research in Tropical Medicine (KCCR), Kumasi, Ghana

Godwin Kwakye-Nuako
Department of Biomedical Sciences, School of Allied Health Sciences, College of Health and Allied Sciences, University of Cape Coast, Cape Coast, Ghana

L. E. Gibbons, R. Fredericksen, M. M. Kitahata, H. M. Crane and P. K. Crane
Department of Medicine, Harborview Medical Center, University of Washington, 325 9th Ave, Box 359931, Seattle, WA, USA

D. S. Batey
Department of Social Work, University of Alabama at Birmingham, 900 13th Street S, Suite 203, Birmingham, AL 35294, USA

L. Dant and K. H. Mayer
Fenway Institute, 1340 Boylston Street, Boston, MA 02215, USA

T. C. Edwards
Department of Health Services, University of Washington, 1208 NE 43rd Street, Seattle, WA 98195, USA

K. H. Mayer
Department of Medicine, Harvard Medical School, Boston, MA, USA

W. C. Mathews and E. Paez
Department of Medicine, University of California at San Diego, 4168 Front Street, San Diego, CA 92103, USA

L. S. Morales
Center for Health Equity, Diversity and Inclusion, School of Medicine, University of Washington, 1959 Pacific Street, Seattle, WA 98195, USA

M. J. Mugavero
Department of Medicine, University of Alabama at Birmingham, 908 20th Street S, Suite 250, Birmingham, AL 35205, USA

F. M. Yang
Department of Biostatistics and Epidemiology, Augusta University, 1120 15th Street, AE-1035, Augusta, GA 30912, USA

L. E. Gibbons
Harborview Medical Center, University of Washington, 325 9th Ave, Seattle, WA 98104, USA

Carmen Hidalgo-Tenorio, Jessica Ramírez-Taboada, Concepción Gil-Anguita, Miguel Lopez-Ruz and Juan Pasquau
Infectious Disease Service, University Hospital Virgen de las Nieves, Granada, Spain

Javier Esquivias
Pathology Service, University Hospital Virgen de las Nieves, Granada, Spain

Mohamed Omar-Mohamed-Balgahata
Infectious Disease Unit of the Hospital Ciudad de Jaén, Jaén, Spain

Antonio SamPedro
Microbiology Service, University Hospital Virgen de las Nieves, Granada, Spain

Catherine Orrell and Robin Wood
Department of Medicine, Desmond Tutu HIV Centre, Institute of Infectious Disease and Molecular Medicine, University of Cape Town, Cape Town, South Africa

Karen Cohen, Rory Leisegang and Gary Maartens
Division of Clinical Pharmacology, Department of Medicine, University of Cape Town, Cape Town, South Africa

David R. Bangsberg
Harvard Medical School, Boston, MA, USA
Massachusetts General Hospital Center for Global Health, Boston, MA, USA
Ragon Institute of Massachusetts General Hospital, Boston, MA, USA

Catherine Orrell
Desmond Tutu HIV Centre, Werner Beit Building North, UCT Faculty of Health Science, Anzio Road, Observatory, Cape Town 7925, South Africa

Faysal Bin Hamid, Jinsun Kim and Cha-Gyun Shin
Department of Systems Biotechnology, Chung-Ang University, Anseong, Kyunggido 456-756, South Korea

M. J. Kruger and T. A. Nell
Department of Physiological Sciences, Stellenbosch University Main Campus, Stellenbosch 7602, Western Cape Province, Republic of South Africa

Tsitsi G. Monera-Penduka and Charles C. Maponga
Drug and Toxicology Information Services (DaTIS), School of Pharmacy, University of Zimbabwe College of Health Sciences, Harare, Zimbabwe

Charles C. Maponga and Gene D. Morse
Center for Integrated Global Biomedical Sciences, University at Buffalo, Buffalo, NY, USA

Alan R. Wolfe
Department of Bioengineering and Therapeutic Sciences, University of California San Francisco, San Francisco, CA, USA

Lubbe Wiesner
Division of Clinical Pharmacology, Department of Medicine, University of Cape Town, Cape Town, South Africa

Charles F. B. Nhachi
Department of Clinical Pharmacology, University of Zimbabwe College of Health Sciences, Harare, Zimbabwe

Teshale Ayele and Girma Mamo
Department of Pharmacy, Jimma University Medical Centre, Institute of Health, Jimma University, Jimma, Ethiopia

Habtemu Jarso
Department of Epidemiology, Public Health Faculty, Institute of Health, Jimma University, Jimma, Ethiopia

Nectarios Sophocles Papavarnavas and Kathryn Manning
Department of Medicine, Old Main Building, J-Floor, Groote Schuur Hospital, University of Cape Town, Observatory, Cape Town 7925, South Africa

Fahd Conrad
Trauma and Emergency Unit, Floor E11A, Management Suite, Groote Schuur Hospital, Main Road, Observatory, Cape Town 7925, South Africa

Milah Govender
Quality and Safety Unit, Groote Schuur Hospital, Main Road, Observatory, Cape Town 7925, South Africa

Gary Maartens
Division of Clinical Pharmacology, Department of Medicine, Groote Schuur Hospital, University of Cape Town, Cape Town 7925, South Africa

Xinli Lu, Hongru Zhao, Yuqi Zhang, Wei Wang, Cuiying Zhao, Yan Li, Lin Ma, Ze Cuis and Suliang Chen
Hebei Provincial Center for Disease Control and Prevention, 97 Huaian East Road, Yuhua District, Shijiazhuang 050021, China

Giovanni Guaraldi, Giovanni Dolci, Stefano Zona, Erica Franceschini, Mauro Codeluppi and Cristina Mussini
Department of Medical and Surgical Sciences for Adults and Children, Clinic of Infectious Diseases, University of Modena and Reggio Emilia, Largo del Pozzo, 71, 41124 Modena, Italy

Giuseppe Tarantino, Valentina Serra and Roberto Ballarin
Department of Medical and Surgical Sciences for Adults and Children, Liver and Multivisceral Transplant Center, University of Modena and Reggio Emilia, Modena, Italy

Thomas D. Brothers
Faculty of Medicine, Dalhousie University, Halifax B3H 2E1, Canada

Oliver T. Stirrup, David T. Dunn and Anna Tostevin
Centre for Clinical Research in Infection and Sexual Health, Institute for Global Health, University College London, London, UK

Caroline A. Sabin
Centre for Clinical Research, Epidemiology, Modelling and Evaluation, Institute for Global Health, University College London, Royal Free Campus, London, UK

Anton Pozniak and David Asboe
Chelsea and Westminster Hospital NHS Foundation Trust, London, UK

Alison Cox
Infection and Immunity laboratory, Charing Cross Hospital, London, UK

Chloe Orkin
Barts Health NHS Trust, London, UK

Fabiola Martin
Hull York Medical School, University of York, York, UK
Faculty of Medicine, University of Queensland, Brisbane, Australia

Patricia Cane
High Containment Microbiology, Public Health England, Salisbury, UK

Suparna Das, Jenevieve Opoku and Adam Allston
Strategic Information Division, HIV/AIDS, Hepatitis, STD and TB Administration (HAHSTA), District of Columbia Department of Health, Government of the District of Columbia, 899 North Capitol St., NE/Fourth Floor, Washington, DC 20002, USA

Michael Kharfen
HIV/AIDS, Hepatitis, STD & TB Administration (HAHSTA), District of Columbia Department of Health, Government of the District of Columbia, 899 N. Capitol St., NE, Washington, DC 20002, USA

Sosthene Tsongo Vululi
Makerere University College of Health Sciences (MakCHS), Kampala, Uganda

Samuel Bugeza
Radiology Department of Mulago Hospital, Lecturer at MakCHS, Kampala Uganda

Muyinda Zeridah
Mulago Hospital, Kampala, Uganda

Henry Ddungu
Uganda Cancer Institute, Kampala, Uganda

Akello Betty Openy
MakCHS, Kampala, Uganda

Mubiru Frank
Stastician-IDI-Kampala, Kampala, Uganda

Rosalind Parkes-Ratanshi
Prevention Care Treatment, Infectious Diseases Institute (IDI), Kampala, Uganda

Graham Toth
Fielding School of Public Health, University of California Los Angeles, Los Angeles, USA

Gitau Mburu
Division of Health Research, Lancaster University, Lancaster, UK

Sovannary Tuot
KHANA Center for Population Health Research, No. 33, Street 71, Phnom Penh, Cambodia

Vohith Khol
National Center for HIV/AIDS, Dermatology and STD, Phnom Penh, Cambodia

Siyan Yi
Center for Global Health Research, Touro University California, Vallejo, USA

Edward R. Cachay and Wm. Christopher Mathews
Department of Medicine-Owen Clinic, University of California at San Diego, 200 W. Arbor Drive, San Diego, CA 92103-8681, USA

Edward R. Cachay, Francesca Torriani and Charles Hicks
Division of Infectious Diseases, University of California at San Diego, 9500 Gilman Drive #0711, La Jolla, CA 92093-0711, USA

Craig Ballard and Bradford Colwell
Skaggs School of Pharmacy and Pharmaceutical Sciences, UC San Diego, 9500 Gilman Drive, La Jolla, CA 92093-0021, USA

Index

A

Abacavir, 11-12, 16-17, 114, 121-122, 149, 152, 157, 168, 178

Antiretroviral Therapy, 1, 4-5, 7-10, 12, 16-17, 23, 25, 32-33, 42-43, 48-50, 61-63, 75-76, 87-88, 92, 97-98, 104, 107, 129, 132, 138, 144, 146, 178-179, 189, 201, 203

Arvs, 12

Assist, 14, 75, 119, 182, 188, 209

Atazanavir, 14, 16, 117, 122, 128, 141, 149, 152, 157, 191

B

Bivariate Analysis, 34-36, 38-40, 80, 82, 192, 194

Body Mass Index, 11, 13, 15-16, 109, 195

Bone Mineral Density, 44, 48, 107-109, 115-116, 118-123

C

Cd4 Cells, 6-7, 218, 222, 229, 231

Chi Square Test, 28, 31, 147

Combined Antiretroviral Therapy, 43, 75, 120

Cytomegalovirus, 161

D

Darunavir, 14, 16, 128

Deep Venous Thrombosis, 190-191, 193, 195-196

Donor Risk Index, 160, 165

Doppler Ultrasound, 190-191, 194, 196

Drug Resistance Mutations, 32, 97, 168, 179

Dual-energy X-ray Absorptiometry, 44, 119, 160

E

Efavirenz, 12, 16-17, 20, 22, 88-94, 96-97, 121-122, 129, 131, 138, 141, 149, 152, 157

Electronic Adherence Monitoring Device, 88, 94

End Stage Liver Disease, 159, 164

Epidemiology, 32, 48, 50, 52, 62, 137, 157, 178, 182, 189, 196, 207

Epstein-barr Virus, 161

Etravirine, 93-94, 149, 152, 157, 179

F

Fisher's Exact Test, 3, 28, 150, 154, 201, 203-204, 206

Frailty Index, 159-165

H

Hcv Treatment, 208-215

Hepatitis B Virus, 81, 144

Hepatocellular Carcinoma, 223

Herpes Simplex Virus, 56

Highly Active Antiretroviral Therapies (HAART), 33, 49-50, 52, 54, 61, 101-104, 106, 111, 113-118, 121-122, 138, 158, 160, 192-193, 195

High Squamous Intraepithelial Lesions (HSIL), 77-78, 80-81, 84-86

Hiv Diagnosis, 13, 15, 33, 43-44, 46, 48, 79, 82, 184-185

Hiv Infection, 9-10, 12-13, 17, 21, 26, 42-44, 48-49, 62-63, 85-86, 97, 105, 113-115, 117, 120-122, 125, 134, 136, 138-139, 144, 147, 157-158, 168, 180, 185, 189, 193, 196

Hodgkin's Lymphoma, 53, 157

Human Papilloma Virus, 81, 87

I

Immune Reconstitution Inflammatory Syndrome, 48

Indinavir, 117, 128

Isoniazid Prophylaxis Therapy, 18, 20, 22

K

Kaplan-meier Survival, 162

Kaposi Sarcoma, 216

L

Lamivudine, 12, 16-17, 93, 97, 116, 121-122, 127, 129, 138, 141, 149-150, 152, 157, 168, 178, 191

Lipodystrophy, 46, 49, 113, 117, 120

Liver Transplantation, 159, 165-166

Logistic Regression Model, 3, 6, 8, 47, 94, 139

Loss to Follow-up (LTFU), 24-27, 29-32, 139-144

M

Magnetic Resonance Imaging, 110, 119

Mann-whitney Test, 3, 38, 80

Moringa Oleifera, 124-125, 127-129

Multicollinearity, 35, 38

Murine Leukemia Virus, 100, 104-106

N

Nevirapine, 90, 93, 97, 124-129, 138, 149, 152, 157, 191

Nnrti, 12, 16, 89-90, 93-94, 146, 150, 155, 171-172, 174-175, 177, 179

Non-infectious Comorbidities (NICM), 43-48

O

Osteopenia, 44, 108, 115, 119, 121-122, 160-161

Osteoporosis, 12, 44, 107-112, 115-116, 118-123, 160-161

P

Pharmacokinetic, 124-129, 131, 136

Plwh, 41, 66-70, 72-74, 182, 208-210, 214-215

Pmtct, 25, 33

Polymerase Chain Reaction, 79, 86-87

Post Exposure Prophylaxis, 139, 144

Pulmonary Embolism, 190, 195

Q

Quadrivalent Hpv Vaccine, 77, 80, 87

R

Reverse Transcriptase, 12, 16, 55, 64, 89, 92, 99, 104, 114, 121, 125, 129, 131, 138, 141, 146, 150-154, 157, 167-171, 174, 176, 178- 180, 191

Rilpivirine, 11-12, 16-17, 93-94, 179

Ritonavir, 14, 16, 116, 121-123, 128, 141, 149-150, 152, 155, 157, 169, 173, 178, 191, 210

S

Saquinavir, 117, 128

Stavudine, 90, 97, 122, 127, 129, 141, 149-150, 152, 157, 167, 178-179

T

Tenofovir, 12, 16-17, 20, 22, 90, 92-93, 114-115, 121-122, 127, 130, 138-140, 144-145, 149, 152, 157, 168, 178, 191

Thymidine Analogue Mutations, 178

Transition Process, 203

V

Variance Inflation Factor, 38

Vincristine, 53

Viral Suppression, 1-7, 9-10, 33, 94, 136, 138, 167-169, 171-178, 181-182, 185, 188, 207, 210

Vocational Training, 197, 199, 202-203

Z

Zidovudine, 90, 97, 121, 127, 130, 138-139, 141, 149-150, 152, 157, 168, 178, 191

Zinc Finger Nuclease, 50, 56, 57

www.ingramcontent.com/pod-product-compliance
Lightning Source LLC
LaVergne TN
LVHW080808220926
848485LV00011B/386